DATE DUE

NOV 30 1993	APR 1 0 2003
JAN 2 5 1994	MAR 2 6 2004
FEB - 7 1994	
MAR 1 4 1994	
APR 1 1 1994	
JAN 2 6 1995	
426	
JAN 2 9 1996	
MAR 1 5 1996	
JUL 1 5 1996	
NOV 1 5 1996	
NOV - 6 1997	
DEC - 5 1997	
OCT 2 3 1998	
DEC - 1 1998	

The Nursing
of Families

The Nursing of Families

Theory / Research
Education / Practice

Suzanne L. Feetham
Susan B. Meister
Janice M. Bell
Catherine L. Gilliss
editors

The information presented by Dr. Feetham in this
volume reflects the opinions and work of the author
and not those of the National Center for Nursing
Research, National Institutes of Health.

SAGE Publications
International Educational and Professional Publisher
Newbury Park   London   New Delhi

For information address:

SAGE Publications, Inc.
2455 Teller Road
Newbury Park, California 91320

SAGE Publications Ltd.
6 Bonhill Street
London EC2A 4PU
United Kingdom

SAGE Publications India Pvt. Ltd.
M-32 Market
Greater Kailash I
New Delhi 110 048 India

Printed in the United States of America

Library of Congress Cataloging-in-Publication Data

Main entry under title:
The nursing of families : theory/research/education/practice
    Suzanne L. Feetham . . . [et al.].
        p.   cm.
    Includes bibliographical references.
    ISBN 0-8039-4715-1. —ISBN 0-8039-4716-X (pbk.)
    1. Family nursing —Congresses.   I. Feetham, Suzanne.
RT120.F3N889   1992
610.73—dc20   92-30712

93 94 95 96   10 9 8 7 6 5 4 3 2 1

Sage Production Editor: Diane S. Foster

Contents

Preface

Barbara A. Durand

Determination of Need

This book is the publication of selected papers from the Second International Family Nursing Conference, held in Portland, Oregon, in 1991. Throughout the conference nurses were challenged to address family needs in a variety of settings and situations across the life cycle and to consider the role of family nursing in relation to those needs. An important consideration in working with families is the frequently missed opportunities with families because of our conception of what *they* need.

The case can be made that all of our professional pursuits evolve from and revolve around our determination of what patients/clients/families need, how that determination is decided, and who decides what families need. Because nursing's mission is to provide services that meet the needs of people, it follows that the determination of those needs shapes the practice of nursing and the education for that practice. Education and practice thus are influenced and formed by the conception of need as explicated in the theoretical models of the discipline.

If our dominant theoretical models are derived traditionally and have as their aim the explanation, prediction, and control of events and phenomena, then it is not surprising that formal rules and models play a major role, conceptually and practically, in nursing care settings. Although the objectivity of formal models is desirable in certain nursing care situations, their use, according to Gordon (1984), is not directed toward the particular desires of the individual patient and family or to the expectations of the nurse.

Although conceptual models attributing agency to the patient have been developed (Riehl & Roy, 1980), in reality, prevailing practice is characterized by professional domination in determining patients' problems and in making plans to solve them. In the inpatient setting, this usually takes the form of the standardized care plan with its listing, by diagnosis, of typical patient problems, recommended interventions, and expected outcomes.

Family Needs in Ambulatory Care

Of concern is that individuals and families do not fit formal plans and guidelines. The following three examples from ambulatory settings reinforce this issue of the discrepancy between family needs and the professional's conceptions of need.

In my early career as a Pediatric Nurse Practitioner (PNP), a 30-year-old primipara came to the clinic with her 2-week-old son for the first well baby visit. At the end of the visit, the mother was told that her son was well. As per the American Academy of Pediatrics Guidelines, she also was told to make an appointment for the next visit in 6 to 8 weeks. Her facial expression changed markedly, and in response to her nonverbal cues, she was asked whether something was wrong. With eyes filling with tears, she said, "I don't think I can wait that long." When asked when she thought she would like to come back, she said, "Would 2 weeks be too soon?"

A second example occurred while observing a patient visit by a master's pediatric nurse practitioner student as part of her clinical evaluation. In this instance an American father and a Thai mother who had recently come to America had brought their 6-week-old infant for a well child visit. When the student asked about any concerns, the mother shyly and hesitantly asked whether it was all right to put oil on the baby's skin. A famous dermatologist had lectured the week before and had advised strongly against putting oil on the skin of infants. The student, visibly brightened by the opportunity to apply new knowledge, immediately said, "No, you should not put oil on the baby's skin," at which point the father looked at the mother and said, "I told you so." The mother looked down at the floor, embarrassed and defeated. At this point I, as faculty, asked the mother what she would be doing if she were home in Thailand. The mother replied that she was following Thai custom and was using special oil that she had brought with her. Of course, the infant's skin was perfect.

The third example comes from PROJECT SERVE (1985). PROJECT SERVE was a 3-year study, funded by a SPRANS grant from the Division of Maternal-Child Health, United States Public Health Service, to improve services for children with chronic illness in Massachusetts. The project surveyed parents and care providers to identify needs of this population. The top five needs listed by professionals were as follows:

1. Counseling services
2. Home health/nursing services
3. Primary outpatient care
4. Respite care
5. Coordination of care/case management

The top five needs listed by parents were as follows:

1. Parent education on rights and entitlement
2. Help in getting needed services
3. Physical therapy
4. Financial help
5. Speech therapy

Respite care, counseling and support services, and home health/nursing services were listed by fewer than 50% of parents as being very important. This finding reinforces the fact that we must exert much effort to decrease the incongruence between what families are telling us they need (if we ask) and what we have been taught or have decided to provide.

Family Needs in Acute Care

The concept of *matching family needs* applies as well in acute, tertiary care settings. After spending 20 years in ambulatory care, I assumed responsibility for nursing care in a 175-bed Department of Maternal-Child Nursing in a major academic medical center. With this change, my focus is now on what children and families face in our hospitals. It is safe to say that every family who has a child admitted to a tertiary care setting experiences severe stress, with many families finding themselves in crisis situations, unable to use normal coping mechanisms effectively.

The expressed needs of families include wanting the following:

- The most competent care available in terms of diagnostic and treatment procedures. Families want the technicians to be skilled in the techniques. From the family's point of view, it does not matter who the technician is as long as he or she is skilled.

- Freedom from pain. The need for appropriate pain management in children is a major issue. At this time a growing cadre of nurse researchers is making impressive strides in this area.

- Skillful and compassionate physical care. It is important to note that what is important to families is the quality of care rather than who the care provider is.

- After the procedures have been performed and the treatments prescribed, someone to help the family manage, someone to help them manipulate the system, someone who can address in a sophisticated manner the impact of the illness on their lives.

The 4 Cs (competence, commitment, collaboration, and communication), though not original to me, are pertinent to the concept of *matching the expressed needs of families to their care*. To meet the needs of families as they see them, all four Cs must occur.

- *Competence* in all clinicians caring for the individual family members and for the family.

- *Commitment* to a philosophy of family nursing. This comes from exposure to conceptual models that include the family as the client, the willingness and the courage to empower the family and to let go of control, respect for the family's primary role as decision maker at all levels of care, and dedication to supporting and strengthening the family because it is the constant in the child's life.

- *Collaboration* that is rooted in the ability to learn from and accept support from others and that is infinitely more difficult than unilateral prescription.

- *Communication* is the critical skill in our ability to identify and meet family needs. This skill hinges on highly developed communication skills, ranging from listening, to the ability to elicit family values, to the ability to anticipate issues of concern to individual families such as attention to their culture and ethnicity.

Although these components are critical in the care of families, it is important to recognize that nurses require institutional and unit support to move from their focus of technical skills to achieving clinical competence in the care of the family. Without such support many nurses will not include the family within their professional role. In one study Brown and Ritchie (1990) documented this lack of family care. They reported that nurses were more involved in gatekeeping and control roles, which overshadowed their provision of family-centered psychosocial care. The authors concluded that this situation will change only if (a) nurses receive primary and ongoing education grounded in a philosophy of family nursing, (b) they practice using nursing and family empowerment models of care, and (c) they practice in environments that actively support and promote nurse-family communication, holistic care, and family empowerment.

In summary, what families need are nurses who have been raised in this philosophy, who have developed the very sophisticated skills required for therapeutic communication, and who practice in environments that support the family. Hirschfeld (1991) stated, "We have to *hear* and to *know* the concerns of families". Acknowledgment of the centrality of the family's concerns and of the family's definition of *needs* must be reflected not only in practice but also in theory, in research, and in policy development. The implications for our care should be obvious.

The contributors to this book provide a unique compilation of the state of the art and science of nursing care with families. The chapters in this volume provide significant directions for crosscutting issues in practice, education, research, and theory to bridge the gap between perceived needs and expectations of families and the practice of nursing of families.

Acknowledgments

This volume began with the vision of the Planning Committee for the Second International Conference on Family Nursing held in May 1991 in Portland, Oregon. The goals of the Planning Committee were to create a forum for the exchange of ideas, information, and expertise, while fostering the continued development of an international community of nurses to improve the health of families throughout the world.

The legacy of collaboration and shared knowledge in nursing of families extends from the two Wingspread conferences on Advancing Family Research in Nursing in Racine, Wisconsin, in 1984 and 1986; the University of Calgary leadership for the First International Conference in 1988 and the subsequent publication, *The Cutting Edge of Family Nursing;* and the direction from the faculty of the four schools of nursing that co-sponsored this Second International Conference. The first international conference formalized the international community while adding to the base of shared knowledge for the nursing of families. The second conference and this volume have significantly expanded that effort.

The chapters in this book are the result of a multistage refereed selection process. First the Scientific Review Committee for the Second International Conference assessed the hundreds of abstracts submitted for presentation. This review resulted in a conference that included 13 symposia, 138 paper presentations, and 82 poster presentations by nurses and other scholars representing the United States, Canada, and 13 other countries. From these presentations the Editorial Advisory Committee selected the 26 chapters published in this volume. These chapters describe the state of the science in nursing of families and demonstrate the relevance of this knowledge for the clinical care of families.

The scholarship and extraordinary work of leaders in clinical practice, research, and theory of nursing of families has resulted in this comprehensive coverage of critical family issues. The preparation of this volume has been supported also by the diligence and commitment of Byron Schneider, Project Assistant for the Department of Family Health Care at the University of California, San Francisco.

This volume is dedicated to the families in our practice and research and to our own families.

The Editors and Authors

Second International Family Nursing Conference—Portland, Oregon
Sponsoring Schools of Nursing

School of Nursing
Oregon Health Sciences University
Portland, Oregon

College of Nursing
Montana State University
Bozeman, Montana

Department of Family Health Care
School of Nursing
University of California
San Francisco, California

Department of Parent & Child Nursing
School of Nursing
University of Washington
Seattle, Washington

Advisory Committee

Dr. Patricia Archbold
Dr. Sheryl T. Boyd[*]
Dr. Mary Ann Curry
Dr. Suzanne Feetham
Dr. Catherine L. Gilliss
Dr. Marcia Killien[*]
Ms. Linda Krentz[*]
Dr. Ida Martinson[*]
Dr. Susan B. Meister
Dr. Clarann Weinert, SC[*]
Dr. Nancy Fugate Woods
[*]Indicates members of Editorial Advisory
Committee for this volume.

Scientific Review Committee

Dr. Catherine L. Gilliss, Chair
Dr. Ida Martinson, Co-Chair
Mr. Byron Schneider, Assistant
Dr. Janice M. Bell
Dr. Yu-Mei Chao
Dr. Catherine A. Chesla
Dr. Elizabeth Davies
Dr. Suzanne L. Feetham
Dr. Maureen A. Frey
Dr. Audrey Grant
Dr. Shirley M. H. Hanson
Dr. Susie Kim
Dr. Tammy Krulik
Dr. Margaret Miles
Dr. Elizabeth Nichols
Dr. Marie-France Thibaudeau
Dr. Judith Vessey
Dr. Clarann Weinert, SC

PART I

The Family's Agents:
Policy and Nursing

Susan B. Meister, Editor

1

The Family's Agents:
Policy and Nursing

Susan B. Meister

Two factors in family well-being have particular consequences for families facing problems: social policies and clinicians. They are interrelated determinants of access to economic, social, health, and education resources. They operate at different levels of aggregation: *social policies* determine access for groups of families, while *clinicians* affect access for individual families.

In this view social policies and nurses are "agents" for their "principals" —families. Three agency relationships result: (a) social policy and families, (b) nursing and families, and (c) nursing and social policy affecting families. These relationships are discussed below and are used to identify crosscutting themes in the interactions of policy and nursing (agents) in relation to family (principal) outcomes. Finally the beginnings of a family nursing agenda for improving agency are introduced.

Principal's Gains and Losses:
Family Outcomes

In any agency relationship, the principal may lose, as well as gain, as a result of the agents' actions. Pratt and Zeckhauser's (1985) innovative analysis of agency relationships pinpointed several determinants of the quality of agency outcomes. They emphasized that *agency loss* is increased when agent/principal relationships include asymmetrical information, divergent incentives, and imperfect abilities for agent and principal to monitor each other. These conditions diminish both the effectiveness and the efficiency of the agent. They are common features of both the development of policies affecting families, as well as health care delivery to families. Some of the undesirable variance in family outcomes therefore may be related directly to imperfections (agency loss) in the agency relationships with policy and nursing.

Agents for Family Well-Being: Status and Implications

At some point the field of family nursing must identify methods for minimizing agency loss associated with all three agency relationships. The status and implications of each relationship are discussed in the following sections. Although evidence of the pervasive influence of policies on all American families is ample, poor families cast the need for thoughtful social policy into particularly sharp relief. Thus data about poor families are used as specific examples of the generic points made below.

Social Policy and Families

Clear analyses of social policy and families are difficult because the range of social policies affecting families is extraordinarily wide and the nature of family vulnerabilities is equally complex. For example, Moynihan (1986) reported that in 1984 half of American households had at least one member participating in one or more government social welfare/insurance programs.

Analyses of social policy and family certainly require complex empirical designs. Family structures vary, some families are at higher risk, policies affecting the same group of families often interact, and extensions to policy may not be clear even for successful programs.

Families in poverty have a number of strikingly different structures. The majority of children born in America will spend some part of their childhood living in a single-parent home and thus are at significant economic risk. Yet half of all children living in poverty are living in two-parent homes with a parent working at least part-time (Edelman, 1987; Ellwood, 1988).

Ellwood's (1988) list of problems related to poverty in the American family illustrates second-order effects of structural differences: After governmental transfers are factored in, the full-time working poor are among the poorest of the poor; single parents must choose between working full-time (and probably still being poor) and being supported by welfare; absent parents usually provide little financial support; and urban ghetto families live in a world without hope. Second-order effects create additional policy issues.

High-risk outliers among families in poverty demonstrate the confounding variables involved in answering the policy question of which characteristics should become the focus of intervention.

Twenty percent of American children live in poverty, and 5% to 10% of the poor live in neighborhoods where at least 40% of the families are poor (Bane & Ellwood, 1989; Ellwood, 1988). In reporting the story of a year in the lives of two young brothers in a Chicago housing project, Kotlowitz (1991) described the unrelenting cultural, developmental, economic, and social factors that become the determinants of family vulnerabilities. The story also illustrated episodic and fragmented incursions of policies into family life. A subgroup of poor families—homeless families—is equally high risk. They account for about 25% of the homeless population, and their numbers are increasing (Wright, 1989). They pose a peculiar policy dilemma in that they might be classified as either homeless or poor.

Poor families are affected by a number of policies, some of which interact poorly. For example, the real value of AFDC benefits decreased 20% between 1972 and 1984, although the number of families needing those benefits rose from about 7% in 1960 to 20% in 1988 (Ellwood, 1988).

The specific problem for poor families is increasing need in a time of decreasing governmental support (Edelman, 1987). In the context of generalized confusion about economic responsibilities and accountability (Zeckhauser, 1986), the magnitude and complexity of these problems are staggering. Further, proposed policy solutions vary according to how the central and peripheral problems are classified and prioritized. For example, Ellwood's (1988) solution begins where health care's might end: to ensure that everyone has medical protection. After folding in that element, Ellwood's solution goes on: to make work pay enough so that working families are not poor; to adopt a uniform child support assurance system; to convert welfare to provide real but transitional and short-term financial, educational, and social support; and to provide minimum wage jobs to people who have exhausted their transitional support. This solution illustrates an approach that would activate agents from various disciplines, along with their divergent views of what is the problem and what is the context.

and innovations abound, but the extensions to policy are noι ⌐or example, although Schorr and Schorr's analysis (1988) demonsu⌐ted that we have a firm grasp on a number of proven programs, social policy development faces substantial and difficult choices. For example, the National Forum on the Future of Children and Families (Both & Garduque, 1989) endorses a policy to stop tinkering with welfare and to get on with the business of overhauling the system. In the meantime families are struggling to find ways of managing their circumstances. For example, increasing numbers of families without health insurance are turning to the school nurse as their source of primary care for their children (Alexander, 1991).

Wilson (1991) and Wright (1989) discussed the urban underclass and the homeless. They emphasized proximate causes: Unemployment causes poverty, and poverty in the context of shortages of low-income housing causes homelessness. They also emphasized, however, the essential role of theoretical frameworks in studies of proximate causes, arguing that such a framework leads to a knowledge base that can clarify policy analyses.

Wilson (1991) emphasized the critical role of theoretical frameworks in analyses of policy and family poverty, and his discussion of the social transformation of the inner city and the increase in ghetto poverty illustrates the point. He carried forward his focus on the underclass and a central problem of joblessness reinforced by social isolation in poor neighborhoods, building a theoretical framework about the structure and determinants of inequality. Wilson noted that the framework prevents the "pollution" of definitions and meanings as research findings are applied to policy development. His framework relates the empirical findings to effects on the structure and function of the truly disadvantaged family. After explaining the vulnerabilities that distinguish that particular group of families, the analysis weighed the merits of race-neutral poverty policies in the context of the theoretical framework.

Nursing and Families

⌐ Nursing has a long history of interest in and involvement with families. Research and practice models are developing and, where possible, benefit from intersection or at least consideration of how to move toward intersection. For example, in 1989, Gilliss et al. introduced a text on the science of family nursing emphasizing the value of moving from a view of the family as the context for the health problems of an individual to a view of the family as the unit of care (Gilliss, 1989b, 1989c). In identifying 10 features of family nursing, Gilliss emphasized the multivariate nature of the relationship between family health and the health of individual members. Summarized here, family nursing is

Concerned with the natural history of the family
Involved with the transaction between family and community
Sensitive to differences between member and group health
Involved with members who are well and ill
Inclusive of care and treatment of individual's health problems
Attuned to the impact of changes in members on the family
Designed to increase family interaction
Focused on individual's symptoms as data about the family
Aimed at mutual support and growth of family and members
A means of defining the family (Gilliss, 1989b)

Having established a basis for intersection between practice and research, Gilliss determined that few nurses had formal preparation in family care, and similarly, few models supported practice (Gilliss, 1989b).

In 1991 Whall and Fawcett confirmed Gilliss's 1989 findings, pointing to the limited work in formalizing explicit sets of concepts and propositions. On the basis of their compilation of the nursing literature related to theory development in family nursing, they concluded that the utility of conceptual models and theories available to family nurse scholars was becoming more evident (Whall & Fawcett, 1991a). Thus they supported the premise of intersection and noted additional development in achieving it.

Feetham (1991a) reported similar findings in her analysis of the development of the concepts and methods of nursing research of families. Despite obstacles posed by limited instruments and by lack of congruence between theoretical frameworks and methods, the field demonstrates an increasing confluence of theory and practice. Feetham's (1991a) purposes of nursing research of families illustrate this emerging intersection: to examine the responses of families and family members to various states of health, as well as expected and unexpected life transitions, to test theories of the effects of nursing on families and their members, and to formulate theories of predictors of family outcomes.

In a later paper, Feetham (1991b) noted that research combining practitioner/family interventions and family outcomes is limited because we first must define and measure family outcomes and family interventions. Nursing offers a foundation from which to build definitions and measures based in practice and science, but much of that work remains to be done.

Nursing and Social Policy Affecting Families

Defining social policy and family nurses/researchers as "agents" of the family is saying in effect that our interest in them lies in what they can do to serve the well-being of families. Further, because they are interactive agents, our interest in the relationships between policy development and nursing science and practice is focused on how those relationships can address family issues.

A concise and thoughtful definition of family issues can be drawn from the National Forum on the Future of Children and Families: education, child health, employment and income, poverty and welfare (Both & Garduque, 1989). For this discussion "child health" has been restated as simply "health and well-being."

Richmond and Kotelchuck's (1983) model of policy development, equally concise and thoughtful, defines one agent (policy) as the outcomes of knowledge base, social strategy, and political will. Bringing the National Forum issues and Richmond's model together creates a 3×4 matrix of the primary relationships between one agent (policy) and the issues of the principal (family). The matrix can be used then to describe what the second agent (nursing) contributes to the primary relationships.

To construct an overlay of what nursing science and practice can contribute, 194 abstracts accepted for the Second International Family Nursing Conference were sorted into the matrix (Table 1.1). Two methodological issues limit the conclusions that may be drawn from this sorting: (a) The papers may not be a representative sample of the state of family science and practice, and (b) the reliability and validity of the sorting method were not tested.

The numbers may be interpreted as follows. The zero in the upper left cell indicates that none of the papers that focused on the knowledge base for practice also focused on the family's issues about education. The next cell to the right indicates that 112 papers that focused on the knowledge base for practice also focused on the family's issues about health and well-being.

Attention to family issues was uneven. Education as a family issue was not addressed in this sample of papers about nursing science and practice. The expected skew toward health and well-being (92% of the papers) was observed. Only 2% of the papers addressed economic family issues.

Almost 75% (141) of the papers addressed both the knowledge base and family health issues. Embedded within that group is the core of the entire distribution; 112 papers (58% of all) focused on the knowledge base about practice and family health issues. This dominant focus on practice and

Table 1.1 Distribution of Family Nursing Practice and Research Within the Policy/Family Matrix

| Determinants of Policy | Education | Issues for Families | | Poverty and welfare | Total (%) |
		Health and Well-Being	Employment and Income		
Knowledge base					
About practice	0	112	3	3	118 (61)
About research	0	29	0	2	31 (16)
Political will	0	10	1	2	13 (7)
Social strategy	0	28	0	4	32 (16)
Total (%)	0 (0)	179 (92)	4 (2)	11 (6)	194 (100)

NOTE: Distribution of 194 abstracts accepted for Second International Conference on Family Nursing.

family health echoes the discussions of Gilliss (1989b, 1989c), Whall and Fawcett (1991b), and Feetham (1991a, 1991b).

In the remaining cells, it is striking that equal numbers of papers focused on the knowledge base about research and family health issues (15%) and social strategies for addressing family health issues (15%). The first group of papers exemplifies Feetham's (1991b) discussion about the emerging confluence of practice and research within the field, while the second illustrates Meister's (1989a, 1989b) premise that the nature of practice endows the field of family nursing with a unique view of strategies for addressing family problems.

In relation to family health issues, the distribution follows the research and policy recommendations made by Kelly and Ramsey (1991). In an analysis of families, poverty, and public policies, they found that policy development must be informed by research that describes the diversity among families. Research that reflects diversity can enlighten policy development by helping separate values from facts and by producing estimates of the potential impact of policies (Kelly & Ramsey, 1991; Wilson, 1991).

One way of ensuring full attention to the diversity of needs is to conduct studies that include and assess the "outliers," as well as families following central tendencies. Chapter 11 in this volume, by Feetham, Perkins, and Carroll, discusses how nursing research of families can capture data about outliers and how the distribution of papers in the matrix suggests that the field is beginning to do so. Multiple facets of the notion of family health are represented: practice, research, political will, and social strategy. Attention to the three other sets of family issues, however, is extremely limited.

Agenda for Reducing Agency Loss

This chapter focuses on the landscape—that is, the context for and larger aims of family nursing. The context is that of the family, not of the nurse. It is complex and heavily affected by social policies shaping education, health care, employment, and income. One aim of family nursing as a field is to foster improvement in how social policies and clinicians serve families. Even this brief discussion of crosscutting themes points to the beginnings of an agenda to reduce agency loss—that is, to improve the performance of policy and nursing as agents of the family. In summary,

1. *Social policy and families:* Design research to clarify policy analyses; use theoretical frameworks to establish definitions and meanings used in empirical work. Design innovations with a plan for extending the findings to policy.

2. *Nursing and families:* Continue efforts to hold work on theory, empiricism, and practice in close association. Increase the overt focus on family outcomes and their sensitivity to the quality of agency relationships.

3. *Nursing and social policy affecting families:* Use nursing science based in practice as a means of developing and refining theoretical frameworks. Make use of the full range of data, especially to understand outliers. Work to relate family health issues to family economic issues. Continue to advance three areas of expertise: practice and family health, research and family health, and social strategies for addressing family health.

Many aspects of these crosscutting themes are tackled in the chapters of this book. In the preface, Barbara Durand discussed the needs of families of a hospitalized child: competent care, the child's freedom from pain, skillful and compassionate physical care, and sophisticated help for the family in managing. This is a clear and comprehensive definition of the components of the agency role of a family nurse clinician. We still need definitions of the components of the agency role of the family nurse scientist, as well as the components of the agency role for clinicians and scientists in relation to social policy. The definitions are worth producing, however, because they will enable unique and vital contributions from the field of family nursing on behalf of its principals.

PART II

Theory Development and Families

Janice M. Bell, Editor

2

Disciplinary Issues Related to Family Theory Development in Nursing

Ann L. Whall

It is always risky business discussing the "state of the art" of anything—both because events/ideas happen so rapidly and because everyone has a different view of the world. Nevertheless, as one who over the past 15 years has been studying and writing about family theory in nursing, about characteristics, problems, and strengths, it is again time to take stock of the state of such development. In essence, discussion on the nature of family theory in nursing began appearing in print in the 1980s (Fawcett, 1975; Whall, 1980). A number of books now are written for this area each year. Much is still left to do. To understand this development further, the views of nurse theorist Rosemary Ellis are used in this discussion. Ellis did not publish most of her ideas in her lifetime. Just as with Harry Stack Sullivan and George Herbert Meade, she left it to her students to publish her ideas after her death. Many of the ideas presented here came from personal discussions with Ellis and with a student of hers, Algase. According to Algase, (1990) Ellis identified four components of a discipline. In reference to family theory in nursing, these four components are used to examine the state of the art.

The first component that Ellis identified is that of a *perspective*—defined here as "an identifiable view, a characteristic approach with persistent themes that can be identified over time." One can trace our nursing perspective on families through our early nursing texts dealing with family, as well as through nursing standards of practice and our only systematically interrelated and examined theory—or the nursing conceptual models.

Evidence points to at least four distinguishing characteristics (Whall, 1982, 1984).

1. A holistic view—nursing is interested not just in family psychic phenomena, for example, but in their physical, social, and other needs.
2. An educational approach—one that seeks to inform families of their options and alternatives and that supports them in making decisions and choices.
3. A focus on changing the environment to bring about health, as first emphasized by Nightingale.
4. A focus on supporting family health rather than on disease or illness primarily. This focus leads us to an optimistic, less negative view.

The second component that Ellis identified is that of *persistent questions.* Our research questions signify the content that nursing addresses with regard to families. Research questions do not exclusively signify this content, but questions addressed in practice with families are a source that informs of such content. In Whall and Loveland-Cherry (in press), several of these persistent questions are identified. Two examples are as follows:

Questions regarding ways to assist families in times of stress
Questions regarding optional support for families during normative growth and developmental events

The study designs are most often associational and descriptive in nature—not at the intervention or prescriptive level at the present time.

The third component is the *domains of knowledge,* or the subjects into which family nursing knowledge is divided—for example, when one describes what needs to be taught to students. The domains or content areas are fairly well understood at the present time, but it is important to note that there are no right or wrong ways to describe these domains, just different ways of separating out our knowledge. Moreover these areas will change or vary somewhat over time.

Meister (1984) described these domains or content areas as theoretical perspectives on family, natural transitions in the family, health and the family, illness and the family, and health policy and its impact on family.

Murphy (1986) described these domains as follows:

Health maintenance and successful coping in healthy families
Family responses to illness
Family transitions and new structures
Family interface with institutions
Public policy and the family
Cross-cultural family research

Whall and Fawcett (1991c) used the following categories to identify the domains:

Changes in family structure
Healthy families
Impact of illness on family

The fourth component is *truth criteria,* or those analytic and evaluative standards that are used to judge nursing's body of knowledge with regard to family. Some of the truth criteria currently used with regard to family theory in nursing are as follows:

- Is research or practice examination of the theory adequate?
- Is this research true to a nursing perspective—for example, focused on supporting health and not solely on disease?
- Is the research examination congruent with the theory; for example, are philosophic assumptions compatible?
- Is a family unit or other meaningful focus involved?
- Can this theory ultimately inform practice?
- Does this theory build on other nursing knowledge or have the potential to build on this knowledge?

These truth criteria still are being developed for nursing's family theory; these criteria also will evolve and change over time as did those evaluative questions asked of the nursing conceptual models. Another disciplinary component that Ellis discussed is a community of scholars, or those who in part produce such nursing knowledge and evaluate it.

The major methods employed in developing family theory in nursing now need to be examined, as well as identification of what still needs to be accomplished in terms of immediate and future goals. First, let us recognize that as Fawcett (1978) suggested, theory without research is trivial, and research without theory is likewise inconsequential. Fawcett cited a double helix relationship, or one in which research produces and tests theory and theory drives and/or is an outcome of research. Second let us recognize that theory development in nursing is a recently recognized endeavor; it does not have a very long history. The theory production methods used in nursing are therefore in their infancy.

In family theory in nursing, however, it appears that primarily three methods are used. First are the borrowed and reformulated (for disciplinary purposes) efforts that have produced theory primarily at the middle range. For example, the stress/coping research and literature are based primarily on borrowed/reformulated theory. This theory is not global or concerned with the universe or with practice application; in other words, it is middle range in nature. One problem with this borrowed reformulation approach is that one may also inadvertently "buy" unrecognized assumptions or one on which the theory is based. One advantage of this method, however, is that it is relatively quick and that this newly formed theory is also relevant to a discipline external to nursing.

The second method used in nursing to date is induction from empirical data usually produced in clinical settings. Inductively developed theory is often related to practice problems. For example, nursing might ask how to help families faced with a given illness. This inductively based theory represents perhaps the largest category of family theory in nursing at the present time.

Some family nursing theory also has been developed from the third method—deduction from nursing conceptual models—and this perhaps distinguishes family theory in nursing from other areas in nursing. This deductively derived theory is not difficult to produce from these models, as the nursing perspective is evident. One problem in this deductive effort, however, is the level of abstraction of nursing conceptual models. Measurement tools often are not available for those abstract concepts, and research examination sometimes lags behind. These epistemological discussions need to continue regarding family theory in nursing. Unless we attend to how family knowledge in nursing is developing, knowledge-building efforts could have unintended outcomes. Such consequences might occur as becoming less congruent with a nursing perspective, and/or the body of knowledge might not build or could become fractionalized, not cumulative and not replicated.

The review article referred to above indicated some problem areas in family research in nursing, such as small sample sizes and mostly descriptive and nonreplicated studies. How should nursing proceed to develop family theory in nursing? A few rhetorical questions might be posed: Why not categorize and classify this theory into domains just as family sociology has? Why not identify the predominant assumptions/propositions and concepts found within each domain? How does the knowledge produced in each domain fit with the prevailing nursing perspective? What other types of family knowledge are needed by nursing, for example, ethical knowledge of cultural variations between groups? Is the current family theory in nursing relevant to various cultural groups?

Since nursing began publishing discussions about the structure of its family theory base, much progress has been made. Back in 1980, few family conferences in nursing were held. Few if any questions were asked about the proper focus of family theory in nursing. The community of scholars who address the development of family theory in nursing need to continue to entertain the disciplinary questions that Ellis explicated—those of perspective, persistent questions, domains, and truth criteria with regard to family theory in nursing. This type of examination will help continue the excellence that is characteristic of the progress to date.

3

Nursing Science in Family Care, 1984-1990

Virginia E. Hayes

This chapter concerns science building, the component Gortner (1983) calls "the consensus of informed opinion obtained usually through research" (p. 1). "The goal of nursing science . . . is to represent nature—in particular human nature—to understand it and to explain it for the benefit of humankind" (Gortner & Schultz, 1988, p. 23). What can be more basic to humankind than the concept of family, the basic socializing unit of the individual in all cultures (Bronfenbrenner, 1979; Gottlieb & Rowat, 1987; Wright & Leahey, 1984)?

With the rise of industrialization and highly technical medical interventions, modern nursing seems to have drifted from the idea of delivering care within and for families (Ham & Chamings, 1983) and has begun to demonstrate revaluing family only during the past 30 years (Whall, 1986). Despite articulated acknowledgements from nurse clinicians and scientists that this is long overdue (Barnard, 1980; Meleis, 1987), published literature remains thin in theory development and research related to the phenomena of family health care.

The purpose of this chapter is to examine the current "state of the science" related to family nursing. I surveyed a selection of major journals in the field to determine the quality and quantity of recent work. The results of this inquiry are presented in three sections: conceptual and literature reviews, instrumentation, and family research. Although the number of family-focused nursing publications has increased slightly since 1984, this critical analysis reveals significant shortcomings in the systematic building of family nursing science. In particular the family as a unit of analysis is in need of clarification, analysis, and investigation. Although there is forward movement in theory development, it is apparent that the discipline has much need for the development of nursing theory related to family and for the testing of theory in research.

Background and Approach to the Review

Two reviews of family nursing research provide landmarks in the progress of knowledge development in family nursing: the first was Feetham's in the *Annual Review of Nursing Research* in 1984; the second was Gilliss's (1989a) chapter in *Toward a Science of Family Nursing* (Gilliss, Highley, Roberts, & Martinson, 1989). Feetham's (1984) critical review analyzed a selection of works up to 1982-1983 by examining conceptual and methodological issues in relation to future directions for family research. She concluded that "nurse researchers have a contribution to make [but] . . . need to continue to build on knowledge and research of other disciplines while developing full theoretical nursing models and examining the family as a unit of analysis" (Feetham, 1984, p. 20). She reinforced the notion that studies should be directed by a full model with internal consistency but did not advocate use of a single model of family care. The work reviewed for this chapter demonstrates that nursing research continues to fall short of Feetham's standard.

Gilliss (1989a), using a taxonomy of research designs adapted from Jacobsen and Meininger (1985), analyzed family nursing research published in six major nursing research journals. She evaluated the content foci and research designs of 76 reports, attributing the preponderance of maternal-child and young family work to "our traditional perspectives on the definition of the family" (Gilliss, 1989a, p. 42). She concluded that the productivity of family nurse researchers was improving, though "startling gaps" were found in nursing knowledge. She further expressed concern about methodological issues in family research, adding that we do not yet know how to capture the different phenomena about families that interest nurses most.

To flesh out an understanding of the state of family nursing science, this chapter examines the scholarly literature from sources not covered by Feetham (1984) and Gilliss (1989a). Table 3.1 summarizes this review: Articles were drawn from the same six journals used by Gilliss (1989a) and

Table 3.1   Articles Reviewed by Source

Type	Name of Journal	No. Issues	Significant	Accepted[*]
Gilliss 1989	*Advances in Nursing Science*	18	5	4
selections	*Journal of Advanced Nursing*	38	18	7
1987-1990	*International Journal of Nursing*			
	Studies	16	0	0
	Nursing Research	24	13	4
	Research in Nursing and Health	24	8	3
	Western Journal of Nursing			
	Research	24	8	5
		144	52	23
Other nonspecialty	*Canadian Journal of Nursing*			
1984-1990	*Research*	24	9	5
	Image	28	6	3
	Nursing Clinics of North America	28	1	0
		80	16	8
Pediatric specialty	*Issues in Comprehensive Pediatric*			
	Nursing	36	12	5
	MCN	42	6	1
	Maternal-Child Nursing Journal	20	2	0
	Pediatric Nursing	42	15	5
		140	35	11
Multidisciplinary	*Children's Health Care*	28	7	4
1984-1990	*Family and Community Health*	28	14	8
		56	21	12
	Total	420	124	54

NOTE: [*]Includes both research and theory articles.

nine additional ones, selected for their acknowledged good quality of works published and for their contributions to the specialty field of care of children and their families, my area of particular interest. Thus all 15 journals were assayed for the same period.

Indexes of 420 issues were examined to ascertain whether the content of articles might be in any way related to family nursing on the basis of Whall's (1986) definition of *family:* "a self-identified group of two or more individuals whose association is characterized by special terms, who may or may not be related by bloodlines or law, but who function in such a way that they consider themselves to be a family" (p. 241). Note the emphasis on the wholeness of the unit and an implied systems approach. An article was not accepted for this review if the unit of analysis or the theoretical concern was restricted to one or more individual family members or dyads.

Table 3.2   Criteria for Inclusion

1. One or more authors a nurse
2. Topic relevant for clinical practice
3. Tested a theoretical framework
   or
   Developed new perspectives
4. Sound method
5. Addressed one aspect of the family group in health or illness:*
   - family role
   - relationship between/among family members
   - relationship between family and larger environs

From "Family Research in Nursing" by C. L. Gilliss (1989a), in C. L. Gilliss, B. L. Highley, B. M. Roberts, & I. M. Martinson (Eds.), *Toward a Science of Family Nursing* (pp. 38-39), Menlo Park, CA: Addison-Wesley.
*It was this criterion that was applied more stringently in this chapter than by Gilliss (1989a).

Approximately 150 such articles were noted, most in the research category. Although it is acknowledged that studies of this kind add to our knowledge about family players, articles were rejected if no effort was made to demonstrate a relationship between the results or argument and family processes or interactions.

The screening criteria of Brown, Tanner, and Padrick (1984) (as modified by Gilliss, 1989a, and shown in Table 3.2) also were used for this review. Abstracts, introductions, summaries, reference lists, and sections devoted to theory and method were appraised for these criteria. This review was more stringent than Gilliss's (1989a) in rejecting articles for authors' failure to articulate even partial family theory as guiding the study or to demonstrate what their studies added to knowledge about families. In total, 54 articles are analyzed here.

Conceptual and Literature Review Articles

Twenty-seven of the 54 articles fit the conceptual or literature review category of Gilliss (1989a). Articles in this section were examined for content, for the nature of explained theory, and for their potential contribution to nursing's knowledge of families.

The dilemma around where family fits into the nursing metaparadigm (Fawcett, 1984b) is addressed by Friedemann (1989). According to this author, all nurses can and should practice family nursing. She suggested that four definitions of family are applicable, necessary, and subsumed in her three-level system approach: the family (a) as environment for the individual (b) as a group of interacting dyads, (c) as a single unit with defined boundaries, and (d) as a unit transacting with the environment. A case is presented for using three levels of theory in practice with families: individually focused, interpersonal family nursing, and family system care. Gill's (1987) premise is similar, supported by her review of the literature about how nurses view the family as a unit of care when children are hospitalized. Although Gill ties her argument concerning nursing education, policies, and attitudes toward parent participation to defined family care, she draws her evidence from studies of parent participation, demonstrating a lapse in logic very common in family nursing. "Legitimizing" family care is also a theme for Reed (1990), who applies the NANDA nursing diagnosis categorization to family care: alteration in family process when a child has cystic fibrosis.

Three articles developed concept analyses important to family nursing science. Primarily interested in practice for communities and nursing administration, Schultz (1987) calls for much-needed research to refine the metaparadigmatic domain concept of *client* and its relationship to health and environment; she develops a persuasive argument for the notion that "client" can be singular or plural, including individuals, groups, families, and aggregates as possible recipients of care. *Role integration* and *social support* are family concepts respectively addressed by Fife (1985) and Kane (1988). Together these three articles demonstrate examples of nurses' attempts to delineate the dynamic, systems-related variables relevant to the study of families and to challenge current scientific thinking about families as the recipients of care.

The remaining 21 articles in this grouping represent a variety of scholarly works in which central theses are based firmly on concepts of family care. Chronic illness in a family member has been documented to precipitate acute and chronic stress or crisis and to disturb family members' relationships and roles and their interactions with the community. Articles that addressed chronic illness focus on coping, power, motivation, resources, and social support within and outside the family (e.g., Ferraro & Longo, 1985; Stengel, Echeveste, & Schmidt, 1985; Stuifbergen, 1987; Woods, Yates, & Primomo, 1989). Interestingly, issues of stress and social support also were raised in articles addressing health promotion and prevention issues. For example, one-parent families are now considered a "legitimate" family type but remain at risk for health problems, according to Duffy (1987), who also published a broader based review of literature on health promotion in the family (Duffy, 1988), pinpointing 12 specific questions for future research in the areas of the family's internal and external environments.

Much valuable direction for future investigators was offered in this analysis, supported as well by Bomar (1990), Dailey (1985), Donnelly (1990), and Puskar (1989).

Two analyses offered specific alternatives for the direction of selected research efforts, both in the area of community-based care. Allen's (1987) advocacy for a critical social theory approach to health care bore on processes and functions related to autonomy and responsibility in families and communities, and Gottlieb and Rowat (1987) outlined the McGill model of nursing. Although these latter authors emphasized how the model directs nurses and students in the care of families in community settings and noted that it requires further theoretical development and testing through research, further publications were not located in the journals reviewed. Such work represents strong potential for middle- and grand-range theory development and directs family nursing research.

The year 1990 produced four clinically based family assessment articles; one of these concerned families of elders (Beckingham & Baumann, 1990, on assessment and decision making in elderly families), a rarely examined clinical group, according to Gilliss (1989a). Other assessment articles are Austin (1990, on parental coping), Lapp, Diemert, and Enestvedt (1990, who presented a theory-based family assessment/intervention tool), and Thomas (1990, an important review of issues central to comprehensive family health care assessment).

Concern is addressed for families whose roles in health care have to expand to encompass care for an ill *child* member: Two similar articles by Rushton (1990a, 1990b) are about family-centered care in the critical care area, though these run close to deteriorating into prescriptions and policies for family members. One article addresses home or hospital care for children with end-stage cancer (Dufour, 1989), and another (Johnson, 1990) is a statement about the position of the Association for the Care of Children's Health concerning the family's changing role in health care, important for its predictions about future directions and hence where nurses might focus research efforts.

Finally, three significant articles concern the complexity of issues and problems facing family nurse researchers: Stuifbergen (1987), Uphold and Strickland (1989), and Moriarty (1990a). They raised questions related to who the best informants are; the size and methods of sampling; measurement design and methods; reliability and validity issues in individual, dyadic, and group measures; the potency of intervening variables in complex research situations; and statistical methods. These authors provided constructive suggestions for future directions and solutions, but as the rest of this review indicates, the current literature provides little actual evidence of movement in family nursing research as called for by Gilliss (1983), Feetham (1984), and Barnard (1984).

Articles on Instrumentation

Six of the 54 articles reviewed concern the appropriate selection or refinement of family measures or the development of new ones. Together they demonstrate promise for research in family nursing and the expertise of family nurse scholars. Speer and Sachs (1985) analyzed the properties of nine existing tools, primarily for their applicability to clinical practice. The description, reliability and validity findings, and pros and cons of each instrument make this a valuable summary for the beginning family researcher, even though the authors said that "most tools have little [reported] empirical validation" (Speer & Sachs, 1985, p. 355). Their challenge regarding validity is addressed for the Family Environment Scale in two papers: a large study by Loveland-Cherry, Youngblut, and Leidy (1989) and another by Munet-Vilaro and Egan (1990). This widely used scale did not perform as well psychometrically as predicted by Moos and Moos (1986), particularly in a group of Vietnamese families. These findings demonstrate both the sophisticated skills of these nurse investigators and the "state of the art" in measurement of family variables. Much caution must be exercised in selecting, using, and interpreting results from existing family measures.

Speer and Sachs's (1985) call for further instrument development was answered in three studies: Reidy and Thibaudeau (1984) have designed and are testing a nine-dimension scale for nurses to use in the evaluation of family competence; Fife, Huhman, and Keck (1986) reported the development and testing of a tool for evaluation of the psychosocial status of families of children with serious illnesses; and Rawlins, Rawlins, and Horner (1990) described instrument development of a family needs assessment tool. All of these authors acknowledged the need for further testing of their instruments.

Family Research Articles

In addition to the five criteria mentioned earlier, the 21 research reports were classified for this review in terms of their content, methods, and design, as presented in Table 3.3.

Table 3.3   Taxonomy of Research Designs

Experiments	Prospective studies in which at least one intervention was manipulated
True experiments	Randomized control trials
Quasi experiments	Nonrandomization, or comparison groups (if any) not concurrent
Observational studies	Naturally occurring events in which no deliberate intervention was made by the investigator
Cross-sectional studies	Observations related to one point in time
Longitudinal studies	Observations related to at least two points in time, even if all data collected simultaneously

Recall that a direct comparison cannot be made with the 76 studies reviewed by Gilliss (1989a) because of the journals sampled, the families-of-young-children bias purposely sought for this review, and the obviously more stringent application of the criterion related to the presence of a family framework for the studies. Because only 21 studies met the inclusion criteria, it seems clear that published research underrepresents the significance of family nursing to practice (Dominica, 1987; Gilliss et al., 1989; Wright & Leahey, 1984). In addition, Gilliss's (1989a) projected trend toward more activity in family nursing research is not borne out in this survey. Although many studies are reported of individuals and dyads located within families, these cannot be construed to be family studies until authors demonstrate a theoretical family focus for exploration or testing and examine the processual, interactional aspects of family responses beyond those generated from family member data.

Content. Variables related to ill adult members were the subject of five studies. Gortner and her colleagues (1988) are studying individual and family health during recovery after heart surgery. Family, stress, and self-efficacy theory were used to develop and manage variables in this ongoing program of research. Heart transplant recipients and their families were the subjects of Mishel and Murdaugh's (1987) grounded theory study; gradually families (partners) "redesigned the dream" during the 12-week postoperative course of discussion groups. Prins's (1989) unique exploratory study of the effects of family visits on intracranial pressure readings of patients in a critical care area integrated data collection with routine nursing monitoring. Rose (1985) took a phenomenological approach to describe families' discomfort, insecurity, isolation, powerlessness, and need for information during a member's psychiatric inpatient admission. Finally a discharge-planning intervention, a family-patient teaching program for psychiatric inpatients, was tested by Youssef (1987).

Two maternal-child health studies were in this category. A sociodemographic (epidemiological) study of the families of low birth weight infants was reported by Brown and colleagues (1989). The baseline data from this study represent framing a model of association with family structure and function variables. Mercer, Ferketich, DeJoseph, May, and Sollid (1988) reported part of a longitudinal study that is testing family developmental theory in couples predelivery, comparing high-risk and low-risk pregnancy groups.

Nine reports concerned the impact of a chronically ill child on the family. Empirical family measures were reported in three of these: family stress and strengths in one- and two-parent families by McCubbin (1989b), as part of her ongoing research program of stress and coping in families; the effects of living with infants with apnea, monitored and nonmonitored, by Sweeney (1988); and Stuifbergen's (1990) use of the FES in a cross-sectional study that demonstrated four clusters of families with a chronically ill parent. Noteworthy is Stuifbergen's conclusion that unidimensional analysis is not sufficiently complex to yield an accurate picture of what is occurring in families.

Parents' concerns of living with a child with diabetes and cystic fibrosis were investigated by Hodges and Parker (1987) and Stullenbarger, Norris, Edgil, and Prosser (1987), respectively. Although parental concerns were cited as the variables of interest in each of these studies, a well-defined family theory link is evident in both. Families whose children had cystic fibrosis were the subject of different aspects of a descriptive study by Canam (1986, 1987). Family information and support needs and intrafamily communication and teaching of young members were investigated.

A group of qualitative studies describe families' coping with a chronically ill child: One (Clements, Copeland, & Loftus, 1990) developed theory about particularly needy times for families from parent data; one studied American Indian families' perceptions of their health care needs (Malach & Segal, 1990); and another looked at relationships between families of children with otitis media with effusion and the Canadian Health Care System (Wuest & Stern, 1990b). Anderson and Elfert (1989), as part of Anderson's research program concerning the impact of having a chronically ill child in families of different cultures, presented caretaking as a women's issue within white Canadian families rather than as the shared family function it is purported to be. Finally one report combined interview data from separate adult and young family studies of the effect of chronic illness in the family. Thorne and Robinson (1988) presented a stage theory of the development of relationships with health care professionals, describing behaviors and reactions of family members at each phase. The rigor of some qualitative research (Sandelowski, 1986) unfortunately is threatened by authors' failure to state clearly who have informed the researcher(s) and what analytic steps (the paper trail) led to the formation of family concepts.

This review contains two Canadian surveys pertinent to family nursing: Clarke (1989) reported use of the Delphi technique in a cross-Canada look at family strengths, and Wright and Bell (1989) assessed the family content in the curricula of Canadian schools of nursing where, they reported, family nursing education is flourishing.

In the reports reviewed, family variables were a mix of independent, dependent, controlled, and uncontrolled. Investigators are not often clear about stating the nature of the family variables within studies, particularly the extraneous ones. Before strong theory can be constructed from independently conducted studies, more clarity will be needed in this area (Barnard, 1984). Noticeably absent are studies of healthy families, especially with community interaction foci. Not one report of completed research addressed elders and their families, despite the widespread concern in nursing about the need to plan for and improve care for this increasing population. Although specialty journals doubtless contain reports of pertinent studies, good studies also should be appearing in the general research journals surveyed for this review. This is one of the "startling gaps" mentioned by Gilliss (1989a).

Design. The bulk of these 21 studies were observational, with a predominance of grounded theory/phenomenological methods; 11 were longitudinal (Anderson & Elfert, 1989; Clarke, 1989; Hodges & Parker, 1987; Malach & Segal, 1990; Mercer et al., 1988; Mishel & Murdaugh, 1987; Prins, 1989; Rose, 1985; Sweeney, 1988; Thorne & Robinson, 1988; Wuest & Stern, 1990b), and 7 were cross-sectional (Brown et al., 1989; Canam, 1986, 1987; Clements et al., 1990; Stuifbergen, 1990; Stullenbarger et al., 1987; Wright & Bell, 1989). Only three represented experimental studies: two true experiments (Gortner et al., 1988; Youssef, 1987), and one quasi experiment (McCubbin, 1989b). This picture reflects the diversity of family problems, dynamics, and health problems that concern nurse researchers, the difficulties presented by naturalistic practice settings, and the ethical dilemmas that often complicate sampling.

Methods. This review identified fewer studies that report the use of multiple methods than was remarked by Gilliss (1989a). Many instruments appear to be under investigation by nurse researchers, most of them designed in related disciplines rather than in nursing. Adequate reliability and validity indicators related to nursing phenomena are sometimes inferred and not reported. Much work needs to be done in the accurate, reliable measurement of family nursing variables, as complex as these may be (Barnard, 1984; Uphold & Strickland, 1989). Phenomenological work continues to investigate and validate family nurses' hunches about significant health-related phenomena from the emic perspective. Although descriptive and explanatory studies are necessary to nursing's understanding of basic family phenomena, prescriptive theory testing is a large gap in work reported to date.

The problems for building of the scientific base of family care are many and diverse. However, we need to work on basic conceptual units for study (variables), approaches (methods), priorities, and identification of nurses' unique contributions in therapeutics and preventive health activities. Compared with the earlier analyses of the issues by Gilliss (1983, 1989a), Feetham (1984), Barnard (1984), and Whall (1986), this review indicates that family nursing research is waning in quantity, though its quality remains sound. Recently more publications have delineated what family nursing is and what concepts are important for theory building and research, but there is much more to do. What are appropriate units of analysis? What are the best methodological and statistical approaches?

Family Nursing Science Revisited

According to Moody et al. (1988), there has been a sixfold increase in the amount of nursing research published in six journals since 1977—sadly this is not apparent in the field of family nursing. The complexities of systems variables, setting issues, ethics, and undeveloped nursing theory no doubt contribute to this lack (Patterson, 1988). Specific types of families are particularly needy of investigation: Nontraditional, families from other cultures (both in North American society and internationally), families of the elderly, and healthy, well-functioning families (Dailey, 1985; Duffy, 1988; Gilliss, 1989a; Meleis, 1987) are examples.

One wonders whether the lack of published activity in the area of family nursing science is related to ongoing debate surrounding the relative values of using "borrowed" or nursing theories to direct family research and practice (Johnson, 1974). Although dissension has abated recently, studies currently appearing in the literature may have been begun when such arguments were more sensitive. Indeed, as programs of research develop with one study building on the findings of its predecessors, the problem of little family research may be perpetuated. We need more thick-skinned innovators to break the mold and to begin systematic examination of issues around the nursing of families in health care.

Another possible inhibition for family investigations may be the meta-paradigmatic discussion of where family falls in the domain concepts (Friedemann, 1989; Murphy, 1986; Schultz, 1987). Perhaps investigators choose to study safer, less risky, less complex topics, testing less controversial nursing theory. Many would argue that nursing families, both as the context for the individual and as the unit of care, is an established concern of nurses and does fall within the domain concepts (Whall, 1986). Effort to enhance nursing's understanding of family care, eloquently demonstrated by such work as Gortner and her colleagues (1988), McCubbin (1989b), Rose (1985), and Thorne and Robinson (1988), is sorely needed.

This is not to discredit individual researchers and theorists or their work. Most of the research published in the credible journals used for this review contributes to an understanding of phenomena in the domains of nursing. In the area of family nursing specifically, there would seem to be need for organization of studies that test and explicate phenomena central to family care and to the development of prescriptive theory that will guide interventions. Family study based on individual frameworks is important, but the field of family care requires integrated studies that contribute to the "particular perspective" of family nursing (Donaldson & Crowley, 1978). Perhaps we are still, as Gilliss said in 1983 and again in 1989, having trouble capturing the phenomena about families that interest nurses most.

To modify a notion from Silva (1977, p. 60), science has fractioned the individual from the family and has not yet reunited them in nursing research. Silva's (1977) characteristics of science are not yet being met in statements about families: Nursing literature does not yet show coherence in facts about families; universal statements that reflect commonalities do not yet occur with frequency or order, and the few investigations and arguments for family-related research published to date are not by and large well explained, elaborated, and linked together or to theory. The holistic, ecological, evolutionary underpinnings of the discipline of nursing provide a mandate for understanding and nursing the family. The standards of good nursing science (Gortner & Schultz, 1988) continue to need specification in the area of family nursing knowledge.

4

A Theoretical Perspective of Family and Child Health Derived From King's Conceptual Framework for Nursing: A Deductive Approach to Theory Building

Maureen A. Frey

The family traditionally and historically has been a central focus in nursing. Whall (1986) traced the elements of the concept of *family* to Nightingale, who recognized the importance of family members, especially wives and children. The role of the family in the care of the sick was included in nursing texts as early as 1890. A more contemporary focus has been on the dynamics of the family in relation to the health and health care of individual members and the unit as a whole.

Despite the centrality of the family to nursing, the development of family theory in nursing has a much shorter history and parallels the development of family theory in the social/family sciences, as well as theory development in nursing in general. Both disciplines—family and nursing—strongly recognize the need for sound theory development with an emphasis on both

AUTHOR'S NOTE: I acknowledge Susan Sereika and Sue V. Fink for assistance with data management and Imogene King and Mary J. Denyes for ongoing assistance with theoretical development.

process and product (Gilliss, Campbell, & Patterson, 1989). At this time family theory in nursing is characterized by various levels of abstraction and approaches to its development.

One approach to the development of nursing theory is the use of nursing's existing conceptual frameworks. The use of a nursing framework has the advantage of providing an explicit nursing perspective, for it is the perspective that distinguishes one discipline from another. The nursing focus on family is characterized by a comprehensive biopsychosocial perspective; an emphasis on wellness, well-being, and quality of life rather than on pathology; and concern for environmental influences on health (Whall & Fawcett, 1991b). This perspective informs a practice that is different from the practice of physicians, social workers, and psychologists.

The process of using a nursing conceptual framework to develop theory is a deductive one that involves specification and empirical testing of a middle-range theory. Excellent guidelines for the process can be found in Acton, Irvin, and Hopkins (1991), Dulock and Holzemer (1991), Fawcett (1989), Louis and Kertvelyessy (1989), and Silva (1986).

In this chapter a program of research built around the development and testing of a theory of family and child health in children with chronic illness and derived from Imogene King's conceptual framework for nursing is presented. The research began with the specification and testing of relationships among five concepts with children with insulin-dependent diabetes mellitus (IDDM) and their families.[1] A smaller study supported the inclusion of a behavioral variable related to illness care and management.[2] Through additional revision and consultation, a refined and considerably more complex theory has been developed. This theory currently is being tested with families who have children with IDDM and asthma.[3] A brief review of each major phase of theory development follows.

The Initial Formulation

In 1985 King's (1981) conceptual framework was used to derive a middle-range theory of social support and health in children with insulin-dependent diabetes mellitus (IDDM). King's conceptual framework consists of three interacting, open systems: (a) individuals as personal systems, (b) two or more individuals forming interpersonal systems, and (c) larger groups with common interests and goals forming social systems. Many concepts borrowed from other disciplines and redefined by King are used to identify relevant knowledge for understanding each system. Conceptual definitions,

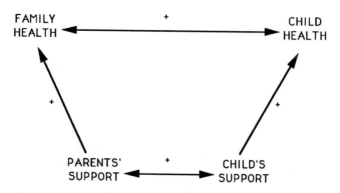

Figure 4.1. Hypothesized Relationships Among Concepts
SOURCE: From "Social Support and Health: A Theoretical Formulation Derived From King's Conceptual Framework" by M. A. Frey, 1989, *Nursing Science Quarterly, 2.* Reprinted with permission of Chestnut House Publications.

empirical indicators, and relationships were derived from King's concepts of health and interaction. The formulation is shown in Figure 4.1. Each arrow represents a hypothesized relationship. These relationships were stipulated in the form of a causal model and were tested with families ($N = 103$) who had children with IDDM. Concepts, indicators, and measures are shown in Table 4.1.

Results of Theory Testing

Several hypotheses were supported: Parents' social support had a direct and positive effect on family health, and parents' and the child's social support were related significantly. An additional hypothesis, which is not shown in Figure 4.1, also was supported: Illness factors had a direct and negative effect on child health. Two hypotheses were not supported: (a) the proposed reciprocal relationship between family health and child health, and (b) the direct effect of the child's social support on child health.

Initial testing of the theory provided empirical support for King's conceptual framework in relation to the effect of interaction on health, at least for adults, to the relationship between available support for parents and available support for children, and to the effect of illness on child health. The nonsignificant findings seemed related primarily to selection and measurement of indicators and to several missing variables that might explain or mediate the relationships and less to the theoretical relationships predicted by King's (1981) conceptual framework. A detailed account of that phase of the research has been published (Frey, 1989).

Table 4.1 Concepts, Indicators, and Measures

Family health	Family functioning	FACES II (Olson, Portner & Lavee, 1985)
	Family composition	Self-report
Parent/Child support	General support	Norebeck Social Support Questionnaire (Norbeck, 1984)
	Diabetes support	Modification of Norbeck Social Support Questionnaire
Child health	Scholastic competence	Self-Perception Profile for Children (Harter, 1985)
	Social acceptance	
	Athletic competence	
	Behavioral competence	
	Physical appearance	
	Global self-worth	
	Metabolic control	Glycosylated hemoglobin

Retesting and Refining the Theory

A 2-year follow-up study with the original sample was done to examine the stability of the traits and measures over time, to improve measurement of child health, and to expand the theoretical model. To improve the measurement of child health, the Brief Symptom Inventory (Derogatis & Melisaratos, 1983), a general measure of physical health symptoms, was used, along with a measure of self-perceived health status (Denyes, 1980).

In rethinking, revising, and extending the model, various aspects of the care and management necessitated by the illness condition were identified as factors that potentially affected and mediated child health. The importance of taking care of and responsibility for one's own health and illness is supported by many theoretical perspectives, the empirical literature, and clinical practice. This behavioral variable has been referred to as *self-care, illness care, adherence,* and *compliance* in the literature.

King (1981) identified that (a) individuals actively promote their own health and manage illness, (b) nurses deal with behavior of individuals pertaining to health and illness, (c) behavior equals actions, (d) interactions influence actions, and (e) actions have a mental (recognition) and physical (operation) component. Accordingly, illness and health self-care were incorporated into the formulation. The concept of illness care was operationalized by the Diabetes Self-Care Practice Instrument (Frey & Denyes, 1989; Frey & Fox, 1990). Behavior related to general health also was measured (Denyes Self-Care Practice Instrument, Denyes, 1980). These instruments, based on Orem's (1985) definition of *self-care,* tap actions that one undertakes to promote health and to manage illness.

At the time of data collection, only 36% ($N = 37$) of the sample was accessible due to an ongoing project at the agency. As a result extensive model testing was not possible. Correlational analysis, however, provided some direction for theory revision. Mother's and father's view of family adaptability were related significantly to several dimensions of child health. General support available to mothers and fathers was related to family cohesion, but diabetes-specific support was not. Support for parents was not related to child general health or to diabetes self-care. The availability of general support and diabetes support for parents was related.

General health and diabetes self-care in youths were related significantly to several dimensions of health status and metabolic control. Youths who reported higher diabetes-related self-care had higher behavioral competence, metabolic control, and perceived health status. Additionally, general health and illness self-care were positively related. Family health and parents' support were not related to the child's general health or to diabetes self-care. The child's diabetes support was not related to general health or diabetes self-care.

The amount of social support available to the child was related to several dimensions of child health. No relationship was found between the type of support and metabolic control or physical symptoms. Children who reported higher levels of general support, however, also reported higher levels of diabetes support. Child's social support and parents' social support were not related in this study.

Overall the findings provided preliminary support for inclusion of the self-care concept and direction for further revision and expansion, especially in terms of indicators and measures. The revised formulation is shown in Figure 4.2.

An Expanded Theory of Family and Child Health

As a result of the two studies, consultation with King, and discussions with colleagues, a more complex theory of families, children, and chronic

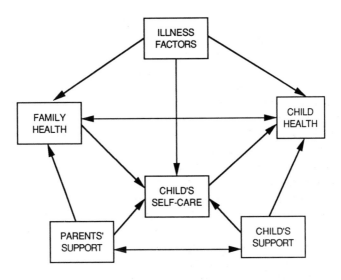

Figure 4.2. Revised Theory of Family and Child Health

illness has been developed (see Figure 4.3). This theory is being tested with families who have children with IDDM and asthma. The project extends previous work in several important ways, primarily in expansion of indicators of concepts, which makes it more theoretically and clinically complete. Direction for selection of indicators came from King's conceptual framework. In addition, self-care has been relabeled "health actions" to be more consistent with the language of King's framework.

Another important extension is the use of a comparison group—in this case, youths with asthma. This application combines a categorical and a noncategorical approach to chronic illness (Stein & Jessop, 1982). The study is designed to examine the common and unique patterns within and between the two illness groups, as well as change over time. Overall this design will maximize the opportunity for further theory refinement, as well as contribute substantive knowledge about the health of families and children with chronic illness.

Evaluation

The use of a nursing conceptual framework to develop family theory has many advantages, as well as a few limitations. In terms of contribution to

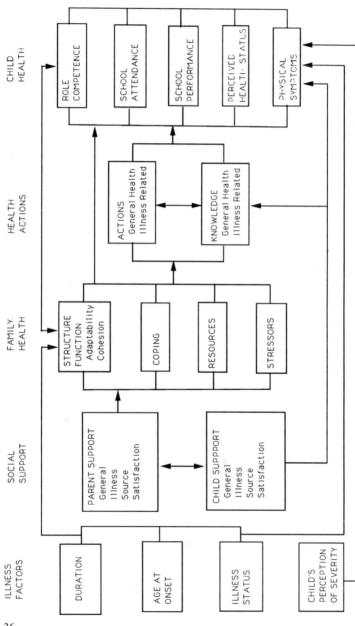

Figure 4.3. Proposed Theory of Families, Children, and Chronic Illness

36

nursing knowledge, use of nursing frameworks to generate middle-range theory is a logical and necessary step. Nursing has gone from debating why the profession needs them, to how many there should be, to identifying strengths and weaknesses via analysis and evaluation. It is now time to address their validity for understanding phenomena and ultimately for informing practice. The approach (a) offers a nursing perspective of important concepts, including but not limited to person, environment, and health; (b) allows nontraditional areas to be opened up; and (c) is applicable to many situations and populations. In addition, extension and testing of conceptual frameworks and theories will address the gaps known to exist.

A major limitation of the use of nursing's conceptual frameworks for the development of family theory is the unit of analysis. Many were developed for individuals. Although most recognize family, the conceptualization of family—that is, as a unit of care or environment—in the middle-range theory needs to be consistent with the conceptualization of the family in the parent framework or theory. Other potential limitations include difficulty in operationalization and identification of nursing interventions. King's conceptual framework has several advantages in these regards because the family is identified explicitly as a system and directions for intervention are clear.

In summary, the paths to theory development in nursing are many. The use of nursing's conceptual frameworks is a challenging process and one that is likely to contribute significantly to the scientific basis of nursing practice with families.

Notes

1. Funded by the American Nurses' Foundation, Michigan Nurses' Association, and a predoctoral fellowship from the American Diabetes Association—Michigan Affiliate, Inc.

2. Funded by Sigma Theta Tau, Inc., and Lambda Chapter, Wayne State University; the Public Health Service (BRSG S07 RR-05796); the School of Nursing, University of Michigan; and the Office of the Vice-President for Research, University of Michigan.

3. Funded by Public Health Service, National Institutes of Health, National Center for Nursing Research 1R29NR02243. Nursing Perspective—Families, Children, & Chronic Illness. M. Frey, Principal Investigator. 7/15/89 to 6/30/94.

5

The Meaning of Caregiving Behaviors:
Inductive Approaches
to Family Theory Development

Janet A. Deatrick

Kathleen A. Knafl

Kim Guyer

Quint (1967) sensitized the nursing community in the late 1960s to the value of theories generated from empirical data. Since that time, such approaches to theory development in family nursing have stemmed in large part from persistent questions regarding the family's experience with illness and disability. The overall goal of these efforts is typically to describe how the family defines, manages, and evaluates their situation when a family member is ill.

AUTHORS' NOTE: This chapter is based on four families in a study funded by the National Center for Nursing Research, Public Health Service Grant #NR01594, awarded to Kathleen Knafl, Bonnie Breitmeyer, Agatha Gallo, and Linda Zoeller in 1987 and 1990, "How Families Define and Manage a Child's Chronic Illness." We wish to thank Dr. Margaret Cotroneo for her contribution to the development of the category of nodal events.

Management behaviors (Deatrick & Knafl, 1990) have been identified as important aspects of the overall family management style (FMS) (Knafl & Deatrick, 1990). These "idiosyncratic procedures and routines related to the child's disability . . . and activities of daily living" (Burke, Costello, & Handley-Derry, 1989, p. 88) were found to be a prime concern of 160 mothers of children ($n = 60$ individually studied and $n = 100$ studied in a group) who were repeatedly hospitalized. These mothers did not feel that nurses and others in the hospital environment adequately understood or valued their management behaviors and that long months of progress in caregiving routines were disrupted by the hospitalization.

The purpose of this chapter is to describe an ongoing process of inductively developing a theory to guide practice, research, and education in family nursing. The process of developing an understanding of management behaviors by applying the concept to reports of all members of four families is highlighted. This process was the first step in an empirical validation of the concept that is being incorporated into a middle-range nursing theory—family-focused pediatric transitional care—which describes "specialist care emanating from tertiary pediatric settings" (Deatrick, Feetham, Hayman, & Perkins, Chapter 16, this volume). Of special interest was the context for these daily attempts to manage caregiving, as most research has focused on the stresses and strains involved in the tasks themselves.

Background

A concept analysis (Knafl & Deatrick, 1986), an exploratory research (Deatrick, Knafl, & Walsh, 1988), and a subsequent concept analysis (Deatrick, 1990; Deatrick & Knafl, 1990; Knafl & Deatrick, 1990) provided a beginning understanding of management behaviors. It was found that the context or meaning of management behaviors can best be explained by their characteristics: their goals, underlying conceptual dimensions, implementors, and foci. The short-term or long-term goal may or may not be discernible to the observer and is the "result toward which the family's effort is directed, such as maintaining and enhancing the affected child's health care . . . goals shape the nature of target behaviors" (Deatrick & Knafl, 1990, pp. 16-17). The underlying conceptual dimension defines the often implicit "descriptive qualities or organizing framework characterizing the management behaviors of interest," which may be primarily cognitive or behavioral in nature. The implementor is the person(s) who "orchestrates or carries out the behaviors necessary to accommodate the needs generated by the child's illness or disability," including a family member or the affected child (Deatrick & Knafl, 1990, p. 17). Three foci or "points of concentration toward which the management behaviors are directed . . . [include the] ill child, family, and social system" (Deatrick & Knafl, 1990, p. 17). The target behaviors are the "actual, observable discreet behavioral accommodations that family members use to manage on a daily basis" (Deatrick & Knafl, 1990, p. 17).

Method

Four cases were selected from the 63 families who were studied in Knafl, Breitmeyer, Gallo, and Zoeller's (1987) research based on the FMS model. Each family had a school-aged child with a chronic condition. The four cases were selected as they represented the range of FMS and management behaviors.

Knafl et al. (1990) identified three provisional FMSs: accommodative, compensatory, and discrepant, based on the parents' views of the ill child and the illness, their parenting philosophy, and their view of their ability to manage the treatment regime. For the *accommodative style,* the ill child and his or her family life is defined as "normal in spite of the illness" (p. 8), but considerable planning and effort may be needed to maintain normal life, including "a degree of self consciousness that had not been there prior to the onset of the illness" (p. 14) and family life that is less flexible and spontaneous than life before the illness. In the *compensatory style,* the child is viewed and treated as a special, sometimes tragic, figure and as different from a normal child. The need to protect the child is the focus of the parents' compensatory efforts. In the *discrepant* style, one parent maintained a compensatory style and the other adapted an accommodative style.

Each case was subjected to intensive case analysis using matrix analysis techniques (Miles & Huberman, 1984). The small number of cases reviewed for this secondary analysis reflects the micro level of analysis of data from all family members across all management behaviors discussed in the interview.

This secondary analysis made use of data gathered for the purposes of a primary research analysis but looked at questions not addressed by the original investigator (McArt & McDougal, 1985). Specifically, the unit of analysis was changed from individual family members to individual management behaviors.

Table 5.1   Sample Family Matrix With Illustrative Characteristics and Categories[a]

Characteristic	Data	Category
Target Strategies		Monitoring diet, treatment, symptoms, and activity
Time 1		
Mother	I peek at her over my shoulder when she's taking the medication.	
Father	I don't get involved in that at all.	
Teenager	I know the names and dosages of my medications and take them myself; at first my parents, especially my mom, reminded me; I communicate with Dr. M. about my medications.	
Time 2		
Mother	I tried to communicate to the new physician that he had prescribed too much Prednisone; we finally had to go to another physician.	
Father	The [third] physician is technically competent but very difficult; I finally had to call her from my law office and insist that she call back.	
Teenager	The [third] physician doesn't talk to me [about medications] like Dr. M.	

NOTE: [a]Case: Lupus, accommodative; no siblings.

Results

Table 5.1 contains a sample matrix of one family in order to display the descriptive and comparative values of the analytic technique. From this analysis the broad characteristics identified in the concept analysis (Deatrick & Knafl, 1990) were refined by descriptions of the content of each characteristic. This refinement yielded various categories for each characteristic and ultimately the target strategies or management behaviors. Tables 5.2 and 5.3 contain those characteristics and categories in the form of a topology.

Validation of Previous Characteristics and Categories

Characteristics. The analysis revealed that all of the characteristics, including the goal, underlying conceptual dimension, implementor, and foci,

Table 5.2   Management Behaviors: Noncategorical Dimensions of Chronic Illness
Management

Characteristics of Management Behaviors	Categories
Goal	[descriptive]
Turning points	Nodal events[a, b]
Underlying conceptual dimension	Cognitive
	Behavioral
	Developmental[a]
Implementor	Child/Adolescent
	Mother
	Father
	Sibling
	Grandparent
	Other relative
	Person outside the family
Foci	Ill child
	Relationships with child
	Family system
	Social system
Target strategies	(See Table 5.3)

NOTE: [a]Reflects a change or addition to previous work.
[b]Bradt (1980)

were confirmed (see Table 5.2). Implementor and foci (see Table 5.3), as
well as the actual target strategies, can involve many options, so the possible permutations and combinations are almost endless; that is, any of the
implementors can manage through use of the strategies focused on the
child, the family, and/or the social system.

Categories. These data also confirmed specific categories of each characteristic. Management behaviors do have cognitive and behavioral conceptual dimensions. Members of the nuclear family, as well as other relatives
and persons outside the family, implement the tasks related to management.
The focus of the management behaviors can be the ill child, in terms of
illness-related or relationship-related activities, the family system, and the
social system (see Table 5.2).

A majority of the categories describing target strategies were validated;
however, categories were added and combined (see Table 5.3). All of the
illness-related activities were supported; however, further refinement
revealed that some illness-related categories could be combined. Treatment was combined with monitoring diet, symptoms, and activities as it
was inextricably related to management. All of the relationship-related

Table 5.3   Foci and Target Strategies

Foci	Target Strategies
Child/Illness-related	Performing activities of daily living
	Monitoring diet, treatment, symptoms, and activity[a]
	Devising routines for ADL's and treatment
	Triaging medical care, self-care, specialists
	Carrying out treatment regimes/therapies
	Obtaining needed equipment and medications[a]
Child/Relationship-related	Showing affection
	Approaching child
	Participating in activities
	Building coping abilities
	Emphasizing appearance and bodily functions
	Participating in decision making[a]
	Participating in treatment regimens
	Sharing information[a]
	Monitoring social activities
Family system	Balancing time schedules
	Traveling distance to health care resources
	Planning couple and family activities
	Finding sitters who are willing and able
	Obtaining financial resources[a]
	Taking responsibility in decision making[a]
	Obtaining, sharing, and controlling information within the family[a]
Social system	Promoting child's acceptance by others
	Obtaining health care
	Conveying impression to others
	Obtaining, sharing, and controlling needed information[a]
	Obtaining help in school
	Participating in outside sporting activities
	Participating in support groups[a]
	Comparing with others[a, b]

NOTE: [a]Reflects a change or addition to previous work.
[b]Affleck, Tennen, Pfeiffer, Fifield, & Rowe, 1987.

activities were supported, as well as the categories related to the family and social systems.

Revisions in the Previous Characteristics and Categories

Characteristics. "Target accommodation" was the only characteristic renamed. It was relabeled "target strategy" to avoid redundancy because one of the provisional FMSs is "accommodation."

Categories. The pattern of presenting the categories also was changed to reflect a more neutral and parsimonious language that would be applicable to a wide range of FMSs. The category "nodal events" was added for the newly developed characteristic of "turning points." This concept is well known in the family systems literature as describing strategic transitions (Bradt, 1980). As such, nodal events necessitate new ways of managing for the family. The family devises new management behaviors largely through trial and error when a threat to present management occurs.

"Developmental" was added to the categories of underlying conceptual dimensions, as it was cited frequently by the parents as an important consideration in the way that they viewed their child as an implementor of his or her care. Parents frequently mentioned that they believed children were now developmentally capable of assuming more self-care.

More substantive changes were made in the target strategies, as reflected in Table 5.3. A category for obtaining equipment and medications was added to the illness-related focus, one for obtaining financial resources was added to the family-related focus, and one for participating in support groups and comparing self with others (Affleck, Tennen, Pfeiffer, Fifield, & Rowe, 1987) was added to the social system-related focus. Two categories were added across more than one focus. An emphasis on participating in treatment decisions was included under relationships with the child and the family-related focus. Information sharing was added to relationships with the child and the family system and the social system.

Discussion

The process of inductively developing the concept of *management behaviors* to further our understanding of the process of caregiving was found to be a productive exercise. The topology of management behaviors helped comprehensively to synthesize concerns related to the daily care of children with chronic conditions from a family perspective. The topology, especially when combined with an understanding of the family management styles model, enables an understanding of the management behaviors of individual family members, as well as the overall management style of the family.

The specificity added to the family-focused pediatric transitional care model through this secondary analysis will enable development of a middle-range theory about families who have children with chronic conditions. This added specificity can lead toward empirical testing or toward further interpretive understandings about children who have chronic conditions and their families.

The narrative of the family provided a context for the management behaviors so that their nature could be understood. For instance, the goal of the management, while not discernible to the observer be he or she another family member or professional, contributes an understanding concerning the behavior of the family member. In fact, in the midst of nodal events, the family member may hold fast to the goal and alter the behaviors in the belief that he or she could more effectively move toward that goal. It then becomes vital for nurses to use the goals of caregiving as the basis of their teaching not only for the goals of individual family members but also for the family as a unit. Otherwise teaching and other interventions may not be seen by the family members as pertinent to the families' situation and may be seen as a threat to their goals (Burke et al., 1989). Through recognizing and valuing the families' goals and solutions, nurses are legitimatized by the family to enter into their problem solving, which eventually may include modification of both the goals and the solutions.

Bowers (1987) also emphasized the importance of the purpose or goal of caregiving activities in her study of intergenerational caregiving (IGC). Her "reconceptualization of caregiving activities—distinguished by purpose rather than by task—is a more accurate representation of the experience, work, and stress of IGC . . . a task-based focus obscured an important aspect of family caregiving work" (p. 24). Although instrumental caregiving, which involves the most observable caregiving activities, is the most frequent focus of our teaching, Bowers found that this emphasis obscured and sabotaged the intent of the family's most ardent focus—anticipatory, preventive, supervisory, and most important, protective caregiving of their cognitively impaired elders. Caregivers may be labeled as "noncompliant" by nurses as they try to protect their parents' self-image or their parent-offspring relationship by focusing away from the tasks of instrumental caregiving. The result may be a reintensification of their protective caregiving.

Thus the context or goal of the management behaviors was identified in this analysis as crucial to planning effective interventions with these families. In addition, the process used over time to develop this conceptual model was described in order to explicate the complexity of such a process. Finally, the usefulness of the model and the process of its development were examined to demonstrate applicability to family phenomenon.

6

Family Stress Theory and the Development of Nursing Knowledge About Family Adaptation

Marilyn A. McCubbin

Family stress theory, as one example of a family theory borrowed from family science, has been used in family nursing research to answer the persistent question of why some family systems adapt and even grow and thrive when faced with normative transitions or situational stressors, while other family units seem to deteriorate and disintegrate under similar circumstances. Because earlier nursing theory development tended to have an individual focus (Murphy, 1986), nurse scientists investigating family phenomena have utilized family science theories to describe, explain, and predict how the family as a unit responds to and manages both developmental transitions and actual and potential threats to the health of its members. The purpose of this chapter is to examine how family stress theory can be viewed within the context of nursing's metaparadigm and to review the development of family stress models and how nursing knowledge about family adaptation is being developed from research using this framework.

Metaparadigm of Nursing
and Family Stress Theory

Nursing's metaparadigm of person, environment, health, and nursing has been used in family theory development in nursing (Fawcett & Whall, 1990). In family stress theory, the family or "person" is viewed as encountering hardships and changes as an inevitable part of family life over the life cycle. Families also develop "strengths and capabilities to enhance the development of individual members and to protect the family unit from major disruption during times of transition and change" (McCubbin & McCubbin, 1989, p. 6). Thus this framework does not focus on psychopathology but rather "de-psychologizes" the family to emphasize such functional family system properties as cohesion, adaptability, family hardiness, coping, and problem-solving communication patterns.

In the environmental context, the family system is viewed as an open system and a component of the larger community and society. It is assumed that families "benefit from and contribute to the network of relationships and resources in the community" (McCubbin & McCubbin, 1989, p. 6), and this is especially applicable during times of stress and crisis.

Health may be defined as "family resiliency" or "the ability of the family to respond to and eventually adapt to the situations and crises encountered over the family life cycle." This does not mean that the family course of adaptation proceeds on a smooth upward course; rather the family's struggles to adjust and adapt to stressful life circumstances may follow what Hill (1958) described as a "roller coaster course of adaptation."

The role of nursing then is not only to promote family members' health, recovery from illness, or maximum functioning within specific health limitations but also to support and enhance family strengths, to assist families in maintaining linkages with community supports, and to aid families in arriving at a realistic appraisal of what is the best "fit" for them in their particular situation. Through these efforts nurses can assist families in the process of adaptation.

Development of Family Stress Models

The first family stress model—Hill's *ABCX model* (Hill, 1949, 1958)—focused on precrisis variables that could differentiate "crisis-prone" families from "crisis-proof" families. Hill depicted a single stressor event (A) interacting with the family's crisis-meeting resources (B) and the family's definition of the event (C) as the critical variables predicting the crisis (X).

The *Double ABCX Model* (McCubbin & Patterson, 1983) linked Hill's precrisis variables with specific postcrisis variables, including the number, type, and cumulative nature of stressors facing the family unit and also the family's resistance resources, appraisal of the stressor event, and coping strategies as facilitators of the family's adaptation over time. Recent investigations have encouraged the further expansion of the model as the *Typology Model of Family Adjustment and Adaptation* (McCubbin & McCubbin, 1989) and the *Resiliency Model of Family Stress, Adjustment, and Adaptation* (McCubbin & McCubbin, in press) to add family types as basic strengths of the family unit, family problem-solving capabilities, and a higher over-all level of family appraisal and meaning as critical factors in family adaptation.

Two phases of family response to life events and changes—family adjustment and family adaptation—are depicted in the Resiliency Model. Families often encounter events, such as an acute illness in a family member, that have a temporary, minimal impact on the family unit. If major hardships are not created for the family system in these situations, the family can attain adaptation by making only minor adjustments or changes in established patterns of family functioning. This represents the adjustment phase in the Resiliency Model (see Figure 6.1).

In this phase the stressor (A) (e.g., an acute illness in an otherwise healthy family member) is interacting with the family's vulnerability (V), or stressors, strains, and transitions already present or occurring along with the illness; and also is interacting with the family typology (T), or established patterns of family functioning; the family's resistance resources (B), such as flexibility in getting tasks done; the family's appraisal (C) (defining the illness as short term, not serious, curable); and the family's problem-solving and coping repertoire (PSC), such as an affirming communication style and seeking immediate care for the illness. The adjustment phase is viewed as one in which the family manages the stressor with relative ease (McCubbin & McCubbin, in press).

Nurses, however, most frequently work with families experiencing major transitions or situational crises, such as the transition to parenthood or the care of family members with serious acute, chronic, or life-threatening illnesses. These families initially attempt to adjust by maintaining the status quo or by making only minor changes in established patterns of family functioning. Over time, however, the family may move into a crisis state or period of family disorganization (Burr, 1973; McCubbin & Patterson, 1983) when previously established patterns of functioning are no longer

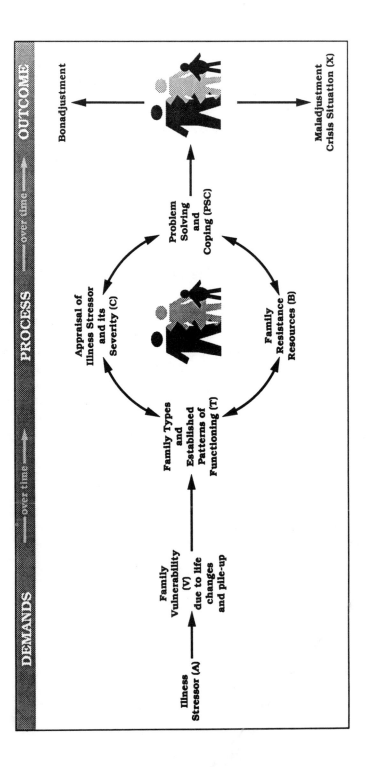

Figure 6.1. Adjustment Phase: Resiliency Model of Family Stress, Adjustment, and Adaptation

SOURCE: From "Family Coping With Illness: The Resiliency Model of Family Stress, Adjustment, and Adaptation" by M. McCubbin and H. McCubbin (in press) in C. Danielson, B. Hamel-Bissell, and P. Winstead-Fry (Eds.), *Families, Health, and Illness*, St. Louis: C. V. Mosby. Reprinted by permission.

adequate to meet the numerous or severe hardships in these situations. The need to change the family system (goals, roles, rules, boundaries) marks the onset of the adaptation phase in the Resiliency Model (see Figure 6.2).

In this phase the ability of the family to recover and adapt from a crisis is depicted as follows: family demands (AA) or the accumulation of family stressors, strains, and transitions interacting with the family's level of re-generativity or resiliency (R) determined in part by the family's established and newly instituted patterns of functioning (adding role as primary care-giver, rearrangement of family routines to accommodate prescribed care regimen), the family resources and social support from the community (BB and BBB) (e.g., assistance received from extended family and health care providers), family's appraisal (CC and CCC) (changes in meaning and reordering of the family's goals and priorities), and problem-solving and coping strategies—PSC—(learning about illness and its management).

Family adaptation is the outcome of the family's efforts over time to bring a fit at two levels: the individual to family, and the family to the community. The continuum of family adaptation ranges from optimal bonad-aptation to maladaptation. *Bonadaptation* involves meeting both the needs of individual family members to enable them to achieve their maximum potential and also the functioning of the family system and its transactions with the community (workplace, school, health care system). Empirical measurement of adaptation in the research has focused on both the individ-ual family members' functioning and the family system by using variables of physical, mental, and emotional health status, actual or ideal family sys-tem functioning, or satisfaction with various areas of family life.

Development of Nursing Knowledge
About Family Adaptation

Empirical evidence of testing the propositions and hypotheses generated from the Resiliency Model of Family Stress, Adjustment, and Adaptation (McCubbin & McCubbin, 1991) and the earlier ABCX (Hill, 1949) and Double ABCX models (McCubbin & Patterson, 1983) has been accumul-ating; the following brief synopsis and discussion, although incomplete, represent a few salient propositions that have been supported by empiri-cally based studies.

Proposition 1. In family crisis situations, the pileup of family demands (stressors, strains, transitions) is related to family adaptation, and this is a negative relationship.

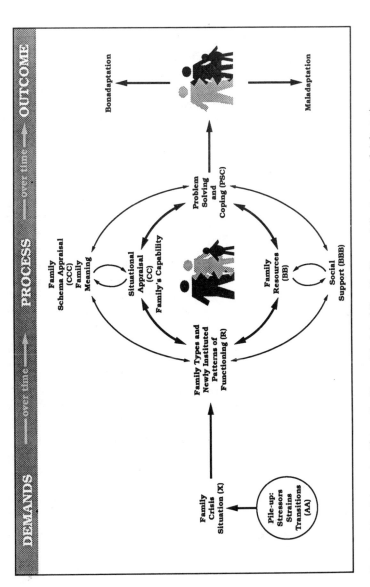

Figure 6.2. Adaptation Phase: Resiliency Model of Family Stress, Adjustment, and Adaptation

SOURCE: From "Family Coping With Illness: The Resiliency Model of Family Stress, Adjustment, and Adaptation" by M. McCubbin and H. McCubbin (in press) in C. Danielson, B. Hamel-Bissell, and P. Winstead-Fry (Eds.), *Families, Health, and Illness*, St. Louis: C. V. Mosby. Reprinted by permission.

In the Resiliency Model it is assumed that families are not only managing the specific event bringing them to the attention of the health care system but also other stressors from all areas of work and family life. Thus the model depicts the pileup of demands related to (a) the initial stressor, such as an illness and its hardships; (b) normative transitions (e.g., a child entering adolescence or a family launching of young adults); (c) preexisting family strains (e.g., difficulty with in-laws or a former spouse); (d) the consequences of family coping efforts (health deterioration of primary family caregiver); and the intrafamilial and societal ambiguity about how the family should respond (McCubbin & Patterson, 1983; McCubbin & McCubbin, 1989).

A negative relationship has been found between the accumulation of family demands and the health status of a child with a chronic illness (McCubbin, 1988, 1989b; Patterson & McCubbin, 1983). Higher levels of family stressors were associated with lower levels of satisfaction with family functioning (Failla & Jones, 1991) in families who had a child with a developmental disability.

The adolescent or launching stage of the family life cycle has been found to be particularly vulnerable to the accumulation of family demands because of the developmental transitions and strains at this time (Olson et al., 1983). A pileup of family demands during the adolescent stage of the family life cycle has been found to be associated with adolescent substance use and abuse (McCubbin, Needle, & Wilson, 1985). In military families relocating overseas, the greater accumulation of demands intensified the strains, reduced the levels of personal well-being in family members, and increased the probability of health, emotional, or relational problems in the family (Lavee, McCubbin, & Patterson, 1985).

Proposition 2. In crisis situations, family typologies based on specific strengths of the family system (cohesion, adaptability, family hardiness, family time and routines) are related to family adaptation, and this is a positive relationship.

Family typologies is defined as "a set of basic attributes about the family system which characterize and explain how a family system typically appraises, operates, and behaves" (McCubbin & McCubbin, 1989, 1991). The creation of family typologies allows the family nurse researcher to examine family system properties in combination to see how these shape the family response to stress and crisis.

In the *Circumplex Model* (Olson, 1989), family types of balanced, midrange, and extreme are constructed by using the dimensions of cohesion and adaptability in the family system. Balanced families who have moderate levels of cohesion and adaptability are hypothesized to be able to adapt to stressors and transitions more adequately over the life cycle due to their ability to change these dimensions in response to stress, to engage in the use of more positive communication skills, and to allow family members to be independent from, yet connected, to their family (Olson, 1989).

Samples of families who had members with schizophrenia or neuroses (Clarke, 1984), mothers or fathers with chemical dependency (Olson & Killorin, 1984), sex offenders (Carnes, 1987), or father absence and adolescent juvenile offenders (Rodick, Henggeler, & Hanson, 1986) were found to have higher numbers of extreme family types than comparison families without these emotional or psychosocial problems. The balanced family type was found to be associated with fewer health problems in the child severely impaired with myelomeningocele (McCubbin, 1988), but in another sample of families of children with cerebral palsy, mid-range and extreme family types with moderate to high levels of cohesion and lower levels of adaptability were found to be associated with improved child health outcomes (McCubbin & Huang, 1989).

The typology of regenerative families using family hardiness and family coherence, and the typology of rhythmic families (McCubbin, McCubbin, & Thompson, 1991) using family time and routines and the valuing of family time and routines also have been introduced to focus on other patterns of family functioning that may be associated with family adaptation.

In a study of families across the life cycle, both of these family typologies were associated with higher levels of satisfaction with the marital relationship, the children's development, the family's overall functioning, and the family's relationships with the community (McCubbin, Thompson, Pirner, & McCubbin, 1988). A significant correlation between the regenerative family typology and children's self-care health behaviors was found by Blecke (1991). Goss (1990) found significant correlations between the rhythmic family typology and the parents' health-promoting life-style in families of school-aged children. These findings represent beginning evidence that family typologies that examine properties of the family system in combination may contribute to a fuller understanding of family adaptation.

Proposition 3. In crisis situations the family resources are related to family adaptation, and this is a positive relationship.

The Resiliency Model depicts resources as being characteristics, traits, or competencies that the family has or develops to manage the stressful event or transition (McCubbin & McCubbin, in press). These resources can be within the individual level (intelligence, self-esteem), the family system (shared adult leadership, family organization), or the community (social support, health care services) in which the family lives.

Comeau (1985) found that family system resources of mastery and health and community resource use of day activity centers and parent organizations were predictors of improved health status in the child with myelomeningocele. Family system resources of esteem/communication, mastery and health, and extended family social support were predictors of improved health outcomes for the child severely impaired with myelomeningocele in another study (McCubbin, 1988). Families of children with epilepsy who had poor psychosocial adaptation (more behavior problems reported by parents and teachers) were found to have lower levels of family esteem/communication, less social support from extended family, and lower financial well-being than families who had children with good psychosocial adaptation (Austin, 1988). These studies of families with chronically ill children underscore the critical role of specific family resources as contributors to the overall health and functioning of the child with a chronic illness.

In more recent research, family hardiness has been conceptualized as a stress-buffering resource for the family system. Building on the work of Kobasa (1979), with the construct of individual hardiness as a personality characteristic with stress-buffering properties, *family hardiness* is characterized as the family working together to solve problems, having a sense of control over the outcomes of life events, a view of change as beneficial and growth producing, and an active rather than a passive orientation in managing stressful situations (McCubbin, McCubbin, & Thompson, 1991).

Family hardiness was found to be associated with the family's mastery of high technology home care regimens for an adult family member with a chronic condition (McCubbin, 1989a). Family hardiness was a significant predictor of satisfaction with family functioning in families with a developmentally disabled child (Failla & Jones, 1991). In a study of individual cancer patients receiving radiotherapy (Oberst, Hughes, Chang, & McCubbin, 1991) and family caregivers of cancer patients receiving chemotherapy (Carey, Oberst, McCubbin, & Hughes, 1991), family hardiness contributed to lower stressful appraisals of the illness and care-giving situation and less mood dysfunction in the patient and caregiver. Thus there is beginning evidence that family hardiness may be a critical family system resource in the management of chronic illness.

Proposition 4. In family crisis situations, the family's positive appraisal of the situation is related to family adaptation, and this is a positive relationship.

Family stress researchers have emphasized the importance of family appraisal in studying family response to crisis (Burr, 1973; Hill, 1958). The Resiliency Model posits three levels of appraisal: *stressor appraisal,* or the family's definition of the specific stressor event; *situational appraisal,* or the family's subjective definition of the total demands they are experiencing in relation to their resources and capabilities; and a third, *global* level of appraisal based on the family's basic beliefs, values, shared identity, and goals. This third level of appraisal is viewed as more stable than stressor and situational appraisals, but it can be shaped, molded, and altered over time, especially in response to severe crisis situations in which the family system has undergone marked changes in its established patterns of family functioning (McCubbin, McCubbin, & Thompson, in press).

Initial findings related to appraisal (Lavee, McCubbin, & Patterson, 1985) revealed that the family's ability to perceive the overall situation as coherent, one that "makes sense" and is a "fit" between the family and their circumstances, was of value to the family in facilitating adaptation. This perception was related to both the accumulation of demands and the resources from the external environment (social support) in relocated military families. Orr, Cameron, and Day (1991) used path analysis to examine the relationship among parenting stress, resources, and appraisal in families of children with developmental disabilities. Results indicated that through the process of perceiving the parenting stressors, families then utilized the resources that they felt they needed, which in turn reduced their stress levels. Thus a linear relationship between the parenting stressors to appraisal and then to the resources and family adaptation was supported by this investigation. In a study of families experiencing occupational stressors and job loss, the families' world view helped facilitate family adaptation and reduce family system distress in the face of economic instability (McCubbin & Thompson, 1989). These findings indicate that appraisal does play a key role in family adaptation; further work is needed to determine the contribution of each level of appraisal and relationships with stressors, family type, resources, coping, and problem solving.

Proposition 5. The range and depth of the family's repertoire of coping and problem-solving strategies when employed to manage a crisis situation are related to the level of family adaptation, and this is a positive relationship.

In the Resiliency Model, coping behaviors are specific strategies used by individual family members or the family system to reduce or manage demands, to acquire additional resources, to manage tension, and to change the meaning of a situation (McCubbin & McCubbin, 1989; in press). Use of coping behaviors was found to be higher in high-conflict families than in low-conflict families (McCubbin et al., 1982), a finding that reflects an active response to manage higher levels of stress and disruption.

Coping behaviors also can be grouped into patterns related to a specific way of responding; coping patterns in families who have chronically ill children have been found to be targeted toward maintaining family integration and an optimistic view; the parents' psychological stability, self-esteem, and use of social support; and understanding the health care situation (McCubbin, 1991). Coping behaviors of mothers and fathers were related to the interpersonal and organizational dimensions of family life respectively and to indexes of health improvement in children with cystic fibrosis (McCubbin et al., 1983). Other work has revealed the critical role of family coping during the transition to parenthood (Ventura, 1986), spousal adaptation to divorce (Berman & Turk, 1981), and chronic illness in the mother (Stetz, Lewis, & Primomo, 1986). Gender differences in coping have been found (Schilling, Schinke, & Kirkham, 1985; Ventura, 1986), which indicates that researchers need to examine similarities and differences in coping among family members.

Family problem-solving communication is another more generalized way of responding that transcends different types of stressful situations and represents the PSC component in the Resiliency Model. Two communication patterns are measured by a recently developed instrument—the Family Problem Solving Communication Index (McCubbin, McCubbin, & Thompson, 1988).

Incendiary communication is communication that is inflammatory in nature and that tends to exacerbate a stressful situation, while *affirming communication* conveys more support and caring for family members and exerts a calming influence. Initial results on these two types of problem-solving communication patterns indicate that incendiary communication is positively related to individual family member and family system distress. Affirming communication was positively related to family member well-being, marital and parent-child subsystem functioning, and overall family well-being (McCubbin & Thompson, 1989). Work in progress (McCubbin, 1990) will examine the role of family problem-solving communication in families who have a child newly diagnosed with a chronic health condition.

Future directions for family nursing research using family stress theory include the following:

1. The development of prediction models of family adaptation, using the Resiliency Model as one of several family stress models, to deter-

mine which dimensions of family life (accumulation of demands, family typologies, resources, appraisal, coping, and problem solving) in what order and combination and under what conditions best explain family adaptation is very critical.

2. Longitudinal studies are needed to depict how Resiliency Model variables remain stable or change over time. Most of the work to date has been cross-sectional. In families experiencing a chronic or life-threatening illness, the characteristics and trajectory of that illness (Rolland, 1988) also can be examined. McCubbin's current work in progress (1990) will examine the family response to the initial diagnosis of a child's chronic condition and will examine model variables over time.

3. Studies of ethnic families based on family stress theory are vitally needed. Are the model variables appropriate for ethnic families? Do the current available instruments accurately measure these constructs in ethnic families? How do the stresses of racism and discrimination relate to family adaptation? Current work by Daniels, Davis, and Sloan (1991) is an important step in this area.

4. With further testing of the ability of the model to describe, explain, and predict family adaptation, the designing and testing of nursing interventions to facilitate family adaptation are indicated. Previous research (Gilliss, Neuhaus, & Hauck, 1990) using randomized clinical trials did not support nursing care and support as a supplement to family resources. The study did confirm the divergent patterns of patient and spouse response following cardiac surgery reported in other research (Oberst & Scott, 1988) with patients and spouses after cancer surgery. Thus interventions that facilitate adaptation for all family members and the family system remain a long-term goal for future research. Meta-analyses of family nursing interventions (Gilliss & Davis, 1991) will greatly facilitate this effort.

The family system is complex, continually changing in an effort to respond to events from within and without, and is charged with the tasks of maintaining both continuity and stability so that members have a sense of security and freedom to grow and to achieve their maximum potential. This challenging complexity supports the use of theories and models from both nursing and family science in family nursing research to capture the dynamic nature of family systems and how nursing might best proceed to support families at all stages of the life cycle. Family stress theory and the models that have been developed from this approach to the family represent but one route to the development of nursing knowledge about the family.

Although many conceptual and methodological issues are yet to be addressed (Feetham, 1990), the findings from well-designed and executed family nursing research investigations will have implications for research, policy, and clinical practice.

PART III

Research Methodological Issues

Suzanne L. Feetham, Editor

7

The Contribution of Qualitative Research to the Study of Families' Experiences With Childhood Illness

Janet A. Deatrick

Sandra A. Faux

Carol Murphy Moore

Researchers using qualitative approaches have made significant contributions to the study of phenomena important to health care professionals who work with acutely and chronically ill children and their families. Calls have been made for additional research using this strategy, in which the meanings or definitions that people use to orient themselves to and make sense of social situations are generated (Munhall & Oiler, 1986). However, the existing body of qualitative research concerning children, adolescents, their families, and their illness experiences needs to be examined thoroughly to determine its current status and how qualitative approaches may contribute to research of families. During this process the "qualitative technique orientation" can be refined to encompass specific interpretive paradigms and the state of the art in family sciences.

Progress has been made during the past 10 years in nursing, as well as in the other family sciences, toward the understanding of the family who has an ill or disabled child. This progress has stemmed from the increasing sophistication of methods used to study families (Moriarity, 1990a; Patterson, 1990).

The sophistication of qualitative methods also has evolved, as has their recognition by the scientific community. These methods are accepted now as contributing toward an understanding of the family's motivations and behaviors in the illness context through discovery and exploration of family processes, relationships, and characteristics. This acceptance followed on the heels of the acceptance of individually oriented qualitative research that had occurred over the previous 10 years (Moriarity, 1990a). In addition, researchers have accepted that children can be reliable, valid informants who can describe their world and their illness experiences, using a variety of qualitative and quantitative methods (Deatrick & Faux, 1991; Faux, Walsh, & Deatrick, 1988).

The purpose of this analysis was to describe the contribution of qualitative research to the study of families' experiences with children who have an illness or disability. In addition, because this type of research methodology is descriptive and question generating, directions for further research also were developed.

Analysis

Studies were included if they met the following criteria:

1. Qualitative methods were used.
2. The focus of the study was the family unit or a family member *other than the ill or disabled child.*
3. The family or family member had a child who was defined as having an acute or chronic illness or disability.

Studies were examined in relation to the factors of study paradigm, purpose, methods, and focus. As Kuhn (1970) used the term *paradigm,* it refers to "the entire constellation of beliefs, values, techniques, shared by the members of a given community" (p. 175), including positivism, interpretivism, and critical theory. Broadly defined, the interpretivist paradigm includes research that is termed *ethnographic, interactive, qualitative, grounded theory, naturalistic, hermeneutic,* or *phenomenological.* All of these interpretivist perspectives were included in this analysis. In this analysis such perspectives were not seen as being ends in themselves (in terms of research methods) or means to another end (future quantification). The perspectives instead were linked to the stated purposes of the research and were classified according to Knafl and Howard's (1984) four purposes for qualitative studies: sensitization, illustration, instrumentation, and theory.

Studies were classified according to their purpose (Knafl & Howard, 1984). The results of qualitative studies can help the reader understand or be sensitized to the viewpoint of a family undergoing an event or process through accurate and complete description of the family's experience. Qualitative data may be used to illustrate the quantitative family data of a study with the qualitative component, usually a small piece of the larger quantitative study. Qualitative data may be used also to develop instruments that measure family phenomena. As an inductive approach to theory development in nursing practice through collection and use of qualitative data, such methods develop theory by using the principles of a specific paradigm (e.g., grounded theory, phenomenology).

Studies were classified also with respect to data collection methods used and the study focus. Qualitative data collection methods included interviews, participant observation, projective techniques, (e.g., Draw a Person), group interviews, and combined methods (e.g, interviews and participant observation), which often included multiple sources (e.g., mother, child, father). The specific research purpose/question also was noted for every study.

Sample

An exhaustive hand search of research and maternal-child journals from 1970 through 1990 was conducted. The research journals included *Nursing Research, Western Journal of Nursing Research, Advances in Nursing Science, Research in Nursing and Health, Canadian Journal of Nursing Research,* and *Journal of Advanced Nursing.* Maternal-child clinical journals reviewed were *Pediatric Nursing, Maternal-Child Nursing Journal, MCN, American Journal of Maternal-Child Nursing, Issues in Comprehensive Pediatric Nursing,* and *Journal of Pediatric Nursing.* In addition, "snowball" techniques were used to make the data base more complete. Article reference lists were checked for additional qualitative studies to be found in journals other than those searched. Finally *Reflections,* the quarterly newsletter of Sigma Theta Tau International, was used to identify doctoral dissertations completed since 1980. Prior to 1980 the abstract section of *Nursing Research* was used to identify potential qualitative studies.

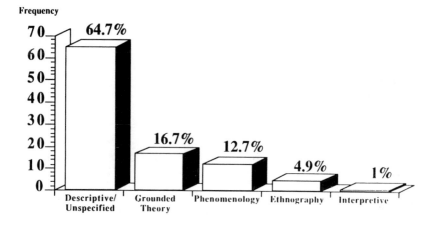

Figure 7.1. Number of Family, Qualitative Publications According to Study Paradigm in 102 Articles, 1970-1990

Findings

Some 102 articles were found that focused on the family unit or members of families who had an ill or disabled child. The majority of articles reflected a single study; however, reports of 9 studies did generate more than one article, and these 9 studies generated 27 articles that focused on various facets of the results.

As seen in Figure 7.1, the articles were tabulated according to the research paradigm. By far the greatest number of studies were labeled as "descriptive" or "unspecified." Only 17 (16.7%) studies had a specific research paradigm guiding the study. Grounded theory was used most frequently (17, or 16.7% of the studies).

The second factor analyzed—study purpose—is seen in Figure 7.2. The four previously described purposes (Knafl & Howard, 1984) were used to categorize the data, and a fifth—intervention—was added to account for three studies that used various qualitative approaches to plan the content of interventions with families. As noted in Figure 7.2, descriptive/sensitization was the dominant category, with 77 (75.6%) of the studies, and the next most frequent category being that of theory development, 18 (17.6%). No examples were found of qualitative data being generated for illustrative purposes.

The primary methods of data collection are displayed in Figure 7.3. Half of the studies used interviews, and 31 (30.4%) used combined approaches,

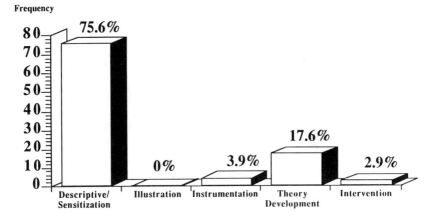

Figure 7.2. Family Qualitative Research: Purpose in 102 Articles of Families With Children Who Have Illnesses and Disabilities, 1970-1990

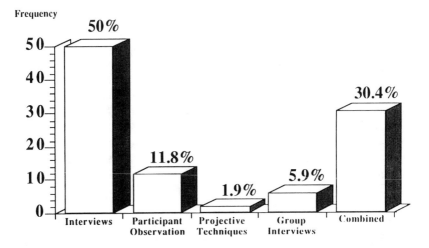

Figure 7.3. Family Qualitative Research: Data Collection Methods in 102 Articles of Families With Children Who Have Illnesses and Disabilities, 1970-1990

with other techniques, such as participant observation, used less frequently. Studies with multiple data sources or methods (including quantitative measures) tended to be used more frequently after 1980, a finding that parallels the development of the concept of *triangulation* in the literature (Denzin, 1970; Mitchell, 1986).

The foci of the research concentrated on the stress of parenting ill/disabled children and their siblings, especially during hospitalization, and how families and their members cope with the experience. Most recently a body of literature has been developed concerning home care of the medically fragile child who requires complex, intensive care in the hospital and home (Anderson, 1990; Aradine, 1980; Hazlett, 1989; Scharer & Dixon, 1989; Stevens, 1990).

Discussion

Initially, the number of qualitative studies that have been done with families during the last 20 years seemed impressive. Additional analysis, however, revealed the challenges concerning understanding and translating the experience of the family with an ill child and how qualitative methods may make unique contributions to that understanding. Although there is a discernible trend for better designed and conducted qualitative research of families, issues were identified (see Table 7.1) related to the design of the studies and to the use of qualitative methods. Feetham's criteria for family and family-related research were helpful in framing the recommendations because the issues became much broader than "methods" issues and "address[ed] the special conceptual issues of research involving families" (Feetham, 1991a, p. 56); that is, Feetham's criteria refer to (a) the framework for the research, (b) the conceptualization of the family and its consistency with the definition of the family, (c) knowledge that is added to an understanding of family functioning and structure, and (d) relevancy to nursing practice. *Family research* refers to the family as a unit of analysis and to the potential contribution made in understanding the family system. *Family-related research* takes into account the responses of individual family members or examines concepts associated with families or their members.

The first recommendation for the design of family qualitative studies is that the overall qualitative approach or paradigmatic orientation needs to be clearly identified by the investigators. It should be noted that the majority of studies conducted with specific paradigmatic orientations were almost exclusively done since 1985. Although the present trend is to refer to a specific paradigmatic orientation, some recent publications still do not do so. The approach needs to be described in detail and substantiated through the use of methods literature or a methods article written by the investigator. For instance, if a "descriptive approach" is being used, it needs to be elaborated. If a "phenomenological orientation" is specified, it needs

Table 7.1 Family Qualitative Research: Design and Methods[a]

1. Specify your overall qualitative approach or paradigmatic orientation.
2. Explicate your conceptual model or sensitizing framework if one is being used.
3. Define family.
4. Indicate the focus of the study as family-related or family research. Specify the sample, unit of data collection, data collection techniques, and analytic techniques, including the unit of analysis.
5. Identify developmental potential of various methods.
6. Describe the implications for how the research adds to nursing's clinical, research, and/or theoretical understanding of families.
7. Develop programs of inquiry that build on previous knowledge bases in the family sciences.
8. Identify gaps in our present understanding of at-risk, high-risk, and surviving families.

NOTE: [a]Adapted from "Conceptual and Methodological Issues in Research of Families" by S. L. Feetham, 1991, in A. Whall & J. Fawcett (Eds.), *Family Theory Development in Nursing: State of the Science and Art,* (pp. 55-68). Philadelphia: F. A. Davis.

to be supported in terms of the research questions and the design of the study.

The second recommendation for the design of family qualitative studies is that the conceptual orientation or sensitizing framework needs to be explicated and substantiated in terms of the rest of the study. For instance, one common pattern that emerged during this review was that studies initially may not specify a conceptual orientation. Then a particular conceptual perspective such as stress and coping is introduced in the "findings" section without being linked to the rest of the study. The reader then is left wondering when and why that particular conceptual perspective entered the research process.

The third recommendation is that the concept of *family* needs to be defined to make clear who is considered to be involved in this "family affair."

The fourth recommendation is that the focus of the study should be indicated as being family-related or family research (Feetham, 1991a), including concerns about specifying the sample, the unit of data collection, data collection techniques, and analytic techniques. Of strategic importance to the specification of the analytic techniques is the unit of analysis being the individual family member or the family unit. For instance, what is the relative contribution of the sibling to the family phenomenon being studied? Although neither family research nor family-related research is seen as being intrinsically stronger research, specification of the focus is seen as integral to the research process. When looking historically at the family literature, the vast majority of studies have been family-related, and very few now can qualify as family research. The earliest exception found to this was Jean Quint Benoliel (1970), who did the first nursing research that was qualitative family research. Presently researchers are beginning to publish the results of studies that qualify as family research (Feetham, 1991a). These investigators include Anderson (1981, 1986, 1990); Anderson and Chung (1982a, 1982b); Anderson, Elfert, and Lai (1989); Knafl (1982, 1985); Knafl, Breitmayer, Gallo, and Zoeller (1987); Knafl, Cavallari, and Dixon (1988); Knafl, Deatrick, and Kodadek (1982); Knafl and Dixon (1983, 1984); Robinson (1984, 1985, 1987); Wuest and Stern (1990a, 1990b, 1991); and Thorne and Robinson (1988). For instance, Knafl's research involving family management styles (Knafl, Breitmayer, Gallo, & Zoeller, 1987) and others such as Thorne and Robinson (1988) are family research studies.

The fifth recommendation for the design of family qualitative studies is consideration of the influence of the child's development on the usefulness of the methods (Deatrick & Faux, 1991; Faux, Walsh, & Deatrick, 1988). The credibility of data collection and analytic techniques for the individuals and, if applicable, the family unit needs to be discussed.

The sixth recommendation for the design of family qualitative studies is that how the research adds to clinical, research, and theoretical understanding of families needs to be considered. A special emphasis can be placed on the potential of inductive approaches for family theory development (Deatrick, Knafl, & Guyer, Chapter 5, this volume).

The seventh recommendation is that programs of inquiry need to build on previous knowledge bases in the family sciences. Neither substantive findings nor the interpretive results have played a major role in planning subsequent studies or in interpreting findings.

The eighth recommendation is that a need exists to increase family and family-related research of at-risk and high-risk families, such as families whose members may be infected by the AIDS virus and may be involved with substance abuse and whose children have survived potentially fatal conditions.

In conclusion, in reviewing the last 20 years of qualitative research concerning the child and family in illness situations, one can see clearly the evolution in the understanding of what is important in developing a coherent, well-defined family study or program of research (Feetham, 1991a). This evolution has brought about more focused programs of family research in which the unit of conceptualization of data collection and analysis is stipulated carefully as the family unit or its members. In addition is an ever-increasing sophistication of qualitative research paradigms, data collection methods, and analytic techniques. This sophistication has helped researchers who have used qualitative approaches to gather and interpret their results and to convince the scientific community of their credibility. Therefore, in the future it is anticipated that those involved in research of families will be able to take advantage of not only the substantive knowledge that has been gained through qualitative studies but also the many methodological advances as well.

8

One Approach to Conceptualizing Family Response to Illness

Kathleen A. Knafl

Agatha M. Gallo

Linda H. Zoeller

Bonnie J. Breitmayer

Lioness Ayres

For family researchers, debates about conceptual issues often focus on the meaning and implications of taking a family perspective. For example, Burr, Herrin, Day, Beutler, and Leigh (1988) stated, "When we start with a familial perspective . . . we see things differently. We ask different questions, focus on different parts of reality, and construct ideas that are different" (p. 190). The importance of a family perspective is grounded in the belief that the family is a unique sphere of human experience (Feetham, 1991; Gilliss, 1983; Moriarty, 1990a). Beutler, Burr, Bahr, and Herrin (1989, p. 806) specified the nature of the family's uniqueness and identified

AUTHORS' NOTE: We gratefully acknowledge the valuable input of Dr. Marion Howard, who reviewed an earlier version of this manuscript.

seven characteristics as defining the family realm: (a) generational nature and permanence of family relationships, (b) concern with total person (not circumscribed role), (c) simultaneous process orientation that grows out of familial caregiving, (d) unique and intense emotionality, (e) emphasis on qualitative purposes and processes, (f) altruistic orientation, and (g) nurturing form of governance. Beutler et al. suggested that these characteristics are most useful when taken together, because they are meant to provide a sensitizing framework for viewing unique aspects of family life. As such these characteristics help identify relevant family research questions and concepts. Although viewing the family as a unique unit is controversial, these characteristics represent an intriguing attempt to explain the position held by many that the family is a unique social entity.

Other authors have attempted to identify defining criteria for family research. In nursing, using the family as the unit of study and analysis is often considered to be the key defining criterion for family research. For example, Feetham (1984, 1991) distinguished between family and family-related research, noting that the former focuses on the family unit as a whole and that the latter focuses on relationships between family members.

Authors also have considered the methodological implications of taking a family perspective and of using the family as the unit of analysis in research (Draper & Marcos, 1990; Feetham, 1991; Gilliss, 1983; Moriarty, 1990a; Thomas, 1987). Discussions about issues and strategies associated with incorporating data from individual family members to reach conclusions about the family unit as a whole have highlighted the dilemmas encountered when using the family as the unit of analysis. For example, Larson and Olson (1990) pointed out that "developing couple and family scores is like dealing with a double-edged sword. The goal is to obtain concise measures that will cut through the complexity of marital and family systems, without destroying the individual components that make up the family system" (p. 29). They suggested incorporating measures and analytic techniques that provide for both pooled and diverse views of family reality (e.g., means and discrepancy scores). Ransom, Fisher, Phillips, Kokes, and Weiss (1990) advocated the use of pattern scores in which scores from individual family members are "juxtaposed in a way that produces a single pattern that is then indexed" (p. 59).

As the chapter title suggests, we have struggled with the issues inherent in trying to conduct research from a family perspective. Of particular interest is conceptualizing family response to illness. This interest has moved us to explain what we mean by *family* response and to determine the methodological implications of that view for all phases of the research. The purpose of this chapter is to share the methodological strategies currently being used to conceptualize how the family as a unit responds to a child's chronic illness. The emphasis is on the words *one approach* in the chapter title. Our approach, which emphasizes comparisons across individual family members to identify family unit responses, is not viewed as the only approach to achieving a family perspective. The intent is both to describe an approach that other researchers may find useful and to stimulate ongoing discussion and debate that will move us forward in efforts to understand families.

Conceptual Underpinnings of Our Research

The study, entitled "How Families Define and Manage a Child's Chronic Illness," was supported by the National Center for Nursing Research (Knafl, Breitmayer, Gallo, & Zoeller, 1987). The study goal was to use naturalistic inquiry to understand and conceptualize how families respond to chronic childhood illness. The study was grounded in a working model of family management style that conceptualizes the family's response to illness as the configuration formed by individual family member's definition of the situation and management behaviors and the sociocultural context in which these occur (Knafl & Deatrick, 1990). *Definition of the situation* is the subjective meaning of the situation to the person. *Management behaviors* are the discrete behavioral accommodations that family members use to manage on a daily basis. Management behaviors and definitions of the situation are inextricably interrelated. Family members' management behaviors are influenced by how they define the situation. Conversely, how they interpret the outcomes of their management behaviors influences the ongoing defining process. Both definitions of the situation and management behaviors are embedded in the family's sociocultural context.

Sampling

Methodological implications of the conceptual framework directed us to obtain data from multiple family members and to use a purposive and non-categorical sample. Specific disease entities were not targeted. Rather, because of interest in illness management, only illnesses that had ongoing treatment regimen requirements were included. Sampling criteria included families with a child between the ages of 7 and 14 who had a major chronic illness but no other major physical or psychological impairments and whose illness required active management by family members to minimize serious consequences. The final sample included 63 families and 210 family members (65 ill children, 62 mothers, 55 fathers, 28 siblings).

Data Collection

The conceptual model of the study provided direction to collect data on how family members defined and saw themselves managing the chronic illness in the context of their family life. Concerning sociocultural context, focus was on the family's interactions with health care and school systems, with particular attention paid to how they defined and managed these interactions. Although a variety of structured and unstructured techniques was used to elicit information on family members' definitions of the situation and management behaviors, the primary data collection technique was intensive semistructured interviews with individual family members. Research assistants, who were doctoral students in nursing, tape-recorded interviews that they conducted in the family's home. Interviewers used an interview guide that included open-ended questions about how families defined and managed their situation. For example, the questions asked of parents about how they defined the situation included, What proportion of your child's days would you estimate are good days versus bad days? and What changes do you anticipate in your child's condition during the next year? Questions asked of parents about managing the situation included, What are your child's responsibilities for managing his or her condition? and What kind of outside help have you received in managing having a child with a chronic illness? We developed separate guides for parents, for children with an illness, and for siblings, and we interviewed them at two points in time 12 months apart.

Data Processing

All interviews were transcribed verbatim and were processed further with *The Ethnograph, Version 3.0* (Seidel, 1988). After transcription, we inductively developed substantive codes to reflect the content of the interviews. In general these codes were descriptive and identified topics talked about in the interviews. All interviews were coded by use of a substantive coding scheme. For example, some codes developed from the interviews with parents included (a) illness course, (b) parenting role, and (c) advice to health care providers. Some codes developed from the interviews with children included (a) knowledge of illness, (b) advice to parents, and (c) career plans. Using *The Ethnograph* allowed us to store and access all data relevant to a specific coding category or combination of categories.

In addition we completed detailed case summaries for each family. These summaries maintained a more integrated overview of each family than was possible when accessing data on individual codes. As such the case summaries balanced the inherently reductionistic coding categories. Case summaries, which the first four authors completed, typically reduced 80 to 100 pages of interview data to 10 to 15 single-spaced pages of narrative summary. Consistent with the conceptual underpinnings of the study, definition of the situation and management behaviors provided the organizing framework for the summaries.

Data Analysis

As previously mentioned, the overall aim of the analysis was to conceptualize how families defined and managed a child's chronic illness. The key terms here are *family,* to go beyond talking about individual family members, and *conceptualize,* to go beyond a description of the content of coding categories or individual family cases. Guided by the conceptual framework, we are looking at the types of configurations formed by the interplay of individual family members' definitions of their situation and their management behaviors. Analysis is ongoing, including the process of identifying and validating a number of distinct family management styles and of exploring the relationship between these styles and various measures of family and individual family member functioning.

Through the review of the case summaries and data from specific codes, a series of defining and managing themes was identified. Table 8.1 lists these themes, which are both broader and more abstract than the substantive codes. Typically they encompass data from more than one coding category. Themes are applicable to all parents and vary from parent to parent. In other words each parent has a "view of the illness," but the content of that view varies from parent to parent. For example, the parent may view the illness as a manageable condition, ominous situation, or hateful restriction. Of particular interest are the subthemes for each of the thematic codes.

A major task of the analysis has been to identify and describe these defining and managing themes and subthemes and the subsequent subtheme classification of family members. The format for classifying and displaying this aspect of the analysis relies heavily on matrix display techniques described by Miles and Huberman (1984).

Matrix displays have facilitated greatly our efforts to compare across family members and to identify configurations of defining and managing subthemes. For example, Table 8.2 shows three mother-father pairs who have been classified on several thematic codes. This example is meant to

Table 8.1 Summary of Defining and Managing Themes for Parents

Themes	*Subthemes and Their Abbreviations*
	Defining themes
View of the child	Normal child (NORM)
	Problem child (PROB)
	Tragic figure (TRAJ)
View of illness	Manageable condition (MC)
	Ominous situation (OS)
	Hateful restriction (HR)
Parenting philosophy	Accommodative/Normalizing focus (ACC)
	Restrictive/Protective focus (RESTR)
	Minimizing/Ignoring focus (MINIM)
	Shifting/No clear focus (SHIFT)
Nature of illness work and associated mind-set	Manageable/Confident (CON)
	Manageable/Burden (BURD)
	Manageable/Confused (CONFS)
	Not my job/Observer (OBS)
	Managing themes
Division of labor	Shared by parents (SH)
	Mother responsible (MO)
	Father responsible (FA)
	Child responsible (CH)
	Comanaged by parents and child (CM)
Illness management approach	Proactive (PRO)
	Reactive (RE)
	Compliant (COMP)
	Uninvolved (UNIN)
Role satisfaction	Satisfied (+)
	Areas of dissatisfaction (+/−)
	Global dissatisfaction (−)

show how the matrix format highlights shared and different views of the situation between parents and at the first and second data collection sessions. As shown in this table, the parents in Families A and B held shared views of the situation, which changed little from the first to the second interview. In contrast the parents in Family C had differing views of their child and the illness work, and their view of the latter changed from the first to the second interview.

Parents from all 63 families have been classified as to their subtheme on the major defining and managing thematic codes for both the first and second interviews. The search for defining and managing configurations that characterize clusters of families is under way.

Table 8.2 Examples of Configurations of Subthemes for Parents in Three Families at Two Points in Time

Time	View of Child		View of Illness		View of Illness Work	
	Mother	Father	Mother	Father	Mother	Father
			Family A			
Interview 1	Normal	Normal	Ominous	Ominous	Confident	Observer
Interview 2	Normal	Normal	Ominous	Ominous	Confident	Confident
			Family B			
Interview 1	Tragic	Tragic	Hateful	Hateful	Burden	Burden
Interview 2	Tragic	Tragic	Hateful	Hateful	Burden	Burden
			Family C			
Interview 1	Problem	Problem	Ominous	Ominous	Confident	Inadequate
Interview 2	Tragic	Tragic	Ominous	Ominous	Observer	Confident

NOTE: See Table 8.1 for the complete key to subthemes.

The use of *dBASE,* a relational data base package, has facilitated greatly the search for configurations of defining and managing subthemes that cluster together. Using *dBASE,* we can see readily whether parents who have one subtheme in common have other subthemes in common as well. To use *dBASE,* the abbreviated thematic codes shown in Table 8.1 are entered into the computer for each subject by using the *dBASE* system. Once these data have been entered, it is possible to generate a wide array of matrices. For example, one can create a thematic matrix for all parents who view their children in a certain way (normal, tragic, or problem) and see whether these parents have other themes in common. Another possibility is to generate separate matrices for families experiencing different illnesses and to inspect these matrices for patterns of commonality and difference.

dBASE allowed great flexibility in displaying data according to specific defining and managing subthemes. In addition to identifying what subthemes clustered together, it facilitated identification of configurations in which parents had different views on certain subthemes, as well as configurations in which parents had a shared view across all the subthemes. For example, all the parents in Table 8.3, which has been adapted from a *dBASE* printout, viewed their children as normal. Although exceptions were found, many of these parents also had an accommodative management philosophy (ACC), viewed the illness as a manageable condition (MC), and presented a confident mind-set when it came to managing the work of the treatment regimen (CON). This configuration contrasts markedly from the one formed by parents who viewed their children with a chronic illness as a problem. These parents typically had a shifting management philosophy, viewed the

Table 8.3   Matrix of Subthemes, Adapted From a *dBASE* Printout of 19 Parents Who Viewed Their Child With an Illness as Normal

Parenting		Parenting philosophy	View of illness	Mind-Set for Managing
Father	1	Accommodative	Manageable condition	Confident
Mother	2	Accommodative	Manageable condition	Confident
Father	2	Accommodative	Manageable condition	Confident
Mother	3	Accommodative	Manageable condition	Confident
Father	3	Accommodative	Manageable condition	Confident
Mother	4	Restrictive	Ominous situation	Burden
Father	5	Minimizing	Manageable condition	Observer
Mother	6	Accommodative	Ominous situation	Burden
Father	6	Accommodative	Ominous situation	Burden
Mother	7	Minimizing	Manageable condition	Confident
Father	7	Minimizing	Ominous situation	Confident
Mother	8	Accommodative	Manageable condition	Confident
Mother	9	Accommodative	Manageable condition	Confident
Mother	10	Accommodative	Manageable condition	Confident
Father	10	Accommodative	Manageable condition	Confident
Mother	11	Accommodative	Manageable condition	Confident
Father	11	Restrictive	Manageable condition	Observer
Mother	12	Accommodative	Ominous situation	Confident
Father	12	Accommodative	Ominous situation	Observer

NOTE: See Table 8.1 for the complete key to subthemes.

illness as an ominous situation or a hateful restriction, and saw the work of managing the illness as a burden.

Like the software packages such as *The Ethnograph* that are specifically designed for processing narrative data, *dBASE* facilitates data analysis. The actual analysis occurred as we inspected the various *dBASE* printouts in an effort to identify clusters of subthemes and patterns of variation across both family units and individual family members. By streamlining matrix construction and manipulation, *dBASE* has freed time for the more important, interpretive aspects of the analysis.

Discussion

Throughout this study, effort has been made to maintain fidelity to the guiding conception of family management style as the configuration formed by simultaneously taking into account individual family members' definitions of the situation and management behaviors. This conception shaped the questions asked in the interviews, as well as strategies used for data processing and analysis.

This "One Approach to Conceptualizing Family Response to Illness" relies heavily on matrix display and analysis as a way to identify clusters of defining and managing themes that characterize family members' responses to chronic illness. The configuration of defining and managing themes across family members will be used to conceptualize the family's management style. Ultimately each family's management style will be compared with that of all other families in the study to identify more general management styles that characterize families with children who are chronically ill. Much of what is presented looks rather far removed from the many pages of intriguing and wonderful interview content. This is more a matter of appearance than reality. The interview summaries and the topical and thematic codes all are closely tied to the data. The classification of the parents as viewing their child as normal, tragic, or a problem was used because this is how parents talked about their children in the interviews. Although reflecting a tremendous reduction of the interview data, the matrices ultimately are grounded in the content of the interviews.

9

Sampling Issues and Family Research: Recruitment and Sampling Strategies

Helene J. Moriarty

Margaret Cotroneo

Nurses view the family as a significant context for each member's health and increasingly as the actual unit of care (Feetham, 1984; Friedman, 1986; Gilliss, 1983, 1989c; Leahey & Wright, 1987a, 1987b; Wright & Leahey, 1987). The body of nursing research on the family has expanded, and as Gilliss and colleagues (Gilliss, Highley, Roberts, & Martinson, 1989) suggest, nursing is moving "toward a science of family nursing." Consequently

AUTHORS' NOTE: This work was partially supported by the following grants to the first author: Individual National Research Service Award (NR06272-01) from the National Institutes of Health, National Center for Nursing Research, 9/1/88-3/31/90; Institutional National Research Service Award (NR07036-01) from the National Institutes of Health, National Center for Nursing Research, 9/1/87-8/31/88; Sigma Theta Tau International Research Award, 1987; and the Lisson Memorial Student Research Fellowship from the National Sudden Infant Death Syndrome Foundation, 1987. The work was also partially supported by the following grants to the second author: Department of Health and Human Services Nursing Research Emphasis Grant, 1984-1985; University of Pennsylvania Center for Nursing Research, Small Grants Program, 1985-1986; grant from the University of Pennsylvania International Programs Fund, 1988.

guidelines for specific aspects of the family research process are surfacing in the nursing literature (Gilliss, 1983; Moriarty, 1990; Uphold & Harper, 1986; Uphold & Strickland, 1989).

Although sampling is a more complex process in family research than in individual research, sampling strategies for family research have received little attention (Kitson et al., 1982; Moriarty, 1990). This chapter first will describe the complexities of sampling in family research and then will discuss recruitment strategies and sampling strategies. Emphasis will be placed on families who are difficult to recruit or who are underrepresented in family nursing research: families confronting severe stressors or sensitive issues (e.g., bereavement, violence, incest) and families with nontraditional forms (e.g., divorced families). Examples of recruitment and sampling strategies will be drawn from previous research with these groups, including research conducted by nurses and those in other disciplines, because we believe that multidisciplinary resources and perspectives are necessary to advance knowledge about recruitment and sampling methods.

Family research in this chapter refers to research that conceptualizes the family system as the unit of analysis (Feetham, 1984, 1991a) and that involves data collection with at least two family members. Researchers working from a family systems perspective contend that measures from multiple family members are necessary to capture the richness of family systems (Cromwell & Olson, 1975; Straus, 1964). Yet gathering data from multiple family members raises methodological, pragmatic, and ethical challenges. Self-report measures, used extensively because they are relatively simple and economical and have some psychometric testing, are designed for adults and adolescents; most are not designed for young children (Moriarty, 1990). Refusal rates in family research are higher (Hagestad, 1981) because one or more family members may choose not to participate. Scheduling data collection at times when all family members are available is often difficult.

Ethical issues in family research are also complex because consent must be obtained from multiple family members. In addition to seeking informed consent from adults and written parental consent for minor children, many family researchers also seek the assent of minor children. The study then must be presented in such a way that parents and children can comprehend the benefits and risks. Precautions also must be taken to protect the voluntariness of family members in their decisions around consent. *Voluntariness* signifies the absence of coercion in choosing whether to participate (Heatherington, Friedlander, & Johnson, 1989). One or more family members, especially children and those who are more vulnerable, may be coerced subtly into participating because of pressure from other family members. To minimize this risk, several family researchers (Heatherington et al., 1989) suggest speaking directly to each family member to request his or her research participation and repeating that the research is voluntary when a family member appears reluctant to take part. In addition parents can be encouraged to monitor their children's responses as the research progresses, and children can be encouraged to ask questions of their parents as concerns develop. Ethical issues in family research, although beginning to receive some attention, require further development (Boss, 1987; Heatherington et al., 1989; LaRossa, Bennett, & Gelles, 1981).

In view of the challenges previously described, some family researchers limit the number of subjects per family to a more manageable number, such as two or three. The process and rationale for sample selection should be outlined in the research report (Moriarty, 1990). For example, Reiss, Gonzalez, and Kramer (1986) defined family and the process for sample selection:

> Each family consisted of at least the patient with renal disease and two other family members living in the same household. . . . When there were more than three members in a household, we picked the three to be tested using the following inclusion rules, in order of priority: 1) patient's spouse over others; 2) oldest child over younger ones; 3) blood relative over foster relative; and 4) member regularly present at the time of first assessment over those away or unavailable. (p. 797)

Although the rationales for this sampling process were not explicit, it appears that the first, third, and fourth rules were designed to include family members who were most significant and available to the person with renal disease (Moriarty, 1990).

Even when measures are gathered from fewer members per family, vigorous efforts to recruit family members are still necessary. Several recruitment strategies will be highlighted in this chapter.

Recruitment Strategies

Making Contact. When recruiting two parents or two or more nonminor family members, the researcher should make contact with all parties. This seems to be an obvious strategy, but it is frequently ignored. Nurse investigators seeking parents and children for family research often approach mothers first because nurses interact more frequently with mothers in many health care settings. Fathers who do not feel as aligned with the nurse or those who feel emotionally distanced from the mother and ill child in a triangular process (Bowen, 1978) may be reluctant to participate in research. These factors could contribute to the underrepresentation of fathers noted in family research and family-related research (on individuals and dyads within the family) in nursing, as well as in other disciplines (Ball, McKenry, & Price-Bonham, 1983; Gilliss, 1989a; Moriarty, 1990). If nurses must approach mothers first about research participation, a letter sent earlier to both parents is helpful in engaging both parents. Telephoning parents at night or at times when both parents are available also increases the probability of engaging both parents (Moriarty, 1990).

Researchers also may attempt to connect with multiple family members through asking for the assistance of persons in the family's ecosystem whom the family trusts. These ecosystem resources include ministers, teachers, neighbors, health clinic staff, community mental health center staff, nurses, physicians, and family practitioners, such as social workers and family therapists. Tapping into an ecosystem resource may be particularly helpful in research recruitment of minority families because the ecosystem resource acts as a liaison between the family and the researcher, and facilitates mutual understanding between parties.

Explaining Benefits. Another recruitment strategy is to explain to the family the potential benefits of research participation for the family itself and for other families. Family members often wish to learn more about each other's needs through the research process (Moriarty, 1990). This wish may be addressed in oral explanations of the study and in the consent form. For example, in our studies (Cotroneo, Hibbs, & Moriarty, 1992; Cotroneo, Moriarty, & Smith, 1992) of relational stressors that influence family decision making in custody litigation, the consent form stated: "Participation in the study may enhance your understanding of the relationship between you and your child." We have observed that the parent-child relationship is the strongest motivator for divorcing parents to be willing to face each other in a research interview.

Family members also welcome the investigator's offer to provide them with a summary of research findings. The summary supplies research families with information on how other families with similar experiences cope and reassures them that they are not alone in confronting particular problems.

Another strong motivator for research participation is the desire to help other families in a similar situation; this may be a positive coping strategy. In Videka-Sherman's (1982) study of bereaved parents, altruistic behavior was related to better psychological adjustment. Similarly, another study (Chodoff, Friedman, & Hamburg, 1964) found that parents of leukemic children benefited from helping other such parents. In Moriarty's (1991) research with bereaved families, almost all bereaved parent participants reported that their motivation for study involvement was to assist other bereaved families. The study also gave parents another opportunity for altruistic behavior: Parents could accept a small "thank-you" payment for participation or could elect to donate it in memory of their child to a national organization for bereaved parents (Moriarty, 1990). This latter option was appealing to many lower-income parents, who noted that they typically could not afford to make such a donation but wished to do so.

Offering Options in the Research Process. Recruitment problems are magnified when research involves families struggling with sensitive problems, affect-laden issues, and painful responses to severe stressors—the very families often in need of the attention of practitioners and researchers. On the one hand, families with sensitive or "taboo" issues may be embarrassed to discuss the issue because of the stigma associated with it. Families with affect-laden issues may be reluctant to share intense affect with a researcher or may be afraid of losing control of overwhelming affect. On the other hand, distressed families often are relieved to share sensitive issues in a research encounter with someone who listens and cares (Boss, 1987).

In Moriarty's (1991) research some bereaved mothers voiced doubt that fathers would take part in the study, stating for example, "He does not like to talk about ___'s death because he doesn't like to show his feelings"; in other couples the roles were reversed. Gender differences and cultural differences in expressions of affect may explain some parents' hesitance to take part in research, particularly research perceived as eliciting intense affect. One strategy to increase recruitment of hesitant parents in the research was to offer options in the research process, thus increasing parents' sense of control over the process, a pressing need for those who feared losing control. Parents were informed that data collection involved the completion of questionnaires by both parents. Parents were presented with options for the research interview, however: A parent could participate, could sit and listen without speaking, and could leave at any time. Just hearing these options appeared to decrease parental anxiety. All parents who were offered these options chose to stay during the interview, and they were quite vocal (Moriarty, 1990).

Home Visits. Use of the home for data collection increases recruitment of families because of the convenience for family members. Furthermore home visits lead to higher response rates in longitudinal studies (McCausland & Burgess, 1989). Home visits also may be instrumental in recruiting families who have experienced sensitive problems and severe stressors, because the home is seen as more private for the discussion of sensitive issues and is the only possible meeting place for families overwhelmed with stress who are too immobilized to travel (Moriarty, 1990). Although additional resources—time and money for data collection and travel—are required for home visits, the investment seems worthwhile in facilitating research recruitment.

Data Collectors/Interviewers. Data collectors play an important role. Considerable evidence (Bradburn, 1983; Kitson et al., 1982) indicates that the training and supervision of data collectors/interviewers influence response rates and response effects (error due to subjects' reluctance to answer question or their misinterpretation of questions) in research with individuals and families. Reviews of research on individuals (Bradburn, 1983; Sudman & Bradburn, 1974) have indicated that other characteristics of the data collectors may increase response effects in certain situations. The data collector's gender and race may alter subjects' responses to questions related to these characteristics. Bradburn and Sudman (1988) recommended matching the interviewer and the subject on race or gender when the topic is about racial relations or sexual behavior and attitudes, respectively.

Whether response effects from the interviewer's race or gender occur in family research has not been documented. Whether the interviewer's gender or race influences response rates in family research is also not clear. Because of the lack of data in these areas, it is critical that family researchers report on differences related to different interviewers. Researchers may ask, for example: Does the gender of the interviewer influence family members' responses to questions about sexual abuse? and Does matching families with interviewers on race influence recruitment or data collection? Moriarty (1990) noted that matching families with data collectors on race appeared to increase the recruitment of families when the data collector had no previous contact with the family and the research concerned painful issues around the loss of a child. When the data collector was known to the family, the response rate of these families was high no matter what the race of the family and interviewer.

We assert that data collectors/interviewers should have, in addition to training in basic research techniques, other qualifications: (a) an understanding of theories of how families function, (b) strong skills in interviewing adults and children, and in conjoint family interviews (all meet together), and (c) skills in making referrals when necessary for the family's well-being. When the investigator has to provide training for data collectors who lack these qualifications, the training may be very costly and time

consuming. It may behoove the investigator to search for data collectors
with the qualifications even if the costs are higher.

Before recruitment begins, the principal investigator also should develop
a good referral network of various disciplines (e.g., a psychologist, psychi-
atrist, nurse or social worker trained in family therapy, a pediatrician or
other medical practitioner) for referrals of families with special needs. An
investigator who has clinical experience with the study population may
better anticipate specific problems in the families that warrant referrals. In
addition she or he has a heightened sensitivity to the general issues and
concerns of the population; this sensitivity promotes recruitment, particularly when families have high conflict or are facing emotionally charged
issues.

Feelings and personal issues of data collectors also may influence recruitment. Conducting research on difficult family issues may elicit data
collectors' anxiety about their own family issues and subsequently may
decrease their willingness to pursue subjects. Data collectors also may
become frustrated after searching unsuccessfully for families or after being
"stood up" for appointments; this too may decrease their enthusiasm for
the project. Investigators in a study of divorced families reported that several staff left the project because these staff experienced painful memories
and increased anxiety during the work (Kitson et al., 1982). Thus debriefing
of data collectors is imperative. Data collectors need an opportunity to
discuss their personal feelings, their concerns for families, and their frus-
trations. They also need consistent supervision to assess whether they are
becoming so anxious or disillusioned by the study problem that recruitment
and interaction with families are affected (Boss, 1987; Kitson et al., 1982;
Moriarty, 1990). Researchers examining families with child abuse (Cautley,
1980) and families who have members with end-stage renal disease (Reiss,
1981) have emphasized the need for team debriefing or co-interviewers to
decrease interviewers' stress when working with these families.

Studying families with sensitive or taboo issues poses special obstacles
because of the difficulty in finding data sources and cooperative subjects.
Selection biases also may occur in particular populations of families, and
prevent random access to the populations. For example, Thomas (1987),
has identified factors, which may be present in populations of families
experiencing very serious physical health problems, that limit direct access
to these populations and thus create sample selection biases. Nonprobability sampling methods are often the most feasible methods for studying
sensitive, relatively low-frequency phenomena, particularly when the researcher has a limited budget. The generalizability of findings from these

studies, however, must be cautiously interpreted. A brief overview of several nonprobability sampling methods will be presented here.

Group Sampling

Researchers may find potential research families through specialized groups in which family members participate—for example, Narcotics Anonymous, Alcoholics Anonymous, Parents Anonymous (for child abusers), and Women Against Abuse (for incest survivors). The major criticism of this approach is self-selection; for example, those who acknowledge abusing their children and seek help for this in a group may be different from those who do not (Gelles, 1978). Studies of these samples, however, are still worthwhile in exploring sensitive topics, in looking at family processes in-depth, and in generating hypotheses for future study. They also may shed some light on the factors that lead family members to become involved in such groups; these data could suggest clinical strategies to increase families' use of such resources. The studies also may illuminate how community groups facilitate healing processes within families, information germane to health professionals who aim to empower families.

Snowball Sampling

In *snowball sampling* the researcher begins with a small sample of families who then refer him or her to other families who are potential research participants. Gelles (1978) cited an example of how a sample of families with a taboo issue could be generated: A woman married to a homosexual identified other families with this situation, who also identified other families, thus creating a pool of potential research families. The disadvantage of this approach is sample bias—families who are known to more people and who have larger social networks have a greater chance of being in the sample than those who are more isolated. This is more of a problem when the sensitive issue under study is related to social isolation. For example, families with abusive parents are often closed family systems, having limited social networks (Gelles, 1978; Strong & Devault, 1989). The advantage of this approach is that the researcher is able to examine connections between people, how people use each other as resources, and what distinguishes connected families from more isolated families.

Use of Public and Private Records

Public documents may be used to locate potential families for research on sensitive topics. For example, police logs of police activities are usually open to the public and are one source of potential families. Gelles (1974, 1987) identified families with possible violence through police records of "family disputes." He acknowledged that this sample might include more urban and lower socioeconomic families because neighbors in closer proximity in poor urban areas would be more apt to see or hear the violence and then contact police. He therefore also sampled from files of a private agency, which would reflect more of a middle-class bias.

Newspapers provide information that may direct researchers to families. Some local papers, for example, list police activities for the week (Gelles, 1978); this list could suggest families in which various types of trauma have occurred. Stories on local fires, other disasters, and murders, as well as the obituaries and birth announcements, may point researchers to specific groups. Researchers interested in bereaved families may gather information on deaths and surviving family members from death certificates and records at the medical examiner's/coroner's office.

In public and private agencies that work with families, such as Children and Youth Services, marital counseling agencies, or hospital clinics, family records are confidential. Researchers may, however, be able to negotiate an arrangement with an agency to gain access to families. For example, agency staff may screen their files for eligible families and then request families' permission to be contacted by the researcher (Gelles, 1978; Kitson et al., 1982). This method was used in our study (Cotroneo, DeFeudis, Moriarty, & Natale, 1992) of families with physical or sexual abuse who were referred by Children and Youth Services; however, it is important to note that Cotroneo, the principal investigator, was known and trusted by the staff as a skilled family therapist. In research with high-risk families, one needs to develop relationships with agencies to gain agency cooperation. The agency also needs to feel that families could benefit from the research and that agency staff could benefit indirectly too by gaining additional resources for aiding families who may drain staff and agency resources.

Mental health therapists in private practice and attorneys specializing in family law also may refer families for research after seeking the families' permission. For example, attorneys referred families for two studies of families in custody disputes (Cotroneo, Hibbs, & Moriarty, 1992; Cotroneo, Moriarty, & Smith, 1992). The principal investigator had worked in the past with these attorneys. The attorneys encouraged their clients to participate because they saw the research interviews as assisting family members to explore their issues around custody and perhaps to avoid repeated litigation.

After Data Collection:
Reporting Response and Refusal Rates

In view of the recruitment problems in family research, it is essential that investigators report on response and refusal rates to enable evaluation of the generalizability of findings and possible systematic biases in sampling (Moriarty, 1990). Yet frequently this does not occur. Kitson et al. (1982) asserted that a serious problem in family research is the lack of a standard procedure for reporting how much of the sample was contacted (sample coverage). Another problem is that response rates and refusal rates are described in different ways, making it difficult to compare family studies. Kitson and other researchers (Alwin, 1977; Kitson et al., 1982; Kviz, 1977) suggested the use of the following definitions. The *response rate* is the number of families who participated divided by the total number of eligible families in the sample. The *refusal rate* is the number of families contacted who refused to participate divided by the total number of eligible families contacted. "The response rate is the more accurate report of sample coverage and should be used, but many studies report refusal rates instead" (Kitson et al., 1982, p. 972). When a large part of a population cannot be found (low sample coverage), the response rate is low. If the researcher does not report the low response rate and only states the refusal rate, then the information is misleading because it gives the impression of a high level of participation. Kitson cited an example in a divorce study: 73% of those contacted agreed to participate, making the refusal rate 27%, but the response rate was only 11% because much of the population was unable to be contacted. The reporting of this low response rate contributed important information on sample coverage and raised questions about the representativeness of the sample. In this situation comparisons between demographic characteristics of participants and nonresponders are necessary to detect potential biases in the sample (Kitson et al., 1982; Moriarty, 1990).

Conclusion

As nurse researchers move toward a science of family nursing, they will test both traditional and novel recruitment strategies and sampling strategies. When the advantages and disadvantages of such strategies are described in research reports, family researchers in nursing and in other disciplines can learn from one another.

It is clear that family research, by its very focus on the family, cannot be done in a professional vacuum. Such research draws on the methods of many fields, such as nursing, medicine, sociology, psychology, family therapy, anthropology, and ethics. Family research, like family practice, is inclined naturally toward multidisciplinary approaches. What cuts across all approaches, however, is a necessary attitude of partnership with families—of shared responsibility for the process and outcomes of research.

Many practitioners of family nursing and other family practitioners, particularly family therapists, have developed skills in joining with family members to work together for the health of individual members and the family as a whole. We believe that family researchers will benefit from collaboration with family practitioners. These practitioners have worked over the years to become partners with families in the care of families. As such these practitioners are invaluable resources to family researchers, who are struggling with sampling and recruitment issues as they strive to become partners with families in research.

10

Scoring Family Data:
An Application With Families With Preterm Infants

Carol J. Loveland-Cherry

Mary Horan

Mary Burman

JoAnne Youngblut

Willard Rodgers

Growing numbers of family researchers conceptualize the family as a system that is more than the sum of its parts. The notion that it is not sufficient to collect information from a single family member, usually the mother, is implicit in this type of approach. Operationalizing family systems concepts in research has proven problematic and has generated a great deal of discussion (Ball, McHenry, & Bonham, 1983; Feetham, 1991a; Schumm, Barnes, Bollman, Jurich, & Milliken, 1985; White & Brinkerhoff, 1977). A major question in these discussions is the collection and scoring of family systems data.

Although observational, projective, and gaming methods exist for measuring the family systems concepts, these techniques are often costly, time consuming, influenced by family age and power structure, and may require bringing the family to a laboratory setting. For the most part, measures of family variables continue to be obtained through assessment of individual members' perceptions of family characteristics. With increasing frequency multiple members are sampled in family studies. To avoid the commission of an individualistic fallacy—that is, ascribing characteristics to the family system on the basis of knowledge of an individual family member—researchers need to measure a collective property or to score data as a collective. Decisions regarding scoring of the data, however, present major problems for family systems researchers. In many cases researchers ignore the issue of difference in units of measurement and fail to address fully the significance of creating a variable that operationalizes the collective from data derived from individuals within the group.

Purpose

The purpose of this chapter is to examine alternative methods of scoring family measures based on data from the Family Adaptability and Cohesion Evaluation Scale (FACES III) (Olson, Portner, & Lavee, 1985) and the Feetham Family Functioning Survey (FFFS) (Roberts & Feetham, 1982) for 125 sets of parents with preterm infants. The specific questions addressed are (a) How are family cohesion, family adaptability, and satisfaction with family relationships related to measures of well-being in mothers and fathers of preterm infants? (b) How do these relationships differ, depending on whether individual, mean, or difference scores for the family variables are used? and (c) What are the implications for interpretations of results relative to the different scoring methods?

First, a brief discussion of the alternative methods of scoring family data that are reported in the literature is presented. Then data from a longitudinal study of families of preterm infants are used to examine the implications and consequences of using three alternative methods of scoring the family data.

Background

Scoring Approaches

A number of reports of alternative methods for scoring family data are available (Ezell, Paolucci, & Bubolz, 1984; Feetham, 1991a; Klein, 1981; Schumm et al., 1985; Uphold & Strickland, 1989; Walters, Pittman, & Norrell, 1984). White and Brinkerhoff's (1977) work provides the basis for this discussion by explicating the concerns regarding the appropriate unit of analysis. Extrapolating from Lazarfeld and Menzel's work (1969), White and Brinkerhoff made the important distinction between individual and collective properties. *Individual properties* characterize individual family members and vary among individuals. They include absolute (e.g., age, education), relational (e.g., one's adjustment to marriage), and comparative (absolute or relational property viewed over the entire collective of which one is a member) properties. It would be inappropriate to devise family scores for measures of such properties. It would, however, be appropriate to consider doing so for *collective properties,* those that vary from one family to another rather than from one individual to another. Three types of collective properties are identified: (a) *analytical properties,* obtained by performing a mathematical operation on a property of individual members (e.g., family income, social class); (b) *structural properties,* obtained by performing a mathematical operation on data about the relations of each member to some or all of the others (e.g., degree of integration, power structure); and (c) *global properties,* not based on information about individual family members but rather that describe family in terms of its role structure (e.g., family typologies or matrices as described by McCubbin and McCubbin [1988] or by Knafl and Deatrick [1990]). The type of property germane to this chapter and most frequently discussed in the family literature is the collective structural property.

The major approaches for creating structural properties for family data have been summarized succinctly by Klein (1981) and more recently by Uphold and Strickland (1989). Generally four basic approaches for creating structural properties are evident in the literature. The first simply is to use each member's discrete scores. This approach assumes multiple realities and may be most appropriate if the underlying conceptualization for the study argues that the perception of the individual is most critical. The major decision is to select the most appropriate respondent.

The second approach is a summative score that may or may not be averaged. The assumption is that each family member's score is equally important and instrumental in creating the family experience. Further it is assumed that extreme reports have equal and off-setting biases or errors. This approach has a number of inherent problems. Two families may have the same total scores when the individual members' scores are quite different. Total summative scores often exceed the upper limit of scales, complicating substantive interpretations. Finally, summative scores do not allow comparison of families of unequal size. In the last instance, taking a mean score for the family allows comparisons across families of different sizes. A major drawback of this approach is the reduction of score variance.

A third major approach is the use of a discrepancy or difference score. The assumption underlying this approach is that families differ, depending on the degree of consensus about aspects of the family. Again the approach has drawbacks. Taking an absolute difference does not indicate the direction of the discrepancy or give information about the relative placement on a scale continuum for families that may have the same discrepancy score. As with mean scores, score variance is reduced.

A fourth approach is to weight individual members' scores by using a variety of techniques. One method is to weight scores by some criterion of adequacy; for example, parents' scores would be given greater weights. Alternatively, individual reports can be weighted by using such statistical techniques as factor analysis, cluster analysis, discriminant function, canonical correlation, or commonality analysis. Although these techniques are appealing, the numbers required would prohibit them for a number of studies. The use of structural modeling techniques employing such programs as LISREL or EQS are currently the vogue for analyzing complex data sets, such as those we often see in family research. Again the sample size is critical and becomes more so as the number of parameters to be estimated increases.

Conceptual Issues

An important consideration that often is overlooked is the fit of the scoring approach with the conceptualization underlying the study. An example from our study of families of preterm infants illustrates this point. Initially we planned to analyze the data using causal modeling via LISREL. In a preliminary examination of measurement models using confirmatory factor analysis, we started with a model that proposed a single latent variable of family functioning with indicators of adaptability for mothers and fathers, cohesion for mothers and fathers, family relationships for mothers and fathers, and the difference scores for each of the three family variables (adaptability, cohesion, and family relationships). The results of the initial confirmatory factor analysis indicated that the fit of the measurement model was poor, χ^2 (9, $N = 125$) = 49.675, $p = < .001$, Bentler-Bonnett normed fit index = .61. Subsequently a second model with three latent variables—adaptability, cohesion, and family relationships—each with three indicators, one for mother, one for father, and a difference score, was evaluated. Although the fit was improved, it was still less than desired, χ^2 (6, $N = 125$) = 37.438, $p = < .001$, Bentler-Bonnett normed fit index = .709. Consequently a third model with two latent variables—mother family functioning and father family functioning, each with three indicators (adaptability, cohesion, and family relationships), was evaluated. The fit of the last model was the best of the three evaluated—χ^2 (8, N = 125) = 22.25, p = .00447, Bentler-Bonnett normed fit index = .827. Even the third model was not all that satisfactory, however; there was a significant lack of fit (p = .00447). A modification of the model in which the unique components for mothers' adaptability and fathers' adaptability were allowed to be correlated improved the fit considerably—χ^2 (7, N = 125) = 11.723, df = 7, p = .11, Bentler-Bonnett normed fit index = .909). That is, the adaptability scores appear to have a variance component that is not captured by the single factor (per parent). When difference scores were added to the model, the fit deteriorated.

Further, a conceptual issue was evident. If separate factors seem to emerge for the two parents, how should difference scores, which reflect both parents, be incorporated into the model? Difference scores consequently were not included in the model. The first model was the one that best fit the original conceptualization for the study. It was the least supported, however, from an analytic perspective. Thus, although the use of structural equation modeling offered the opportunity of using a measurement approach that was congruent with the study conceptualization of family, a dilemma resulted: the lack of empirical support for the original conceptualization. The measurement model supported by the confirmatory factor analysis indicates that mothers and fathers have separate but related perceptions of family variables. This is consistent with both other reports in the literature (see, for example, Mercer, Ferkitich, DeJoseph, May, & Sollid, 1988) and with subsequent analyses for our own work. Difference scores further appear to measure yet another dimension of family functioning, different from individuals' perceptions.

The various approaches for scoring family data are described clearly in the literature and the strengths and limitations of each discussed (Ezell et al., 1984; Feetham, 1991a; Klein, 1981; Schumm et al., 1985; Uphold & Strickland, 1989; Walters et al., 1984). Each researcher needs to consider carefully what will be gained or sacrificed through the use of the various approaches.

Methods

The results reported here are from preliminary analyses performed during the early stages of a longitudinal study of the impact of parental and family factors on preterm infant development. The focus at this point was on exploration of various approaches for scoring data on family variables collected from 125 sets of mothers and fathers of preterm infants. The infants were less than 38 weeks gestation and appropriate for gestational age and were patients in a level III neonatal intensive care nursery for at least 1 week but not more than 3 months. These results are based on wave one data collected through the use of structured interviews and self-completed questionnaires in the family home when the infant was 3 months old.

Family measures included the Family Adaptability and Cohesion Evaluation Scales III (FACES III) and the Feetham Family Functioning Survey (FFFS). The FACES III (Olson et al., 1985) is a 20-item scale with two 10-item subscales—Adaptability and Cohesion. Item responses are made on a 5-point scale ranging from *almost never* (1) to *almost always* (5), and resulting values are summed for each subscale. Estimates of internal consistency reported in the literature were .77 for cohesion and .62 for adaptability (Olson et al., 1985). For the current study sample, alphas for cohesion and adaptability for mothers were .80 and .63, and for fathers, .79 and .67, respectively. The revised FFFS (Feetham & Humenick, 1982; Roberts & Feetham, 1982) has 25 scorable items, each measured on three subscales (How much is there now? How much should there be? and How important is this to you?) using a 7-point scale. A total discrepancy score is computed by summing the absolute differences between "what should be" from "what is" for each item. An alpha of .81 was reported (Roberts & Feetham, 1982). For the current sample, the alphas were .80 for fathers and .79 for mothers.

Parental well-being was measured by using the Affects Balance Scale (ABS) and a single-item 5-centimeter visual analog scale with the anchors of *poor* and *excellent* asking respondents to rate their own health. The ABS is a 40-item checklist that measures affective status. Responses for items range from *never* (0) to *always* (4) and reflect the degree to which a specific emotion is experienced in a specified time period. The overall score on the test reflects the balance between positive and negative affects, expressed in standardized scores. The alpha for the negative scale was reported as .92 and for the positive scale as .94 (Derogatis, Abeloff, & Melisaratos, 1979). For the current study, alphas for both the negative and positive scales were .89 for both mothers and fathers.

Individual scores for mothers and fathers were computed for the three family variables (adaptability, cohesion, and family relationships) and the ABS. Family mean scores and difference scores were computed for each set of parents for each of the family variables. Bivariate correlations were calculated between ABS scores and the self-rating of health scores and (a) the individual scores, (b) the mean scores, and (c) the difference scores for the three family variables. Finally, the ABS scores were regressed on adaptability, cohesion, and family relationship scores by using the three alternative methods of scoring. Separate analyses were run for mothers and fathers. Thus three multiple regressions were run for mothers and three for fathers.

Results

The mothers ranged in age from 18 to 41 ($M = 28.23$, $sd = 5.26$) and the fathers from 18 to 47 ($M = 30.73$, $sd = 5.99$). The sample consisted of generally white (93%), middle-class individuals. The infants' gestational age ranged from 27 to 36.5 weeks ($M = 32.57$, $sd = 2.28$). The parents in the study were generally healthy.

The descriptive statistics for the family variables are summarized in Table 10.1. Although the means and standard deviations are very similar for mothers and fathers, mothers' cohesion scores and FFFS scores were significantly higher than those of fathers—$t(122) = 1.40$, $p = < .05$, and $t(108) = 3.12$, $p = < .05$, respectively. Adaptability scores were not significantly different for mothers and fathers. Mothers' and fathers' adaptability, $r = .32$, $p = < .01$, cohesion, $r = .21$, $p = < .05$, and FFFS, $r = .21$, $p = < .05$, scores were significantly correlated.

The results of the correlational analyses were similar using either individual scores or mean family scores. Individual and mean adaptability scores were related positively to mothers' ABS scores—$r = .29$, $p = .001$; $r = .41$, $p = < .001$, respectively. For cohesion, individual and mean scores were related positively to mothers' ABS scores—$r = .39$, $p = < .001$; $r = .39$, $p = < .001$, respectively—and fathers' ABS scores—$r = .29$, $p = .001$; $r = .23$, $p = < .01$, respectively—and to fathers' self-rating of health—$r = .16$, $p = < .05$; $r = .16$, $p = < .05$, respectively. Individual and mean FFFS scores were related negatively to mothers' ABS scores—$r = -.47$, $p = < .001$; $r = -.48$, $p = < .001$, respectively—and fathers' ABS scores—$r = -.38$, $p = < .001$; $r(101) = -.42$, $p = < .001$, respectively—and mean FFFS scores to mothers' self-rating of health—$r = -.18$, $p = < .05$. Negative correlations between FFFS scores and measures of well-being were expected because higher scores indicate less satisfaction. Dissatisfaction with significant relationships can produce stress and thereby negatively affect well-being.

Adaptability difference scores were related negatively only to mothers' self-rating of health—$r = -.16$, $p = < .05$). Cohesion difference scores were related negatively to mothers' ABS scores—$r = -.32$, $p = < .001$—and fathers' ABS scores—$r = -.21$, $p = < .01$. FFFS difference scores were related negatively to mothers' ABS scores—$r = -.28$, $p = < .01$—and to

Table 10.1 Descriptive Statistics: Adaptability, Cohesion, and Family Relationships for Individual Mothers' and Fathers' Scores, Family Mean Scores, and Family Difference Scores

Variable	Potential Range	Actual Range	M	sd
Adaptability				
Mothers	10-50	17-42	30.96	5.24
Fathers	10-50	17-46	30.52	5.20
Family mean	10-50	21.5-45	35.76	4.85
Difference	0-40	3-20	10.15	3.49
Cohesion				
Mothers	10-50	15-50	40.67	6.06
Fathers	10-50	24-49	39.28	5.63
Family mean	10-50	23-47	39.97	4.56
Difference	0-40	2-22	9.19	3.93
FFFS				
Mothers	0-150	3-59	25.36	12.38
Fathers	0-150	1-62	22.16	11.35
Family mean	0-150	3.5-50	23.61	9.23
Difference	0-150	7-56	26.18	8.72

NOTE: $N = 125$

mothers' self-rating of health—$r = -.17$, $p = < .05$. Overall the magnitude of the correlations was greater for mothers than for fathers.

For mothers, regression analyses for predicting ABS scores were significant with individual (adjusted $R^2 = .26$; $F = 12.79$, $p = < .01$), mean (adjusted $R^2 = .27$; $F = 13.08$, $p = < .01$), and difference scores (adjusted $R^2 = .13$; $F = 5.76$, $p = < .01$). FFFS scores were significant predictors with individual (Beta $= -.36$, $t = -3.69$, $p = < .001$) and mean (Beta $= -.38$, $t = -3.77$, $p = < .001$) scores. Mean adaptability scores were also significant predictors of ABS scores (Beta $= .29$, $t = 2.21$, $p = .03$). When difference scores were used as predictors, FFFS and cohesion scores were significant (Beta $= -.27$, $t = -2.44$, $p = < .05$; Beta $= -.25$, $t = -2.41$, $p = < .05$; respectively).

For fathers, regression analyses for predicting ABS scores were significant with individual (adjusted $R^2 = .17$; $F = 8.34$, $p = < .01$) and mean scores (adjusted $R^2 = .17$; $F = 7.54$, $p = < .01$). FFFS scores were the significant independent variable for individual (Beta $= -.33$, $t = -3.50$, $p = < .001$) and mean (Beta $= -.35$, $t = -3.30$, $p = < .01$) scores.

Discussion

The family characteristics measured in the current study meet the criteria of collective structural properties; all focus on relations among family members. Use of individual scores gives information about the different realities of family perceived by mothers and fathers. The effects of the family variables were different for the two parents when individual scores were used. Although relationship dimensions were explanatory in predicting well-being in both parents, adaptability was influential only for mothers. Adaptability was related similarly to only mothers' well-being when a mean score was used. Further, individual and mean scores accounted for more of the variance in parents' ABS scores than did difference scores. It appears that individual and mean scores may be more significant when looking at individual well-being measures.

Different results clearly are obtained if one uses difference scores versus either individual or mean scores. Difference scores seem to represent a collective structural property that is quite different from the individual or mean scores of the same family property. A difference among family members' scores reflects a lack of consensus that may or may not be dysfunctional for the family. It may be that the critical issue is not the difference or the incongruence but rather the family dimension. For this sample of families with preterm infants, it appears that relationship dimensions are more critical to well-being than the adaptability of the family and that differences between the parents negatively affect their well-being. Further, difference scores are better predictors of well-being for mothers than for fathers. Thus difference scores reveal something different about predictors of well-being than do individual measures. Finally, it is important not to lose sight of the conceptual meaning when interpreting family scores.

11

Exploratory Analysis:
A Technique for the
Analysis of Dyadic Data
in Research of Families

Suzanne L. Feetham

Mary Perkins

Ruth Carroll

Decisions for data analysis is one issue in research of families when more than one family member is the focus of the research. The analysis plan should be consistent with the conceptualization of the research, the research questions, and the methodology. Because data are gathered from multiple family members, the analysis plans are supported more solidly when they include methods to review the scores of family members from several standpoints. In spite of it being unfamiliar to many researchers, exploratory data analysis (EDA) is a technique that can help array family

AUTHORS' NOTE: Appreciation is given to Dr. Ramona Mercer for the data used for analysis in this chapter. Data are from the project *Antepartum Stress: Effect on Family Health and Functioning*, Grant Number NR01064, National Center for Nursing Research, National Institutes of Health, Ramona T. Mercer, principal investigator.

member's scores in a number of ways and therefore evaluate the analysis plan and the associated theoretical frameworks.

Exploratory data analysis provides information about the characteristics of the sample to confirm the appropriateness of the planned analysis (Ferketich & Verran, 1986; Hartwig & Dearing, 1985: Tukey, 1977; Verran & Ferketich, 1987). Through the ability to examine responses between family members, EDA also may result in the need to alter or propose new theory and possibly new hypotheses. EDA, a technique consistent with the conceptual and methodological rigors required in research of families, also can yield information about the characteristics of the sample to give direction for further research and for clinical practice. In this chapter the analysis of a subset of data from 73 pregnant high-risk women and their partners is presented to demonstrate the process, characteristics, and applications of EDA.

Data Analysis

With recent advances in the conceptualization and measurement in research of families, the issue of data sources has received considerable attention. Issues include the identification of which elements of the family are to be examined and the determination, through analysis, of the characteristics and contributions of family members' responses (data), both individually and collectively (Larsen & Olson, 1990; Loveland-Cherry, Horan, Burman, Youngblut, & Rodgers, Chapter 10, this volume).

Basic mathematical and theoretical assumptions are applied at each decision phase of data analysis. Fisher and colleagues (Fisher, Terry, & Ransom, 1990) recommended that no method of assessment, data management tool, or design strategy should be excluded from consideration in family and health research as long as (a) the method is logically consistent with the construct being assessed, (b) the data management procedure maintains the logic, and (c) the design strategy and units of analysis are derived adequately from that portion of the theory that underlies the research.

Having obtained information from individuals of interest to family research, the investigator's usual statistical option in research of families is to take the data "as they are" and to subject them to analysis as aggregate data. A second option is to obtain data from additional family members on the same instrument or series of instruments and to combine the scores in some way or to compare and contrast the interfamily member patterns across family members to produce a conjoint index. A third option is to determine dyadic scores from the data from family members and to treat the data as relational data (Feetham, 1984, 1991; Fisher et al., 1990; Schumm, Barnes, Bollman, Jurich, & Milliken, 1985; Uphold & Strickland, 1989).

Following the selection of one of these options, the usual sequence in a quantitative study is to use descriptive statistics to characterize the sample and then to use inferential techniques, such as confirmatory analysis, to test predetermined hypotheses. The application of traditional quantitative techniques in research of families, however, may yield less information about family members because attention is not focused on the patterns of similarities or differences between and among family members. Traditionally the mean and the standard deviation are used as measures of location and spread. These statistical summaries are not resistant to the influence of outlying data points or distributions other than bell shaped. The use of the mean as a measure of central tendency may obscure the identification of extreme values or the tendency toward bimodal distribution. To understand family data, the shape of a distribution is as important as location and spread. Traditional inferential techniques that numerically summarize variables can hide or misrepresent important patterns in the data between and among family members.

It is the opinion of some family scientists that differences in scores between family members are due to problems with self-reporting and with research instruments resulting in random measurement error. Other scientists contend that true differences exist between the perceptions of individual family members (Larsen & Olson, 1990; Schumm et al., 1985). It is known that the type of analysis conducted affects the size or amount of the discrepancy or difference between responses of family members. For example, aggregate analysis will result in a smaller difference. This influence reinforces the potential of exploratory analysis. It is important that the investigator know what information may be lost in aggregate analysis.

At the time of analysis, researchers should consider carefully the conceptual framework of the study before proceeding with traditional statistical tests of data (Schumm, 1982; Schumm et al., 1985). The characteristics of data from multiple family members, such as the underlying family variance factor and the positive intercorrelation of the scores of each family member, are additional reasons to consider using EDA before the traditional analyses (Schumm et al., 1985).

Exploratory Data Analysis:
An Aid for Confirmatory Data Analysis

In recognition of the complex issues of analysis of family data, exploratory techniques will assist the family researcher in ensuring the appropriateness of the planned confirmatory analysis, such as discriminate analysis and multivariate multiple regression (Verran & Ferketich, 1987). The step of using EDA to confirm the appropriateness of the planned analysis is necessary because research of families involves the capture of human re- sponses that may vary between and among family members. The objective of exploring the data is to sensitize the researcher to patterns that may go undetected with only the application of traditional analysis. The identification of these patterns may have been part of the original rationale for collecting data from more than one family member.

Exploratory data analysis is an interactive approach to data analysis that allows the researcher to use visual displays and graphs of data concurrently with numeric summaries and theoretical considerations (Tukey, 1977). Because of the subjectivity involved in interpreting the visual displays, some investigators consider this technique to be somewhat unscientific. The subjective element in interpreting graphs and visual displays decreases, however, when a series of displays shows consistent evidence of the same patterns in the data (Ferketich & Verran, 1986).

Examinations of outlier data points or distributions other than the normal distribution curve are performed through the use of visual displays and graphs. A determination of what information is contained in the data is made as the spread and location of the distribution and patterning effects of outliers are examined (Verran & Ferketich, 1987).

The analysis presented here demonstrates the use of EDA in the study of families and the contributions of this technique in determining patterns and unique characteristics of the family member's responses. The analysis was conducted for this chapter and is not reported in other publications of the research. The data were collected in a longitudinal study of pregnant women and their partners. Subjects were followed from the 24th to the 34th week of pregnancy and for 8 months after the birth of their infants. Subjects were 18 years or older and, if unmarried, were living with their partners and planning to parent with the partners. The women were categorized as high- or low-risk on the basis of stress indicators from life events, antenatal hospitalization, and pregnancy risk scores. The total sample of pregnant women and their partners was 593 (Mercer & Ferketich, 1990; Mercer, Ferketich, DeJoseph, May, & Sollid, 1988; Mercer, May, Ferketich, & DeJoseph, 1986). A subset of all of the high-risk partners (73 high-risk women [HRW] and 73 high-risk men [HRM]) was selected for this analysis.

The data analyzed were for the family functioning variable as measured by the original version of the Feetham Family Functioning Survey (FFFS). The FFFS measures family functioning across three areas of relationships. The instrument score is calculated from the difference between the perceived and expected occurrence of 23 family functions. The FFFS has reported reliability and validity across multiple samples, including families of healthy children, families of children with health problems, and families with adult children (Roberts & Feetham, 1982; Thomas & Barnard, 1986). The Cronbach alphas for this sample ranged from .78 to .82.

Scatter diagram plots, box plots, stem and leaf displays, and graphic displays were used to examine the single distributions of the HRW and their partners (HRM) and their score relationships on the FFFS variable. The scatter diagram in Figure 11.1, which is a visual representation of the raw scores, shows a positive relationship between the HRW and HRM scores. The Pearson r ($r = .167$, df = 72, $p < .157$) indicates a statistically insignificant small positive relationship. The difference between the paired means ($t = .91$, $p < .365$) is also insignificant statistically. This is because the average scores of the HRW (19.12) are similar to those of the HRM (17.45). Because the statistical analyses show neither a significant correlation nor means difference, the researcher may conclude no association between the pairs of scores or any difference between the groups. On visual examination of the data, however, unique and revealing characteristics of the data are uncovered. For example, approximately half of the scores fall between 10 and 30; the other half are outliers and extreme value points. In family research and in particular for the family functioning variable, dyadic behaviors of these types may be clinically significant. When significant numbers of outlier or extreme values are evidenced in visual displays of data, the examination of residuals will assist the researcher in answering questions of association, concordance, or difference for those data points. The questions of interest in this study include concordance or discordance between partners or the differences and similarities among and between couples in the 10-30 scoring range and couples who are in the outlier or extreme range.

Additional information is revealed when the shape of the distribution, as well as location and spread, is examined in visual representations of the data. "Evaluation of shape is necessary to determine which numeric summaries of location and spread are appropriate, and to explore significant features leading to theory construction and explication" (Verran & Ferketich, 1987, p. 142). Stem and leaf displays and box plots are used to visualize the differences between the shapes of distribution, characteristics of location, spread, and presence of outliers. The stem and leaf technique displayed in Figure 11.2 was used to order the data and to obtain a visual view of the distribution shape and pattern (Hoaglin, Mosteller, & Tukey, 1983).

The possible range of scores on the FFFS is 0-150; the usual reported range is 0-59. The scores on the FFFS for the HRW ranged from 0-66, with

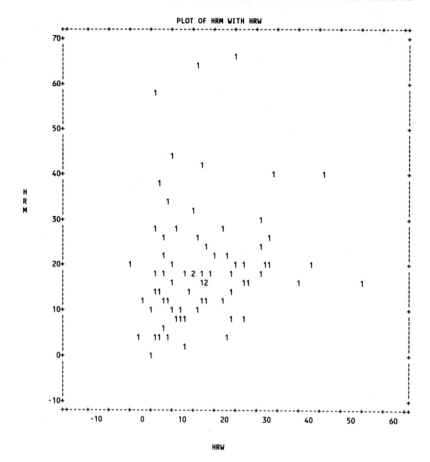

Figure 11.1. Scatter Diagram of High-Risk Dyads
NOTE: HRM mean = 17.45, *SD* = 11.06; HRW mean = 19.12, *SD* = 13.09, *r* = .167, *df* = 72, *p* = .157, *paired t* = .91, *p* = .365

a mean of 19.2; scores for the HRM ranged from 0 to 55, with a mean of 17.45. These results are consistent with other reports of the FFFS (Feetham & Humenick, 1982; Thomas & Barnard, 1986).

Both stem and leaf displays (Figure 11.2) depict a right-skewed distribution with evidence of gaps in the data. For the HRW no scores occur at 29, 32, 33, 35, 36, 40, 42, and 44-58. For the HRM no scores occur at 21, 26, 29, 30, 35-39, and 47-54. The bulk of data points for both the HRW and HRM are between 0-28. When these kinds of patterns are detected, one may question how similar or different the scores of the partners are and

Stem-and-Leaf Display for High-Risk Women

```
0 .023344467888899
1 .0011122233345566666677777788899
2 .000011234566788
3 .014799
4 .13
5 .8
6 .36
```

Stem-and-Leaf Display for High-Risk Men

```
0 .02355666667778888888999
1 .000011223334555666777788889
2 .02233444557778
3 .1112334
```

Figure 11.2. Stem-and-Leaf Displays for High-Risk Women and Men

whether both partner scores are concordant at the extreme or outlier end of the distributions. This information would not be detectable in a typical frequency histogram.

To further visualize such prominent characteristics in the data as spread, symmetry, and presence of outliers, box plots were used. In the box plots of the HRW and HRM (Figure 11.3), the asymmetrical nature of the distributions is obvious. In the HRW scores, the spread of the distribution (length of the box) is more condensed than that of the HRM. The median, which summarizes location (indicated by an asterisk in the box), is near the midsection of the box for the HRW and near the upper section of the box for the HRM. Again in Figure 11.3, the length of the box and the location of the median, along with the vertical dashes or tails of the plot, are equal and indicate a symmetrical distribution for the HRW. These data, however, show more outlier and extreme values at the upper end of the distribution. The box plot of the HRM indicates a somewhat asymmetrical distribution. The vertical dashes are unequal and result in an extension of the upper tail. The distribution for the HRM does not show as many extreme and outlier values at the upper end of the distribution.

These three EDA techniques show that the distributional behavior of two family member responses on the FFFS differed. The dissimilar distribution characteristics of the HRW and HRM as seen in box plots and stem-and-leaf displays warranted additional visualization of paired data. Therefore,

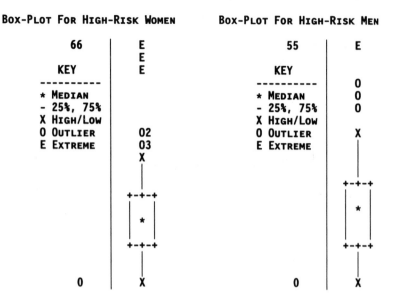

Figure 11.3. Box Plots for High-Risk Women and Men

to further visualize the contrast in behaviors of individual couples on the FFFS variable, the couple scores were plotted on a graph (see Figure 11.4). HRW scores were plotted in ascending order with their partners' scores and confirm, in a simple graphic depiction, the variability between and among multiple data sources. An examination of the subset at the HRW mean of 19.17 reveals major differences between the HRW scores and those of their partners. The depiction not only shows the variation between partners but also between couples with the same or comparable FFFS scores; that is, few couples look alike. These displays reinforce the variability of family members' responses and the importance of visually examining data characteristics.

Regardless of whether the visual displays and the statistics show agreement, it is a matter of the researcher's judgment how the group scores will be summarized. There is no simple prescription to justify the construction of couple or family scores from individual responses. The decision to create group scores, however, should be based on a solid set of decision guidelines with recognition of any trade-offs (Jacobsen, Tulman, & Lowrey, 1991; Larsen & Olson, 1990; Ransom, Fisher, Phillips, Kokes, & Weiss, 1990). The decision is strengthened when individual scores are reviewed carefully

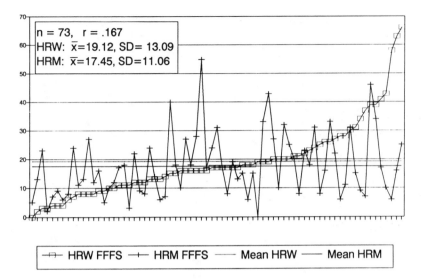

Figure 11.4. Comparison of FFFS Scores of High-Risk Women (HRW) and High-Risk Men (HRM) Sorted by Women's Scores in Ascending Order

from several standpoints, questions to be asked of the data are stated clearly, and explanations for specific decisions are provided.

In summary, decisions on scores from more than one family member can be facilitated through the use of EDA. The decisions for these scores should be made from consistent guidelines and a full understanding of the pattern of distribution of data between and among family members. EDA allows the researcher to visualize and confirm variability in distributional behaviors of individual responses and therefore confirms the appropriateness of the planned analysis. In addition EDA provides information related to the patterns of outliers within and between dyads. It is anticipated that the examination, through visual displays, over time and across multiple studies, of family members who are outliers or at the extremes, may provide information about predictors of family outcomes (Filsinger, 1990). The determination of these predictors may give direction for nursing interventions that address the entire range of family member responses and promote positive outcomes for families.

PART IV

Practice

Janice M. Bell, Editor

12

The Nonexistence of Noncompliant Families: The Influence of Humberto Maturana

Lorraine M. Wright

Anne Marie C. Levac

In the nursing of families, the expectations are that families will comply with ideas and advice that could promote, maintain, and/or restore their health. When families are not compliant to nursing interventions, nurses frequently interpret this behavior as an unwillingness or a lack of readiness to change. This linear view implies that problems with adherence to treatment regimens reside within individuals and families, not within the interactions or relationships between individuals. In our opinion it is arrogant, insulting, and violent to label families as "noncompliant."

If nurses choose to apply some of the ideas of Chilean biologist Humberto Maturana, however, descriptions such as "noncompliant," "resistant," "dysfunctional," and "unmotivated" are questioned. On the basis of the science of biology, Maturana (1978, 1983, 1985, 1988) offered an intriguing metatheory of cognition. When this theory is applied to nursing practice,

AUTHORS NOTE: this chapter was previously published as follows: Wright, L. M., & Levac, A. M. (1992). The noncomliant families: The influence of Humberto Maturana. *Journal of Advanced Nursing, 17,* (913-917). Reprinted with permission.

the nursing diagnosis of "noncompliance" is not only an epistemological error but a biological impossibility. This revolutionary theory invites nurses to reexamine their assumptions about the existence of noncompliance and challenges the relevance of the North American Nursing Diagnostic Association's (NANDA) classification system.

Although many interrelated sets of theoretical concepts are inherent in the theory, the definitions and significant implications of structural determinism and objectivity-in-parenthesis are highlighted in this chapter. The application of these concepts reveals the impossibility of "instructive interaction," leading us to conclude the nonexistence of noncompliant families.

Structural Determinism

A major proposition of this theory is that all living systems, including humans, are structurally determined. It is the individual's structure and history of interactions that determine change in his or her state or behavior. It is not nurses who determine or direct change.

Maturana's metatheory of cognition evolved from the most unlikely of experiments—experiments examining the structural mechanism of perception in frogs. Maturana, Lettvin, McCulloch, and Pitts (1960) discovered that the "function of the retina in the frog is not to transmit information" and further concluded that "the transformation of the image (not transmission of the image) constitutes the fundamental function of the retina" (p. 170). What a frog perceives visually has been transformed by the retina in a manner that is specific to the organization of the frog's nervous system. Thus perception is not a picture of the world coming in and recording on the frog's brain (Simon, 1985), but rather it is the frog's structure that determines its own reality.

Maturana, Uribe, and Frenk (1968), when describing a biological theory of color coding in the primate retina, concluded that the activities of a nervous system do not reflect an independent environment and therefore do not reflect an absolute external world. Maturana and his colleagues also concluded that an animal's interactions with an environment are best represented by the animal's own organization and not by an independent external reality. Because the basic architecture of the nervous system is universal, Maturana extended his earlier ideas related to the visual perception of frogs to the perceptual process of primates, which includes human beings. Consequently what is perceived by an individual is always a result of transformation within the structure of the individual.

The revelation that all living systems cannot refer to an external, independent reality becomes not only a philosophical reflection but also a constitutive biological condition of humanity (Mendez, Coddou, & Maturana, 1988). The uniqueness of this theory is that it reflects an epistemology in which individuals (living systems) draw forth reality—they do not construct it nor does it exist independently of them (Maturana, 1988). Therefore change or learning occurs in humans from moment to moment, either as a change triggered by interaction(s) or "perturbations" coming from the environment in which it exists or as a result of its own internal dynamics. It is the history and structure of the living system that determine which perturbations can trigger changes of state.

Explanations of Our World: Objectivity and Objectivity-in-Parenthesis

Maturana offered the idea of two possible avenues for explaining our world: objectivity and objectivity-in-parentheses.

Objectivity. This view assumes one ultimate domain of reference for explaining our world. Within this domain, entities are assumed to exist independently of the individual. These entities are used to justify and validate explanations. Such entities are as numerous and broad as imagination might allow and may be identified explicitly or implicitly as objects such as "truth," "mind," "knowledge," and so on. In this avenue of explanation, we come to believe that we have access to an objective reality.

Knowledge about the "truth" by one person becomes a demand for obedience by another—for example, a nurse's expectation of compliance by families. Maturana (1987) claimed that the view of an objective reality entails the possibility of conflict (a mutual negation) that may lead to emotional contradiction. An act of "violence" that is "holding one's opinion to be true such that another's must change" (Maturana, 1987) may result from conversation based on descriptions of "truth."

The label of "noncompliant" arises in this domain of explanation. "Noncompliance" is one of the NANDA-approved nursing diagnoses under the category of "Choosing" (Carpenito, 1991; Carroll-Johnson, 1989). Specifically it has been defined as "a person's informed decision not to adhere to a therapeutic recommendation" (Carroll-Johnson, 1989, p. 541). When we operate in the domain of objectivity or empiricism, nurses believe and behave as if they have access to an objective reality—that is, that our observations/assessment of a family member's behaviors are "true." Consequently, within this domain, nurses can fall into the trap of believing that individuals and families are noncompliant and that families should adhere to our advice and opinions. We also invite the possibility of conflict and violence between ourselves and our patients.

Objectivity-in-Parenthesis. When objectivity is placed in parenthesis, nurses recognize that objects do exist but are not independent of the living system that brings them forth. The only truths that exist are those drawn forth by observers such as nurses. "The observer brings forth the objects that he or she distinguishes with his or her operations of distinction as distinctions of distinctions in language" (Maturana, 1988, p. 30). Distinctions made by an observer of what appears to be stimulus (input) and response (output) of the nervous system is not a property of the nervous system but rather a property of the domain of observations. Thus brain and behavior are linked only in the eyes of the observer. As Maturana (1985) states, "The mind is not in the head, it is in the behavior" (p. 311).

Drawing distinctions is the basic cognitive operation of the observer. *Cognition* may be defined as "the act or process of knowing, including both awareness and judgment." Cognition is not a representation of the world "out there" but rather an ongoing bringing forth of a world through the process of living itself. Therefore it is always in our coexistence with others that we are bringing forth reality. Humans literally create the world in which they live, while coexisting and co-drifting with other human beings. It is human activity that brings forth and validates human activity.

Maturana (1988) claimed that we exist in domains that we bring forth through living and that "they are domains of realities, domains of explanations that we present for explaining our experience, in the understanding that we cannot claim anything about an independent reality" (p. 29). Every explanation is a reformulation of our experience. Our explanations are conveyed through narratives that embed the meanings (beliefs) that we have about our experiences. It is these beliefs that our clients have about their experiences—such as chronic or life-threatening illness—that are central to how they cope with them. In applying this idea to the nursing of families, every family member has his or her own reality or perspective of his or her experience of illness. Nurses need to encourage the expression of each family member's reality. For example, if each family member is asked, "What is your point of view on how your mother is coping with her MS?" many different perspectives or realities will be drawn forth. On the basis of the concept of *structural determinism,* each reality must be considered as "true," valid, and legitimate.

The idea that humans bring different perspectives to their understanding of events is not new. But Maturana's perspective on observations is much more radical: It is based on biology and physiology, not philosophy.

Maturana stated that not only do we have different views or perspectives on a given event but also the event itself has no existence separate from our ability to distinguish it in words and symbols. One's view is not a distortion of some presumably correct interpretation. Instead of one objective universe waiting to be discovered or to be correctly described, Maturana proposed a "multiverse," where many observer "verses" coexist, each valid in its own right.

Mendez et al. (1988) state:

> If . . . we claim that the biology of the phenomenon of cognition demands that we operate with objectivity-in-parenthesis, then we can no longer keep the notion that we have a legitimate transconsensual authority of power to decide what happens to another human being, based on the demand for obedience that the claim of objective knowledge entails. . . . Indeed, putting objectivity in parenthesis entails the explicit recognition that the desirability or undesirability of any given behavior is socially determined, and that we cannot go claiming that something is good or bad, healthy or unhealthy in itself, as if these were intrinsic constitutive features of it. (p. 151)

Within the domain of objectivity-in-parenthesis, we cannot claim that a family is noncompliant. Therefore nursing assessments are based on observer perspectives, not on ultimate truths.

The Impossibility of Instructive Interaction

Instructive interaction implies that a living system is able to receive instructions from the environment, in the form of information to be processed (Aboitiz, 1985). It assumes that individuals can specify structural changes in other individuals through instruction. For example, as nurses we believe and are invested in the idea that what we teach our clients is what they will learn. Maturana and Varela (1987) made the startling declaration that there cannot be any instructive interaction. This notion emerges from the central assumption that living systems are structurally determined. Furthermore the nervous system is an informationally and operationally closed system. As a closed system, it is the nervous system that determines the changes of relative neuronal activity; it is not the perturbation or information that determines the state of the nervous system. If living systems were "instructable," they all would respond in the same way to a given perturbation. Information or instruction cannot be imparted onto someone; it can be offered only as part of an interaction. It is the system in constant interaction with its medium, not the information or instruction, that specifies how it will behave.

Structural changes in living systems are unique and dependent on the phylogenic history (genetic or evolutionary history) or the ontogenic history (all the past structural changes or history of interactions) in the life of the organism. Thus changes in family members are determined by their own structures, not by others. Therefore nurses are not change agents; we cannot and do not change anyone.

Consider the following scenario: A cardiovascular clinical nurse specialist (CNS) conducts a weekly smoking cessation clinic for cardiovascular patients and their families. The CNS provides relevant literature informing her cardiac patients about the risks of smoking and promotes a variety of strategies for patients to decrease and eliminate smoking behavior. She is puzzled by the wide range of responses to her nursing interventions: Some patients quit smoking almost immediately, others decrease their smoking behavior, and still others remain firm in old smoking habits. Clients who fall into this latter category may be diagnosed quickly as "noncompliant." An implication of Maturana and Varela's (1987) theory, however, is to recognize that such clients are not noncompliant but rather have not selected a particular novel perturbation that invites them to decrease their smoking.

The Possibility of Collaborative Interaction

If instructive interaction cannot exist, how can we as nurses impart ideas about health promotion and health restoration? Maturana offered the following suggestion: "You will never be able to do instructive interaction. The most that you can do is to talk to the patient and invite this person to a reflection that will allow the realization that there is an illness and that there are certain actions that he or she has to take. You cannot force the other to an understanding" (H. R. Maturana, personal communication, October, 1988). Inviting individuals and families to a reflection can be accomplished by (a) creating a context for change, (b) creating an environment in which persons change themselves, and (c) offering ideas, advice, and suggestions that can serve as useful perturbations. By remaining curious about family members' beliefs about their illness, nurses can help patients and their families discover which perturbations (interventions) will trigger structural changes that will result in more effective responses to health problems.

Through collaborative interaction with families, nurses also can eliminate what has been called the "language of loathing" (Szasz, 1973, p. 27) and can liberate themselves and families from the language of pathologizing. Labels such as "noncompliant," "resistant," and "dysfunctional" become irrelevant, disrespectful, and insulting descriptors. More important, when applying Maturana's theory of metacognition to nursing practice, these behavioral descriptors are biologically impossible.

One of the assumptions of noncompliance is that relationships between nurses and families are hierarchical (Stanitis & Ryan, 1982). It would be more respectful and more humble for us to think of ourselves in non-hierarchical, collaborative relationships with families—that we are involved in co-drifting with families, creating a context for change rather than believing that we can be change agents.

To move toward more collaborative relationships with families, we often find it useful in our clinical practice to ask families what they want to conserve rather than what they want to change. This is also a very useful intervention on ourselves as family nurse clinicians (Wright, Watson, & Bell, 1990). We attempt to design interventions that invite families to a reflection (Wright & Nagy, in press; Wright & Simpson, 1991; Wright & Watson, 1988). Interventions that invite reflection have the potential of being selected as perturbations. Family members who respond to particular perturbations (therapeutic interventions) do so because of the fit between the perturbation and their structure.

Conclusion

One question still remains: Are there risks of being too enraptured with Maturana's metatheory of cognition? We believe one risk of embracing Maturana's theory with overwhelming enthusiasm to be that we would behave with too much certainty. If we are too enthusiastic or certain about Maturana's theory, it becomes too "true." This "truth" becomes a tyranny because we end up submitting to an external "truth," which is the very idea that Maturana is challenging. On one occasion, though, we need to embrace wholeheartedly Maturana's theory: whenever we encounter the impulse to pathologize families as noncompliant.

13

Ethical Decision Making
With Families in Crisis

Teresa A. Savage

Barbara A. Durand

Judy Friedrichs

Jeanne F. Slack

Introduction

Parents experiencing the serious illness of a child are faced with many decisions. The nurse is frequently the health care professional with whom the family has extended contact. This chapter will describe the nurse's role in facilitating ethical decision making by families who have a seriously ill child. A clinical scenario will illustrate the parallel processes performed by nurses to assess the family's adaptation and coping and to facilitate ethical decision making.

Theoretical Framework

The double ABCX model (McCubbin, Patterson, & Cauble, 1981) from family stress theory provides a framework for understanding how stress affects the family system and its adaptation to the illness. The nurse employs this model to appreciate the family's experience from their perspective and to gain insight into their values, which must be clarified in the ethical decision-making process.

The double ABCX model looks beyond the immediate stressor that has produced the crisis and examines postcrisis family behavior and changes that make family adaptation more difficult. It contributes to understanding (from the family's perspective) the nature of the crisis, to identifying resources that families use to deal with the crisis, and to assisting families toward decision making that will achieve bonadaptation and balance in the family.

Two forms of the family's perception are critical components of family coping: (a) the family's perception of the most significant stressor event, and (b) the family's perception of its total crisis situation, which includes estimates of what needs to be done to bring the family back into balance. This "redefining" of the situation is critical in facilitating family problem solving and adaptation and lends itself naturally to nursing assessment and intervention.

The Nurse's Role
in Facilitating Ethical Decision Making

In the case of critical illness, the tertiary care hospital is often the setting for the crisis, the assessment of the family's perceptions, and the analysis and facilitation of ethical decision making by the family. Although decisions about clinical management of the child must involve the health care team, the impetus for decision making often comes from the nurse. These decisions involve analysis of the medical condition of the patient, feasibility of treatment options, clarification of family values, and identification of the obligations owed to the patient. In a meeting with the parents, the physician usually gives an overview of the situation, outlines the options, presents the questions to be faced, and suggests a course of action. Nurses may be merely witnesses to this process or may become involved integrally.

Nurses have been socialized to believe that they have no role in ethical decision making and have been taught to reinforce information given by the physician. The process of ethical decision making by families requires more than reinforcement of information. It requires facilitation of the process through therapeutic communication. Clarifying and articulating family values and strengths, thinking through possible consequences, and working through parental guilt, shame, and fears are part of the process. Nurses are well prepared for this process because they have more extended contact with the patient and family than any other health care provider and thus have an extensive data base of the family's values, expectations, coping styles, and support systems. Further, the family may find nurses particularly approachable; finally, nursing actions depend on the treatment plan, and nurses often push for treatment decisions.

Nurses are moral agents in a covenantal relationship with the patient and family. Obligations are implicit—to care for the patient with compassion and respect for the patient's and family's dignity. This relationship is an avenue for communication for goal setting, for sharing emotion, and for rehearsing negotiations. May (1983), Veatch (1981), and Gadow (1980) described this relationship as one of mutuality and reciprocity, essential for therapeutic communication.

The Process of Ethical Analysis

Nurses acquire the skills to analyze ethical issues and to facilitate decision making through formal study and through the modeling of more experienced nurses, ethicists, chaplains, or other professionals. Knowing the frameworks for decision making is a beginning; being able to implement those frameworks in a compassionate way is an art acquired by practice. Many frameworks, all reflecting a systematic approach to problem solving, include a clarification of the values of key players (patient, family, health care providers, institution) and application of ethical principles (beneficence, nonmaleficence, justice, autonomy). Most frameworks suggest these steps:

1. Gather and confirm information
2. Clarify the values of the key players
3. Identify the conflicts in values and determine the overriding values
4. Examine all options and the possible consequences of each option
5. Examine the ethical ramifications of each option
6. Choose the option most consistent with the values of the key players
7. Implement the option
8. Evaluate the process

The nurse can facilitate decision making by helping the family focus their questions or by assisting them to formulate questions that they need to ask themselves in clarifying their values. The family needs to identify their available resources to face the prognosis. The nurse can assist the family by identifying additional resources. Exploration of the family's options and the analysis of "benefit versus burden" to the infant or child may be helpful. It is often necessary to repeat information and to be especially clear, honest, and diplomatic in sharing harsh information. The nurse can further facilitate ethical decision making by discussing the facts as they are known, the values that the family has expressed, the options available, and the course the family wishes to pursue.

The goal of facilitation is to move the family toward resolution of an issue. Feedback from families, other members of the health care team, nursing management, and self-evaluation helps shape the nurse's style in facilitating ethical decision making. Although the outcomes in these difficult and complex cases are often sad, the process of dealing with the issues and of working with the family is gratifying.

Movement toward primary nursing mandates the role of facilitator. The nurse has a duty to acquire the skills and to be realistic about his or her abilities. The nurse may best facilitate decision making by seeking an ethics consultant or ethics committee assistance.

Organizational Environment

Today the hospital is a complex human arena containing a network of reaction and interaction among professionals, patients, and families. Creating an environment that fosters accountability, responsibility, interdependence, and patient advocacy on the part of individual health care professionals is the responsibility of organizations that support nurses and families during complex and critical illness situations.

In most cases health care ethical issues require a decision or action. An ethical decision-making framework facilitates the assessment, analysis, and resolution of ethical dilemmas. It should be flexible and lend itself to both clinical and institutional decision making. No matter which decision-making framework is selected, it should meet the following criteria identified by Silva (1990, p. 110): adequacy, consistency, coherency, comprehensiveness, and practicality. The use of a systematic process by which ethical issues can be reviewed enables administrators to create an environment supportive to nurses and families confronted with ethical decisions. Organizational support systems cannot guarantee infallibility or dictate the action to be taken on the part of health care providers but are essential to creating an environment that enables health care providers and families to resolve ethical dilemmas.

A variety of resources is available for institutions to consider in an effort to provide a system of support for ethical decision making. These include bioethics committees, in-house counsel, ethics consultants, and policies that define exactly what must be documented. The documentation usually includes the patient problem; the decision to be made; the possible choices; the advice given to the family; their response; the decision made, including the rationale; and who was involved in the decision-making process. Decisions to withhold life support or to withdraw care are best discussed with all staff involved in the care of the child. The health care team should consider not only the child's medical condition but also the psychosocial considerations within the context of the family. Mechanisms should be in place for continuous assessment of the appropriateness of ethical decisions as the child's condition changes.

To orchestrate effective support systems, it is necessary to understand the family's perception of the situation and identification of their needs. In the following sections, the double ABCX model will be applied to a clinical scenario.

Clinical Scenario and Application of Model

Two parallel processes are occurring: assessment and facilitation. The nurse assesses the needs of the family faced with an ethical decision and the differences in expectations between parents and health care professionals (Figure 13.1). The nurse facilitates both clinical and ethical decision making by developing interventions grounded in parental perceptions, needs, and goals and by examining the ethical ramifications of the interventions they may choose (Figure 13.2).

Family Assessment

At the time of the birth of a critically ill infant, all existing inputs of the family change. Parents describe the sensation of moving in slow motion, yet everything is happening so quickly. The nurse's role during the family's struggle to maintain equilibrium is one of a two-way filter, helping the family pace their energies. During the initial week of admission, the nurse should interview the family to "take stock." This assessment is meant to provide a basis on which all actions can be planned. The nurse must assess how parents have dealt with crises in the past, what their expectations of hospitals and health care providers have been, what their financial situation is, and what type of family and community supports they have.

Entry into the health care system distorts usual inputs for the family. Their financial, emotional, and social structures are altered. Explanations are hard to understand, and the parents are in shock, faced with decisions that need to be made quickly. The parents experience confusion, frustration, and anger. These emotions and thoughts are very common, and the outcome

Clinical Scenario: Part I

After a normal pregnancy, Mrs. L. was admitted in active labor at 34 weeks gestation. Within 4 hours, Baby Boy L. was born requiring mechanical ventilation. It was evident that he would become oxygen-dependent secondary to bronchopulmonary dysplasia. This baby was the third child for his parents; they visited daily during his first week of life. The father returned to work, and the mother's visits decreased to twice per week. She would ask about the baby's weight and ventilator settings. She called for updates, but visits decreased after a diagnosis of a degenerative neuromuscular disorder was made. Nurses made appointments to begin teaching the mother how to care for her baby. She missed appointments. The staff continued to call, but these calls were more often a report of setbacks. They tried to encourage the parents to visit: "Their baby needed them." Staff became focused on the need for long-term care, which would require a gastrostomy tube. When the family was contacted by the physician, they refused consent for surgery because they did not want their baby to be transferred to an "institution." At the same time, they did not feel able to take the baby home and became hostile toward the staff for the pressure they felt.

Model Application: Family's Perspective
Double ABCX Model

a. Stressor—normal pregnancy, preterm labor

b. Existing resources (inputs)—husband/wife, neonatal intensive care

c. Perception of a. (Perception is reality)—expecting a normal delivery, denying long-term problems

X. Crisis—usually inputs are distorted Husband's support drops off. New set of rules confined to neonatal intensive care unit. Demanding immediate decisions affecting lifetime of family. Tentative diagnosis of degenerative neuromuscular disorder. Continuous setbacks.

aA. Pileup—new information; need to decide; no perceived support; unable to take on the parenting role

bB. Existing and new resources—Staff are present but not yet utilized; clinical specialist consulted by staff. Strong faith of husband and wife.

Coping-avoiding decision making and discharge teaching. Feelings kept in control by keeping them within.

cC. Perception on X + aA + bB—overwhelming, unable to prioritize; easier to avoid, delay, deny

Figure 13.1. Clinical Scenario: Part I and Model Application: Family's Perspective

is dependent on the interventions of the health professionals with the family and acceptance of interventions by family in this stage.

The Nurse's Role as Supporter

The family may need assistance in identifying the effect that this crisis is having on them. The nurse as supporter reassures them and does not offer false hope or overwhelm them with facts. The nurse's focus should be on immediate needs. According to Thorne and Robinson (1989), the first wave

Clinical Scenario: Part II

C. L. was discharged to home at age 2 months, oxygen-dependent, no voluntary movement, and requiring round-the-clock care for positioning and suctioning. Gastrostomy tube placement again was recommended. During follow-up visits, discussion occurred with the clinical nurse specialist about the ethical consideration of choosing or forgoing the gastrostomy tube. The parents elected to have the gastrostomy tube placed. He had a choking episode in which he became quite cyanotic. After this incident the home health nurse and her supervisor contacted the physician to request an order for an ambu bag and airway or a Do Not Resuscitate order (DNR). The physician refused to write an order until he met with the parents. They canceled appointments. Mr. L. sought information on residential placement; Mrs. L. refused to consider placement. She feared that C. L. would die shortly after being placed. Although the parents understood that C. L.'s condition would only deteriorate, they avoided discussions with the health care team about C. L.'s inevitable death. Mrs. L. was angry with the nurse and supervisor for pushing the issue of DNR. A few weeks later, C. L. presented in the emergency room in respiratory distress, with unstable vital signs. In discussion with the parents, clinical nurse specialist, and physician, a decision was made to admit him to the intermediate care unit and to write a Do Not Resuscitate order. Requiring 100% oxygen and frequent suctioning, C. L. stabilized and 1 week later remained on 100% oxygen.

Model Application: Nurse's Role in Ethical Decision Making

Double ABCX Model

a. Stressor—current illness; does "burden" now outweigh "benefit" of living? Consider child's best interests apart from family's best interests. Help focus questions for family.

b. Existing resources—family support (friends, clergy), state financial assistance, long-term relationship with health care providers. Mobilize resources for family.

c. Perception of a.—Mrs. L. denying death could occur. Mrs. L. seeking residential placement. Nurse should be clear, honest, diplomatic, sensitive.

X. Crisis—no improvement or deterioration; status quo with intensive support. Nurse should help plan for possible course of disease process and various options for family to consider.

aA. Pileup—resuscitation discussion occurred in emergency room and again in hospital; each problem required ethical reflection and decision.

bB. Existing and new resources—nurses in hospital; plan for continuing care outside hospital. Patient care conferences with both hospital and home health agency staff.

cC. Perception of X, aA, bB—Is this terminal event vs. deterioration? Required analysis of balance of benefit and burden to child; all options must be explored and all consequences discussed.

Figure 13.2. Clinical Scenario: Part II and Model Application: Nurse's Role in Ethical Decision Making

of questions from a family will focus on how it happened and what and how they will tell others. The second wave will be a period of stepping back, regrouping, and letting it "sink in." The third wave will be filled with emotions, depression, anger, and testing. At this point they need help to identify and ventilate feelings and frustration. Nurses, along with other members of the health care team, can assist the family in identifying and ventilating their frustration.

Strategies for Facilitating Family Coping

Family coping includes reduction or elimination of stressors and facilitation of adaptation. Parents grasp at whatever is available. Doubting caretakers but fearing to challenge, parents feel angry, resentful, hostile, and eventually frightened and exhausted. Caplan (1960) identified some patterns to assist in evaluating parental response:

1. How actively do they seek information?
2. How are feelings handled? If feelings are freely expressed, does that result in relief from tension?
3. Do they actively seek help with the tasks required? Are they receptive to help that is offered? How much help do they actually accept?

An individual in crisis can function at a high level for a short period of time. After the initial peak of adrenalin, however, according to Davidson (1990), there is a resistance to stimuli: The body shuts down, thinking actually cannot occur, the ability to absorb and assimilate information drops dramatically, and the ability to make "informed" decisions does not exist. The nurse needs to be aware of this in advance and be able to care for the family to decrease anxiety before decisions are required. The nurse should provide the family with immediate facts that will help them develop a plan.

The parents need to be recognized as parents with immediate responsibilities. One way to assist them is to point out the specific features that the baby has in order to help them find the baby in amongst the machinery. It may take days of repeated explanation until they touch their baby without fear of disturbing some vital piece of equipment. Barnard (1990) stated that parents cannot recognize support if they are not able or allowed to reciprocate. If the nurse helps them identify and fulfill their role as parents no matter how sick the child is, they will begin to feel some usefulness and begin to accept a level of responsibility and planning for their child.

By using some of these strategies, those involved in ethical decision making can better understand the needs of the family in crisis so that an informed decision is possible and mutual goal setting becomes a reality. The parallel process of assessing the family's adaptation and coping abilities and of facilitating ethical decision making is an art and a science.

Nurses refine these abilities in clinical practice. First they must learn these skills. Educators have a responsibility for incorporating critical thinking skills, therapeutic communication skills, ethical analysis, and clinical opportunities or role playing into the curriculum to hone these skills. Health care organizations have the responsibility to structure the environment to support and nurture the nurse in this role. Ultimately the nurse has an obligation to keep faithful to the covenantal relationship with the patient and family. That requires commitment. As Florence Nightingale said:

> Nursing is an art; and if it is to be made an art, requires as exclusive a devotion, as hard a preparation, as any painter's or sculptor's work; for what is having to do with dead canvas or cold marble, compared with having to do with the living body—the temple of God's spirit . . . It is one of the fine arts; I have almost said the finest of the fine arts. (Donahue, 1985, p. 469)

14

Family Nursing Diagnosis
as a Framework
for Family Assessment

Robin B. Thomas

Kathryn E. Barnard

Georgina A. Sumner

Family-Centered Care

Family-centered care emphasizes mutual respect and cooperation between family members and providers. It is an approach that recognizes a family's rights and responsibilities and their central role in guiding the person's selection and use of health care services, as well as compliance with recommendations from health care providers.

Family-centered care is defined as helping the family achieve their best possible condition for promoting growth and development of individual members of the family (Thomas, Barnard, & Sumner, 1989). The role of the provider is to offer support for the family to care for their member. One essential ingredient in family-centered care is grounding all interventions in accurate family assessments. The purpose of this chapter is to present a framework for family assessment, to briefly discuss some issues in family assessment, and to offer suggestions for family assessment tool selection.

What Do We Assess in Families?

The family assessment framework was created to support nurses and other professionals who provide family-centered care. It is grounded in the belief that health care interventions are most effective when offered in the context of understanding and respecting the family's central role in the health care of their members. Our first goal was to develop a structure for nurses to use in tailoring their assessment of the family to their purpose for intervention, the families' needs, and the nurse's skills. Our second goal was to offer concrete suggestions for appropriate tools for accurate family assessment as the foundation to family-centered care.

A major concern among clinicians is to identify the components of the family that are appropriate and accessible for assessment. Each category or component should target a specific set of functions in family life that can be assessed independently as needed. In this approach to categorizing areas for family assessment, we looked to the work done in nursing diagnosis. That work was reviewed and compared to the knowledge base of family nursing and family assessment. Five areas of family functioning that we believe are appropriate and important to assess when working with families were identified. These areas are based on the work of the North American Nursing Diagnosis Association (NANDA); the *Handbook of Nursing Diagnosis,* by Lynda Carpenito (1989); and the *Manual of Nursing Diagnosis,* by Marjory Gordon (1989). Although these areas for assessment are derived from the field of nursing, we believe that they have relevance to professionals in other disciplines. The areas are family processes, family coping, parenting, health maintenance and management, and home maintenance and management.

The "family processes" category is broad and addresses basic functional patterns of the family. Assessments in this area give nurses information about how the family acts as a family and how they approach the world. It includes relationships among members, how they communicate with each other, and how they make decisions or solve problems. Individual satisfaction with family is another element in this category. A key component for nurses is how the family adjusts to the changes and challenges that health care and other problems present. Finally, the family's approach to relationships with other people and how they choose to use organizations and resources outside the family are a part of this area. Assessment of all these elements is not necessary for most families. Interview and observation of the family will guide the nurse to probe further into only those areas that the family identifies as problematic and requests assistance with or that interfere with the family's ability to care for their members.

"Family coping" is central to supporting the family as they deal with a health care crisis. How a family copes with a health problem affects treatment outcome, the family's ability to function in other areas, and the family's relationships with friends and professionals. First, the timing of assessment is critical in family coping. In the early stages of adjustment to the problem, the family will use old or practiced ways to cope with a new problem and gradually will learn novel ways to cope. The professional's assessment of the family's coping will be different at the beginning versus latter stages. A second issue is that families and professionals often disagree about the success of family coping. Some families may choose a coping style that interferes with the professional's work or that is different from the professional's coping style. A family's efforts do not have to be successful according to the professional's standards to be recognized as coping. The use of an objective measure for assessing family coping is helpful in avoiding bias in evaluation of family coping. Also, simply asking the family how they prefer to cope with a situation and their own evaluation of the coping strategy's effectiveness might help the professional see the strategy differently and offers an excellent point for intervention.

"Parenting" is a specific area of family functioning that revolves around the care of and stimulation provided for children. Family nursing is concerned with how children are encouraged and permitted to grow. This category includes physical, emotional, and social growth-enhancing activities on the part of the parents. An important concept is the parent's ability, on some occasions, to place their own need fulfillment on hold in order to support the child. An obvious example of this is ensuring that the child has adequate food before purchasing alcohol or drugs for the parents.

Nurses have a long tradition of concern with the fourth category, "health maintenance and management" skills in families. This category encompasses the family's knowledge of and investment in ordinary health care practices such as good nutrition, dental and medical care, and adequate sleep patterns. Also important are the family's knowledge about current health problems and necessary treatment, and their skills for providing and willingness to carry out prescribed treatments. Nurses involved with a family around any health care concern will assess the family's functioning in this category.

Finally "home maintenance and management" is an area of long-standing concern for nurses. Included in this area are (a) the environment in which the family lives (safety, water, etc.) and (b) the family's financial resources (ability to obtain enough food, clothing and medical supplies). As with the health maintenance and management category, nurses will

Table 14.1 Five Areas for Family Assessment

Family processes

    Family patterns of living and communication that create an environment to meet members' physical, emotional, and spiritual needs as far as is possible to support individual growth and functioning.

Family coping

    The collective behaviors and/or thought processes of family members for the purpose of dealing with an identified threat or challenge to the family or a member.

Parenting

    The ability to recognize a child's physical, emotional, and developmental needs and capacity and to delay one's own need gratification to meet the child's needs to foster the child's growth and development.

Health maintenance and management

    The ability to develop and use patterns of daily living that support health and/or health-seeking behavior and the knowledge, skills, and willingness to carry out illness-related regimens.

Home maintenance and management

    The acquisition and use of financial and other resources to satisfy family needs and to provide a safe home environment.

---

assess the family's functioning in this area frequently. The categories are defined in Table 14.1.

Issues in Family Assessment

Observer Objectivity

Obtaining an accurate assessment of the family is challenging in part due to biases in the process. Two of the bias problems are (a) a lack of observer objectivity and (b) the timing and frequency of family assessment. It is difficult to be objective in assessing families. Each of us is an expert on the subject of the family, having grown up in one, and each holds strong beliefs about how a family should function. The beliefs that we hold serve as our model for ideal or adequate family functioning that is compared with the families seen in private and professional life. This comparison process biases the provider's assessment of client families. If the comparison is unconscious, it will affect the accuracy of family assessment. To counteract this bias, the provider needs to use objective assessment tools when possible and to remain aware of the pull of her or his own family model.

Timing and Frequency of Family Assessment

Nurses usually assess families at a time of disruption or crisis in their lives, when they are facing a health care problem. The stress of the problem causes changes in the family's ordinary functioning and coping. The family's fit with the environment changes. New demands are placed on the family, and the family's previous functioning is compromised. Over time most families adjust to their situation and gain new coping skills.

An example of these changes was found in a study of family coping and adjustment when a child had a severe chronic condition. The families in this study described a series of stages that they experienced in coping with and adapting to their child's chronic condition (Thomas, 1986). Not all families traveled through the stages at the same pace or necessarily in the same order. The concept of stages in response to health care concerns is important to the process of family assessment. The stages are shock, denial, grief, and reorganization (Thomas, 1986). The family's functioning and coping differed in each stage. Assessment of the family in an earlier stage of shock or denial clearly leads to different conclusions about a family than assessment of the same family as they reorganize their functioning. The interventions resulting from the two assessments would differ dramatically. To enhance the accuracy of family assessment, it is essential to note where the family is in their adjustment to the health care problem, to understand that the family's functioning will change over time, and to assess the family at more than one time.

Methods for Family Assessment

With this framework as a foundation, there are many methods are available for nurses to use in clinically assessing families. The first assessment method is the *interview,* both structured and unstructured, a method well known to nurses.

The second assessment method is *observation.* Available strategies can reduce the bias that observation may inadvertently contain. Examples of these strategies are the Nursing Child Assessment Feeding Scale and the Nursing Child Assessment Teaching Scale (Barnard, 1978a, 1978b), which train observers to collect reliable observations in specific areas of parent-child interaction.

A third method available to the provider for family assessment is the use of *unstandardized surveys, questionnaires, or checklists.* Usually these tools have been created for use in one setting and were not intended to be used widely. Unstandardized measures have not undergone rigorous development and may not generalize well in either administration or interpretation to a different population. They must be evaluated on their face validity and must be used with some caution and awareness of their limitations.

The fourth and best known family assessment method is the use of *published standardized questionnaires or measures.* Each of these instruments is designed to measure a specific area of the family, and all are usually published with psychometric information and norms against which other families can be compared. Many of these tools are research tools and must be used with that awareness. Others are tools developed for clinical use or are research tools acceptable for clinical use.

Finally, the fifth assessment method is the *interpretive measures.* These include kinetic family drawings and other techniques. All of the interpretive measures require extensive training and frequent reliability testing to enhance accuracy in their use.

Adequacy of Family Assessment Tools

It is useful to know that some published tools have not been well crafted and may not perform as advertised. Sometimes measures are developed not on research or an analysis of the literature but from one person's ideas or hunches about what is important. With this as a basis, the tool will collect information in only a limited and possibly inappropriate area. Other tools may purport to measure an area, such as family coping, yet have internal biases that ignore family strengths. Several tools offer a list of coping strategies from which the family may choose. If this list contains only harmful coping strategies, such as drinking or excessive eating, the family will appear weak in coping, and only a negative assessment of their coping will be possible through use of that tool. The design of the tool makes it impossible to find out whether the family is using other, more healthy coping practices. If the questionnaire gives "faulty" information, and if the provider uses the information to intervene with a family or to build a program for intervention, both efforts are likely to be less successful than they might be with accurate information. One goal of this framework is to evaluate tools presented as clinical family assessment tools and to provide clinicians with a list of acceptable tools.

Family Assessment Versus Family Research

A distinction should be made between clinical assessment and research-oriented instruments. *Research* is concerned with in-depth examination or explanation of an entire event or interest area. It is broad, all-inclusive, and exists to explore an area as fully as possible. In contrast, *clinical assessment* is a more limited activity that serves as a tool for the provider and family to plan specific activities around specific client needs. It is an appraisal of one characteristic or concern. To engage in family assessment beyond that necessary for working with the family is an invasion of the family's privacy.

Well-meaning clinicians, in an attempt to assess families, often have adopted research strategies or tools for clinical assessment. These research questionnaires are comprehensive, often intrusive, and request information from families that is intimate and highly charged. For example, many research tools ask participants for information about their marital or sexual relationships. Clinical assessment tools are more limited and collect information related to the reason for the professional's involvement with the family. It is inappropriate to gather information not directly related to the provider's interventions unless the family has requested help in some other area. We believe that providers have the right to assess the family only in areas (a) that are directly related to the individual's health care concern or (b) in which the health care concern has stressed the family and has led the family to request help coping with it, and particularly (c) that fall within the area of expertise of the health care provider.

Assessment of the Family Diagnostic Categories

Once the family diagnosis categories listed above were created, we thought it useful to cite selected family assessment tools appropriate for each area. An extensive review of the "family" literature was undertaken to identify and review family assessment strategies and tools. The list of tools and strategies generated by the review became the basis for selection of clinical family assessment measures. Criteria for selection included a clinical rather than a research focus, availability of psychometric information about the tool when appropriate, accessibility in the literature or from the author, and available training when required. We then evaluated the selected measures, using a standard format, and categorized them according to our definitions.

The list is a resource for nurses in completing their assessment of the family. It comprises the best clinical assessment tools that we found. The process that we suggest for using this list is based on traditional nursing skills of interview and observation of the family, diagnosis of areas of concern for the family, and negotiation with the family to use appropriate assessment tools. Unfortunately, adequate tools for assessing all elements

Table 14.2 Family Assessment Tools Categorized by Family Nursing Diagnoses

Family Processes

The Eco-Map (Hartman, 1978, 1979)
> Offers information about people or organizations in the family's life, the type and amount of resources available to the family, and the family's perception of how much stress and support their social environment offers.

Family APGAR (Smilkstein, 1978)
> Developed as a clinical screening tool for assessing an individual's satisfaction with his or her family's functioning.

Family Genogram (Hartman, 1978, 1979)
> Organizes information about the intergenerational family system and family health history and identifies available family resources.

Family Support Scale (Dunst, Trivette, & Jenkins, 1988)
> Assesses the family's perception of the social support that they receive in raising their child(ren).

Prenatal and Child Health Nursing Standards for Role Relationships (Region X Nursing Network, 1990)
> Standards for assessing and intervening with mothers and children up to the age of 3 years.

Parenting

Home Observation for Measurement of the Environment (Caldwell & Bradley, 1978)
> Developed to measure the physical environment and the quality of interpersonal interaction available to the child.

Infant Care Survey (Froman & Owen, 1989)
> Developed to assess a mother's confidence and knowledge of caring for her infant.

Knowledge of Infant Development Inventory (MacPhee, 1984)
> *Created to assess parents' and providers' knowledge about infants.*

Nursing Child Assessment Feeding Scale (Barnard, 1978a)
> Assesses the quality of the mother-child interaction during feeding.

Nursing Child Assessment Teaching Scale (Barnard, 1978b)
> Assesses the parent-child interaction while the parent teaches the child a defined task.

Parenting Daily Hassles (Crnic & Greenberg, 1989)
> Developed to measure the daily hassles of parenting that affect the quality of the parent-child relationship and the family.

(Continued)

of the family do not exist. Until appropriate measures for all areas are developed, nurses must depend on their skills in interview and observation to assess areas for which tools have yet to be constructed. In addition, some tools assess family functioning in more than one category. We grouped those tools into the health maintenance and management area (Table 14.2).

Table 14.2 Continued

Family Coping

Coping Health Inventory for Parents (McCubbin, M., 1987)
    Designed to assess parental coping when a child has a chronic condition.

Difficult Life Circumstances (Barnard, 1988b)
    Used to assess major problems of families living in poverty or in stressful life circumstances.

F-COPES (McCubbin, H., Olson, & Larsen, 1987)
    Developed to assess general family coping; not restricted to health-related problems.

Family Hardiness Index (McCubbin, M., McCubbin, H., & Thompson, 1987)
    Created to assess the internal strength of families for meeting challenges and stress.

Postpartum Adjustment (Lederman, Weingarten, & Lederman, 1981)
    Assesses a women's adjustment to her new role as a mother.

Prenatal and Child Health Nursing Standards for Coping (Region X Nursing Network, 1990)
    Standards for assessing and intervening with mothers and children up to the age of 3 years.

Health Maintenance and Management

Family Needs Scale (Dunst, Cooper, Weeldreyer, Snyder, & Chase, (1988)
    Identifies family needs for resources and support when a child has special needs.

Family Needs Survey (Bailey & Simeonsson, 1988)
    Designed to assess family needs when a child has special needs.

Family Resource Scale (Leet & Dunst, 1988)
    Assesses the family's perception of available resources to support them as a family with a child who has special health care needs.

Health-Promoting Lifestyle (Walker, Sechrist, & Pender, 1987)
    Measures a person's health-promoting behaviors.

Nursing Child Assessment Sleep/Activity Record (Barnard, 1979)
    Used to collect information and identify patterns about sleep patterns or other activities or behaviors.

Prenatal and Child Health Nursing Standards for Health Perception/Health Management (Region X Nursing Network, 1990)
    Standards for assessing and intervening with mothers and children up to the age of 3 years.

Home Maintenance and Management

Community Life Skills Scale (Barnard, 1988a)
    Designed to measure the mother's ability to use community and interpersonal resources.

Summary

In summary we believe that respecting the importance of the family in the life of the individual is central to effective interventions. Family-centered care as an approach to care delivery is a promising method of care delivery.

To practice family-centered care, providers must learn to objectively assess family processes, parenting, family coping, health maintenance and management, and home maintenance and management. The tools for family assessment included in this chapter are excellent supplements to good nursing interviews and observation. They serve to support family-centered care by providing accurate family assessment as a foundation for interventions.

15

Family Nursing Approach for a Clinical Ladder

Sharon Jackson Barton

Arlene M. Sperhac

Sheila A. Haas

Introduction

Family involvement can be supported in many ways: Policies and procedures can allow families to room-in, and surveys can assess parental needs and wishes regarding their child's care. These strategies create a family-centered environment but do little to foster creation of partnerships or major changes in practice. This chapter describes the use of a clinical ladder as a means of formalizing professional and family partnerships. The setting for this development was the nursing department at Children's Memorial Hospital, Chicago, Illinois.

Development of the Clinical Ladder

The nursing department began work on a clinical ladder system in the early 1980s. A nursing retention committee identified the clinical ladder as one way to promote retention, to enhance satisfaction, and to reward nurses who chose to develop their expertise at the bedside.

The clinical ladder committee work moved rapidly once a professional practice model and a philosophy of nursing were put into place. The professional practice family ladder model and philosophy of nursing were developed through use of the concepts of family-centered care outlined by the Association for the Care of Children's Health (Shelton, Jeppson, & Johnson, 1987) and Fawcett's (1984a) metaparadigm of nursing. The philosophy and practice model stated that the patient was the family. This strong statement became the basis for the development of levels of family nursing practice operationalized through the clinical ladder.

Geary's (1979) research, as well as our own observations of practice at Children's, made clear the need for a change in language to reflect the family focus. Words used to describe practice influence the perceived importance of that practice. We wanted to develop words that would describe family practice and to use those words on a daily basis. Dance (1979) described this as the "acoustic trigger to conceptualization." If words are used often enough, they begin to have value and significance. Nursing practice and daily activities can be influenced greatly by the words that people use to describe their actions.

The Practice Model

The *practice model* was based on Fawcett's (1984a) metaparadigm of nursing. The four components of the practice model are nursing, patient, health-illness, and the environment. Each of the four definitions is based on nursing theory or research. The most important definition for family nursing practice is the definition that the patient is the family.

Implementation of the Clinical Ladder

After the practice model was adopted, the clinical ladder/retention committee moved forward with the development of levels of practice based on the model. The nurse advances on the ladder in two ways: by assuming more responsibilities for coordination of family care and by advancing in education. The ladder has four levels: family care nurse, family care coordinator, family care consultant, and family care specialist. Beginning in 1995 the family care consultant will be open only to nurses with a bachelor's degree, and the family care specialist will require a master's degree. Any nurses achieving these levels prior to 1995 may stay at those levels regardless of their educational degree.

**Family Nursing Behaviors
at Each Level of the Clinical Ladder**

Each level of the clinical ladder contains behaviors related to the nurse as clinician, teacher, manager-leader, and researcher.

Level 1. The *family care nurse* coordinates nursing care as an associate nurse on the primary nursing team. Interactions and assessment with the family are conducted primarily around illness issues. The family care nurse is concerned with the family in the hospital environment.

Level 2. The *family care coordinator* acts as a primary nurse. She or he is concerned with the family as they care for their ill child in the hospital and in the home.

Level 3. The *family care consultant* has an identified area of expertise in nursing practice. This expertise may be on an illness or diagnostic area or in a specific skill such as anticipatory guidance for school-age children and their families. The family care consultant enables families to connect with other resources within the hospital and the community.

Level 4. The *family care specialist* is a resource for the hospital and the community. She or he has a readily identifiable area of expertise, coordinates a broad base of resources for families, and is a mentor for nurses at other levels of practice. (Only those behaviors related to the family are included in this chapter.)

**Family Nursing Behaviors
for the Clinical Ladder**

Family Care Nurse (Level 1)

(Clinician behaviors)

1. Documents actual health care needs of child and family within 8 hours of admission
2. Begins to document goals appropriate for child and family for a plan of care based on nursing diagnoses within 24 hours of admission
3. Relays routine information to child and family in terms they can understand
4. Relays clearly and concisely the status of child and family to co-workers
5. Identifies immediate learning needs of patient and family

(Teacher behaviors)

1. Communicates basic information about such things as nursing activities, environment, and illness to patient and family

(Leadership behaviors)

1. Creates an atmosphere of respect and concern during family and visitor interactions

Family Care Coordinator (Level 2)

(Clinician behaviors)

1. Documents physical and obvious psychosocial nursing care needs of child and family within 8 hours
2. Documents goals appropriate for child and family for a plan of nursing care based on nursing diagnoses in conjunction with family
3. Maintains a safe environment and anticipates alterations in family, patient, and/or environment that may impair safety
4. Acts as advocate by enabling families to identify basic health care needs
5. Communicates effectively to facilitate exchange of information with families

(Teacher behaviors)

1. Identifies intermediate and complex learning needs of families
2. Assesses child's and family's readiness to learn self-care skills
3. Develops and individualizes teaching plan to meet immediate and routine learning needs of child and family
4. Modifies approaches to standard teaching plans or checklists to meet complex learning needs of child and family
5. Documents individualized teaching to meet immediate and routine learning needs of child and family
6. Documents actions taken to implement standard teaching plans or checklists to meet complex learning needs of child and family
7. Provides anticipatory guidance to family consistent with child's developmental status and in relation to risk situations and their management

(Researcher behaviors)

1. Reads research articles related to family care topics when available on the unit

(Leadership behaviors)

1. Is flexible in creating a warm, comfortable environment by listening and anticipating needs of families and visitors

Family Care Consultant (Level 3)

(Clinician behaviors)

1. Documents actual and potential nursing care needs (physical, psychosocial, developmental, family dynamics, cultural, spiritual) of family
2. Builds plan of care based on family strengths
3. Documents mutually agreed-upon goals in collaboration with families
4. Writes comprehensive nursing care plan encompassing admission to post-discharge involving continuous collaboration with family
5. Creates a climate that facilitates therapeutic relationship with families
6. Acts as advocate by enabling families to develop action plans to reach their highest level of functioning
7. Coordinates family care conferences
8. Collaborates with family on an ongoing basis to change plan of care
9. Documents patient's and family's response to alterations in plan of care

(Teacher behaviors)

1. Assesses ability of family to assimilate complex teaching plan
2. Identifies cultural and belief systems that influence health practices and teaching plan
3. Assesses family's learning needs related to developmental stages, parenting skills, family role transitions, and family interaction patterns
4. Develops teaching plans to meet identified complex learning needs of child and family
5. Individualizes teaching plans to make them consistent with family members' identified learning abilities
6. Individualizes teaching plans in consideration of family members' identified cultural and belief systems
7. Develops teaching plans to meet identified family learning needs related to life-styles or environments that minimize identified health risks
8. Provides anticipatory guidance with understanding of developmental status of child and family

9. Documents family teaching strategies that enhance parenting skills, family role transitions, and family interaction patterns
10. Documents evaluation of learner's comprehension of anticipatory guidance
11. Documents evaluation of learner's comprehension of developmental stages and strategies to enhance parenting skills, family role transitions, or family interaction patterns
12. Documents family's comprehension of necessary changes in life-styles or environments that minimize health risks

(Leadership behaviors)

1. Actively promotes and markets nursing by educating patients and families about nursing role
2. Responds to complex needs of families and visitors by seeking alternatives

Family Care Specialist (Level 4)

(Clinician behaviors)

1. Assesses whether health care delivery method is flexible, accessible, and responsive to family's needs
2. Documents goals that reflect ongoing assessments and family collaboration
3. Writes comprehensive plan of care employing creative strategies based on assessment of total family dynamics
4. Communicates with families and staff in supportive manner, while simultaneously performing direct patient care activities
5. Acts as advocate by empowering families to reach their own highest levels of functioning in meeting their health care needs in hospital and community
6. Initiates family care conferences
7. Documents family response to empowering activities

(Teacher behaviors)

1. Assesses family's need for anticipatory guidance related to life-style and environmental factors that create health risks
2. Consults with family to develop teaching plans to meet identified complex learning needs of child and family
3. Individualizes teaching plans to make them consistent with family members' identified learning needs and abilities·
4. Individualizes teaching plans in consideration of family members' identified cultural and belief systems

5. Develops teaching plans to meet identified family learning needs related to life-style and environmental factors that create health risks
6. Facilitates implementation of individualized teaching plans to meet complex learning needs of family
7. Documents creative teaching strategies consistent with learning abilities of family members

(Leadership behaviors)

1. Proposes system changes that are flexible and responsive to needs of families and visitors

Evaluation of the Clinical Ladder

Because clinical ladders are complex and multiple outcomes are expected, little research has been done on their impact. With the exception of Medicus (1980), Haas (1986), Barhyte (1987), and Porter (1987), no empirical research on the impact of clinical ladders exists.

To evaluate the impact of implementation and maintenance of the clinical ladder performance appraisal system at Children's Memorial Hospital, a time series design was used with pretest measures of staff nurse perceptions of each of the clinical ladder's proposed outcomes before the implementation of the clinical ladder. The study design also measured nurse perceptions after the clinical ladder was implemented. Posttests were given 1 and 2 years after the clinical ladder was introduced. The repeated measures study of impact is in progress at this time.

Conclusion

A clinical ladder performance appraisal system structures the workplace and work processes. Development of a clinical ladder requires review and analysis of nursing work from the Department of Nursing's philosophy and mission statements, through the model of care delivery, and down to nursing policies and procedures. At Children's Memorial Hospital, the commitment to family as client is the thrust of all department of nursing activities and is obvious in the performance expectations for all nursing personnel. The behavioral objectives on the clinical ladder tools and the charges given to nurse peer reviewers in the hospital peer review committee reflect the commitment to family as client.

PART V

Education

Catherine L. Gilliss, Editor

16

Development of a Model to Guide Advanced Practice in Family Nursing

Janet A. Deatrick

Suzanne L. Feetham

Laura Hayman

Mary Perkins

Family-focused pediatric transitional care is being developed as a model to guide educational curricula, clinical programs, and research activities. The basis of the model, its components, and educational application will be described to explore its usefulness for today's challenges in family nursing and advanced practice in pediatric nursing. Family-focused interventions, advanced skills in clinical decision making, and continuity of care will be analyzed as they relate to this model, which has been derived from two ongoing programs of research.

AUTHORS' NOTE: Preparation of this chapter was supported in part by Division of Nursing Advanced Nurse Training Grant 1D23NU00970-01 to Janet Deatrick and by a grant from the Clinical Collaboration Program of the University of Pennsylvania School of Nursing to Janet A. Deatrick, Kimberly Mason, and Richard Davidson.

The site of caring for ill children and the individuals caring for them has evolved over the past century concomitant with advances in society and technology. When the care of seriously ill children was removed from the home and became institutionalized in hospital settings, families virtually were excluded from their care. Expert health care workers employed by the hospital took the place of the family and nurses who worked in the home and community.

Due to the efforts of families and health professionals, families were able to reverse these patterns dramatically during the 1970s. By the 1980s family involvement in the care of the hospitalized child had become a cornerstone of quality care (Shelton, Jeppson, & Johnson, 1987). At the same time, advanced care technologies led to a decrease in overall childhood mortality but to an increase in the sustained morbidity. A shift to include family care in the home, as well as in the hospital, resulted from concern over the cost of hospital care for these children and the quality of their lives as they survived in compromised states for prolonged periods of time in hospital settings.

Once home, children who had been hospitalized for long periods of time thrived developmentally. Care in the home was also sometimes found to be less expensive than hospital care and was accepted by more third-party payers and federal entitlement programs. Therefore both the family and the home once again became important in the care of children with health problems (Dowd & Vlastuin, 1990; Feetham, 1986; Martinson, 1976; Stein & Jessop, 1984).

Throughout this evolution "family-centered" became the ideal model of care; that is, the family was recognized as either the context for the child's care or the actual client (Gilliss, 1991). Professionals, institutions, programs, standards, and policies became increasingly family-centered. This "gold standard" began with clinical programs for children with minor illnesses and moved to encompass children with virtually every kind and degree of health care problem (Shelton et al., 1987). Enthusiasm for "the family movement" was influenced by research results indicating that the presence of parents helped hospitalized children recover faster with decreased morbidity and mortality (Thompson, 1985).

At the same time, a variety of social changes brought about an expansion of the definition of *family*. Health care professionals, along with the rest of society, struggled to adjust interventions to new family structures and ways to accomplish family functions. No longer was the two-parent family necessarily made up of the child's biological parents, nor was the mother always the primary caregiver available around the clock for unpaid labor in the home (Olson & Hanson, 1990). Throughout these evolutionary changes, nurses concentrated on the involvement of the family in the care of their hospitalized child (Barnsteiner & Gillis-Donovan, 1990; Deatrick & Knafl, 1988; Deatrick, Stull, Dixon, Puczynksi, & Jackson, 1986; Stull & Deatrick, 1986).

The challenge for the next decade is that of effectively helping children and families manage across systems of care. The related challenge for education is how to effectively prepare nurses with the competencies to support families' management across these systems. To date, nurses have been prepared primarily to function with children and their families within the context of the tertiary care environment. Clinical decision-making skills and continuity of care capacities have been included in the preparation of nurses but have not been emphasized. In addition, their education has not always prepared them to intervene effectively with the contemporary family unit in the home and community. The aim of this chapter is to provide an overview of a model that addresses some of these challenges, as well as to explore implications for graduate education.

The Conceptual Model

Today the empirical basis for providing nursing interventions for families is becoming available in the research literature pertaining to families (Barnes, 1985; Gilliss, 1990; Rose & Thomas, 1987; Wright & Leahey, 1984). This newly evolving knowledge has been incorporated into a conceptual model for educational curricula, clinical programs, and research activities known as *family-focused pediatric transitional care* (FFPTC) (see Figure 16.1). The purpose of the model is to provide a basis for advanced practice nursing intervention that promotes continuity among the family, home, school, and health care systems needed to effectively accommodate and treat children who have health care problems.

The FFPTC model is based on the synthesis of two models: the nurse specialist transitional care follow-up model (Brooten et al., 1988) and the family management styles (FMS) (Knafl & Deatrick, 1990) model. The synthesis of these two models describes specialist care emanating from tertiary pediatric settings and incorporates family intervention skills, continuity of care, and advanced skills in clinical decision making.

Needs of the family unit are conceptualized on the basis of their family management styles (FMSs). Although families are not seen as responding in any one fashion to illness situations, they are seen as responding in ways consistent with how they define their situation and their sociocultural

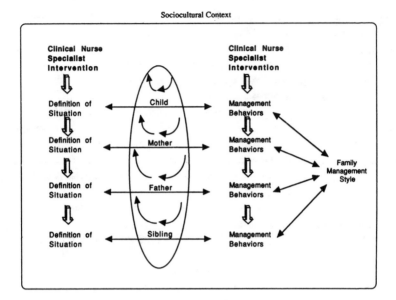

Figure 16.1. Family-Focused Pediatric Transitional Care

context, as depicted in the reciprocal elements of the model. The sociocultural context is the set of "culturally, ethnically, and religiously influenced values and beliefs" (Knafl & Deatrick, 1990, p. 9) that frame the family's ideology. Definition of the situation includes the "identification and interpretation of significant aspects of environment and constitutes the basis for action or behavior" (Deatrick & Knafl, 1990, p. 15). FMSs are the configuration of the defining and managing behaviors across family members (Knafl & Deatrick, 1990).

Of particular note are the management behaviors of the child, mother, father, sibling, and/or other individuals who comprise the family of the child or who serve as caregivers (Perkins, 1988). The management behaviors are based on how the family and its members define their situation. The behaviors are the "discrete accommodations made to the child's condition on a daily basis" (Knafl & Deatrick, 1990, p. 9) by family members that relate to the child's illness, to their family system, and to the social system (Deatrick & Knafl, 1990). The *clinical nurse specialist interventions* are best focused at the level of the management behaviors and the way that the family and its members define their situations. The interventions are based on the needs of the family and its members in terms of their transitional care requirements (Brooten et al., 1988).

On the basis of a symbolic interactionist perspective, *family* is defined as the membership defines itself. Furthermore the FFPTC model is based on the assumption that the family is able to actively formulate solutions to daily management issues and that collaborative intervention with the child and family can assist with the recognition of these solutions.

Family-Focused Interventions

The FFPTC offers the clinical specialist a unique entrée into the family for negotiating the child's health-related care, for assisting the family to maintain family life, and for providing continuity of care by acknowledging the family's current management behaviors, as well as how they define their situation. The family remains the unit of analysis and care, as the family management style conceptualizes the usual response of the family unit. This includes the family member's management behaviors, which may have a differential focus on the child, the family, or the social system, depending on the needs of the family and its members (Deatrick & Knafl, 1990). This perspective then is consistent with family systems nursing (Friedemann, 1989; Wright & Leahey, 1990) and with a specialist approach (Gilliss, 1991) to practice that is grounded in work with children and their families.

Interventions consistent with the FFPTC can be viewed as systematic family interventions (Doherty & Baird, 1986) or the fourth level of a five-level categorization of family involvement with families that ranges from *minimal emphasis* (Level 1) to *family therapy* (Level 5). Skills on this level include "reframing the family's definition of their problem in a way that makes problem solving more achievable . . . helping family members view their difficulty as requiring new forms of collaborative efforts . . . helping family members generate alternative, mutually acceptable ways to cope" (Doherty & Baird, 1986, p. 154). If these efforts are not successful, the professional is directed toward making an effective transition to an individual qualified to do family therapy.

The FFPTC anticipates that nodal events, or turning points where present management behaviors are threatened, will occur. At those times, established routines become unsuitable, and problem solving by the family and its members attempts to identify new solutions or management behaviors (Deatrick, Knafl, & Guyer, Chapter 5, this volume). Systematic interventions by a specialist may be needed at this juncture. For instance, the mother of a 10-year-old girl with spina bifida reported that she could no longer lift her daughter. Further assessment revealed that during the past 6 months her daughter had gained 10 pounds. She ate snacks from the time she got home from school to the time she ate dinner. In addition, she was not using her crutches but was remaining in her wheelchair. The specialist needs to be sensitive to the fact that the mother and daughter socialize in the kitchen as the mother prepares dinner and that the daughter does not move out of the kitchen during that time even when other family members arrive home. Initial attempts at changing the behavior revealed that the daughter had been ill 6 months earlier, and since that time the mother had been having a great deal of difficulty separating from her daughter. The mother stated, "I find our after-school discussions very comforting."

The FFPTC views the specialist as having a unique supplemental and/or substitutive role with such a child and family. In this role the specialist does not prescribe management behaviors or tasks per se but rather puts those management behaviors in the context of the family member's overall goal for that particular way of managing. This may represent a shift in paradigms for the specialist who typically would prescribe a change in diet or exercise for this 10-year-old girl without explicitly acknowledging the goals of the family members. According to the FFPTC, the interventions would be focused on helping the girl and her mother arrive at new ways to accomplish the girl's weight reduction, while still respecting their underlying goals. If the specialist thought that new goals were necessary, the previous goals would be respected and would be the starting point of negotiation.

Wright and Leahey (1984) warned, "In some cases, the more serious problem is at the interface of the family with other health care professionals rather than *within* the family itself. Thus, interventions [would] need to be targeted at the family-professional system *before* addressing problems at the family system level" (p. 175). Through family interventions consistent with the FFPTC, however, specialists can see themselves as facilitating the child and the family's movement through the stages of establishing a relationship with themselves and other health care professionals. In addition, they help the child and the family establish trust in their own competence (Robinson & Thorne, 1984; Thorne & Robinson, 1988, 1989).

Continuity of Care

Reflected in this model are the transitions of seriously and chronically ill and impaired infants, children, and adolescents and their families along a continuum of care in home, hospital, community, and school settings throughout the cycle of illness (Rolland, 1987). All transition points serve as potential periods of intervention by master's-prepared clinical nurse specialists because these turning points are usually when the family perceives their present ways of managing to be unsuitable or defines their child or their own situation differently. Trial and error may result in the formation of new ways to manage that may or may not be consistent with optimal treatment and continuity of their child's care. One of the primary roles of the pediatric clinical nurse specialist is to provide interventions that enable children and families to make effective transitions and thus improve the continuity of the children's care.

For example, when a child with asthma is rehospitalized after a severe attack, that child and family are often most open to exploring with the specialist preventive management in the home, community, and schools to avert another hospitalization. Or, in the case of a child with HIV infection-related diseases, caretakers may be most motivated to become more knowledgeable about daily treatments that may help prevent further pulmonary opportunistic infections.

Advanced Skills in Clinical Decision Making

Skills in clinical decision making are necessary to care for these populations within and across the continuum of care throughout the various phases of an illness (Lipman & Deatrick, in progress). Clinical decision making involves a process of gathering data about the physical, developmental, behavioral, psychological, and social status of an infant, child, or adolescent; drawing a conclusion; and making a plan for nursing interventions based on these findings. In some clinical situations, the decisions seem fairly straightforward; however, conditions of uncertainty greatly increase the complexity of making decisions (Weinstein & Fineberg, 1980). Therefore graduate education must focus on the scientific base of practice, as well as on the mastery gained through experience and personal reflection. The competencies related to the work of clinical decision making from this perspective include clinical judgment, scholarly inquiry, and leadership (Diers, 1985; Lipman & Deatrick, in progress). The curriculum related to clinical judgment includes both specialty-specific assessment skills, as well as the scientific basis for specialty-specific practice. Through scholarly inquiry, advanced practitioners develop a spirit of inquiry to question clinical practice and to investigate alternatives within nursing and other disciplines. Leadership skills coupled with knowledge of social and health policy enable the clinical nurse specialist to make use of resources that may be available to the child and family.

Pilot for Curriculum Development

Presently an intervention project based on the FFPTC is being conducted with children undergoing limb repair by use of an Ilizarov device (Deatrick,

Mason, & Davidson, 1990). The overall goal of the project is to improve the care outcomes of these children and families, as well as to prepare for application of the model to other populations. A prepilot project analyzed management behaviors typically used by children and families undergoing this procedure. These behaviors then were used to plan a protocol, consisting of a collaborative intervention by a clinical nurse specialist, an orthopedic surgeon, and a physical therapist with subsequent children and their families, that anticipates nodal events in treatment and offers anticipatory guidance at these junctures.

Preliminary results indicate that the approach has resulted in positive patient outcomes, as well as in increasing the confidence of the primary caretaker. The project also has enabled the faculty to visualize how the model can be applied in a clinical situation and to further define and develop the model for application to the graduate curriculum.

Summary

To prepare advanced practice specialists who can work effectively with children and their families, the FFPTC can be used as a model for curriculum development. Didactic content emphasizes family interventions, continuity of care, and advanced skills in clinical decision making. Clinical experiences are concentrated in tertiary care settings but also include collateral community experiences. Such experiences will enhance the student's understanding of home and community settings to prepare them for effective role functioning between and within the settings.

The potential exists for the use of this model in other educational initiatives, such as current work in the undergraduate and doctoral curricula. In addition the model could be used to guide staff development curricula in hospitals to prepare nurses for parent participation in caregiving. Such a program could lead to an atmosphere of respect for the parent's skills, as well as to an understanding of how these skills could be transferred to the home setting.

17

Education for Family Health Care in Clinical Settings: Nursing Focus

Mary Perkins

Kathy Rigney

Family-centered care has been a part of the philosophy of community health care (Frost, 1939) and has become a persistent goal among pediatric health professionals over the past 10 years. Impetus to accept this health care trend as a necessity is influenced by the increase in children with chronic illnesses and the advent of multiple specialty services. It is apparent that during any one hospitalization of a child, the services and health care professionals change, while the family remains as the only constant during and after the experience (Shelton, Jeppson, & Johnson, 1987). Nonetheless revealing such facts has not been enough to ensure that family needs are addressed or that family interventions are carried out during the hospital stay of one of its members. The process of integrating family interventions into health care delivery models has been difficult because it requires concerted efforts on behalf of both the institution and the care providers.

The purpose of this chapter is to describe a conceptual framework for a hospital staff development curriculum that includes family nursing education. Descriptions of the framework and the utility of its components to support a continuum of learning in the clinical or hospital setting are presented. Family content elements are identified. The process of integrating the family content elements into a pediatric health care staff development curriculum is addressed.

The Conceptual Framework

The inclusion of family content in university nursing curricula has proliferated over the last decade (Wright & Leahey, 1990). Despite the drive to include family theory and family assessment content, however, little emphasis has been given to family intervention models and to intervention outcomes. Family interventions and intervention outcomes are the primary practice foci expected of professionals in clinical settings. Therefore, to help professionals assess and respond to the unique needs of families, a learning/reinforcement continuum between academia and service institutions must be established.

The conceptual framework presented in this chapter is a product of the communication established between colleagues in academia—the Nursing of Children Division of the University of Pennsylvania School of Nursing —and service—the Nursing Education, Staff Development, and Training (NESDT) Department of Children's National Medical Center (CNMC) in Washington, DC. Colleagues at the university shared pediatric and family course objectives with the educators at Children's Hospital. The materials were examined to determine the emphasis placed on family in pediatric nursing courses and were compared to family intervention expectations delineated in the job descriptions for each level of practitioner at Children's Hospital. The intent of these efforts was to establish a bridge between academia and service that allows both environments of learning to keep pace with one another. It was determined that the essential characteristics of the curricula, particularly the core family content, are the same regardless of discipline or setting. A continuum of learning was needed, however, to reinforce basic nursing education and to foster clinician role development in the area of planning and implementing family-focused interventions.

Shared materials, such as the university course outlines, NESDT department philosophy, CNMC's Division of Nursing's career ladder job descriptions, and selected theoretical models, provided the basis on which the curriculum components were identified in Figure 17.1. The postulates of two theoretical models—developmental and interaction (Fawcett, 1984a) —were adopted by the department as underlying support of the curriculum. The assumptions of the models support the dynamics of interactive learning

Curriculum Component of NESDT Curriculum

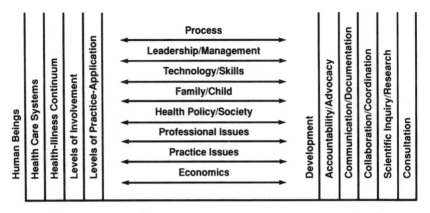

Figure 17.1. Nursing Education, Staff Development, and Training (NESDT) Curriculum Components Based on the Theoretical Framework and Job Expectations for All Levels of Practice

processes and a progressive continuum of learning and development. The primary thrusts of these models are change, social relationships, processes of growth, development and maturation of individuals, perception, communication, role, and self-concept (Fawcett, 1984a). The characteristics of the models provided additional support for the curriculum framework and facilitated the identification of major curriculum components.

The major components are the structural foundation for all course and program development and evaluation. The components listed horizontally in Figure 17.1 relate to clinical nursing practice. The components listed vertically relate to systems, interactive processes, and role development. The identified curriculum components are organizing concepts that guide the selection of substantive content relevant for expected job requirements of clinicians, from entry/beginner to mastery level. The specificity, breadth, and depth of substantive content included in courses or programs are dependent on assessed learning needs of the clinician.

In sum, the curriculum framework and its components illustrate a unifying link between academic and clinical settings. The components of the hospital curriculum provide the professional nurse with a planned and integrated approach to continuing education. This curriculum was designed to supply the nurse with access to content and information, to reinforce principles learned in preparatory courses, and to enhance learned experiences.

Core Family Curriculum Components

Family content elements are integrated throughout the curriculum. Core family content elements relevant in both service and academic environments include family theories, interactional phenomena, developmental patterns, family health and illness cycle (Doherty & McCubbin, 1985), family assessment and interventions, multidisciplinary collaboration, parent caregiving role (Perkins, 1988), and professional role development. The major family content elements for professionals are presented in Table 17.1.

Family content elements stemming from select curriculum components are identified in Table 17.1. The content elements were selected to provide professional nurses with information, both reinforced and new, needed to communicate with and make comprehensive assessments of the child and the family, based on parental concerns and desires. To enhance family involvement, corollary education programs with similar content for parents and ancillary personnel are also necessary in service environments.

Family content elements identified in Table 17.1 are the same for all levels of professional practitioners. Content may be shared through the use of many teaching strategies, but the main emphasis of learning in the service arena is on clinical applications. For example, theoretical content on family functioning and adaptation is provided within the context of case scenarios of families of children with chronic conditions. The contextual experience provides nurses with clinically relevant materials grounded in reality.

Teaching strategies focus on the analysis of family-clinician involvement strategies. Real-life situations are used as professionals are encouraged to discuss and/or role-play issues related to family-professional dynamics. Consequently techniques to assess and identify individual and family strengths and resources that enable the family are discussed. The professional actively engages in examining ways to ensure responsible practices to achieve patient and family outcomes.

Although content may be presented through similar teaching strategies for all levels of nurses, as the professional nurse progresses along the role development continuum, it is expected that the nurse will become engaged more actively in educational endeavors. The more experienced nurse is expected to design education materials that deal with relationships among colleagues (within nursing or other disciplines), the family, and the child, which are shared with their nurse colleagues.

In classes consisting of experienced nurse participants, specific professional-parent collaboration techniques are discussed, and strategic plans are developed to establish standards of practice for professional-parent

Table 17.1 Family Content Elements in a Pediatric Hospital Curriculum

Curriculum Components	Systems	Practice Issues	Health	Professional Issues
Content presented in family courses	Society/Government Family Individuals (Child) Health care Trends Economics Legislative policy Inter/Intra- group dynamics Cultural systems Hospital systems Community systems	Dynamics of interactions Technology/Skills Personal/Professional skills Collaboration • Multidiscipline • Professional • Client-nurse • Family-nurse Consultation	Wellness-illness Stressors Adaptation Caregiving Management Resource accessing Levels of involvement Advocacy • Ethnicity and health/illness Levels of intervention	Decision making Problem solving Role development Facilitation Leadership/Management Documentation Accountability Research Risk management Legal issues
Supporting theories	Systems Needs Change Organization Conflict Human development Family development • Structure • Functioning • Adaptation	Teaching/Learning Ethics Cultural Personality Interaction Conflict Exchange	Continuum of care Crises Coping	Role Change agent Development Interpersonal communication Involvement Strategies Appropriate care • Developmental • Cultural

collaboration. Discussions about the professional self, attitudes, and parental caregiver behaviors are explored as they relate to clinical decision making.

The appropriateness of selected family content and teaching strategies is supported by fundamental organizational structures of the hospital. Background assessments were performed to ensure that the appropriate structures were in place. Such structural features are important to ensure the success of curriculum implementation.

Integration of Family Health Care
Education Components in the Service Curriculum

The success of the nursing curriculum implementation in a service setting depends on the supportive structures and values of the broader system or hospital as a whole. Documents such as the hospital's philosophy on care and its goals and strategic plans were reviewed for supportive evidence and consistency within the overall goals of the education plan.

The review resulted in the identification of structures already in place at CNMC that support the curriculum designed to develop practitioners who work collaboratively with families to improve patient outcomes. These supportive structures include (a) a philosophy that emphasizes family-focused care, (b) a professional nurses' career ladder (Program for Professional Advancement) that states expectations of family-focused interventions, and (c) forums in which medical staff and staff from other disciplines, such as nursing, meet as colleagues to discuss family needs. In addition, results of the staff nurse questionnaires, parent feedback obtained in a focus group, and satisfaction surveys were incorporated into the curriculum design. The parents' and nurses' comments supported the inclusion of family content in planned education activities.

Comments from nurses and parents were descriptive of the levels of professional involvement with families in health as outlined by Doherty and Baird (1986), which range from *minimal involvement* (Level 1) to *family therapy* (Level 5).

Nurses in the survey stated that they enjoyed intervening with and on behalf of families (Level 2). They declared that they were most satisfied when they could see patient outcomes based on planned and coordinated care (Level 4). Parents revealed that the hospitalization event was most satisfying when nurses and doctors were concerned with the effects of the child's illness on the family, when the parents' emotional needs were addressed, and when they could easily share information with and receive information from all members of the health care team. These findings are analogous to Doherty's Level 3 of professional involvement. The information obtained from nurses and parents highlights the disparity between their views on professional involvement in the hospital care of children. These findings provided additional support for including family content in a hospital staff development curriculum.

Although the aim of most preparatory curricula in nursing is for nurses to intervene with families at Level 3, most beginning practitioners feel ill-prepared to intervene at that level. The priority for the beginner nurse is to attain competencies in performing psychomotor skills. Thus the framework of the curriculum was designed to focus on role development content, with varying degrees of emphasis on psychomotor skills and therapeutic interactions. Benner's (1984) role proficiency theory easily is tied to the CNMC career ladder and was used to project the levels of clinician development for involvement with families. Family content components of the curriculum were delineated for each level of practice. Examples of core family content are presented in Figure 17.2, using Benner's (1984) model and the Children's Hospital career ladder. The significant feature about Figure 17.2 is that family course content at each level is designed to be a building block for the upper levels and at times is connected to previous course offerings.

Discussion

Pediatric hospitals or service education departments are struggling constantly to identify ways to develop nursing professionals who can address competently and comfortably the needs of families of hospitalized children. Because hospitals hire graduates from schools of nursing, continuous collaboration between service and academia is necessary to enable hospital education programs to build on the graduates' background knowledge. Although academia has provided students with theoretical knowledge about families, few if any service environments have designed curricula that include family nursing care knowledge. Through establishing a continuum of learning such as the curriculum described in this chapter, professional nurses are enabled to attain competence in intervening with families. Designing this curriculum is just one step toward creating open collaborative relationships with colleagues in academia.

Core Family Content

CN IV (Expert)*

Consultation
Advocacy for families
in clinical care

CN III (Proficient)*

Multidisciplinary Coordination
Professional-parent Collaboration
Accountability

CN II (Competent)*

Enabling parents/families in clinical
    setting - contracting for care
Compromised parental caregiving role
Accessing supports for families
Family centered discharge packets/conferences
    (Information/education)
Developmental/emotional needs of family

CNI (Advanced Beginner)*

Family theories
Facilitating positive coping
Family needs assessment
Identifying family strengths
Values clarification

CN (Novice)*

Family as unit of care
Introduction to family centered care concepts
Influence of families on child responses
Coping with hospitalization

Figure 17.2. Examples of Core Family Content for Each Level of Nurse Care
Provider at Children's National Medical Center
NOTE: *Benner, 1984, Levels of Proficiency

18

Preparing Specialists in Family Nursing: The Benefits of Live Supervision

Catherine A. Chesla

Catherine L. Gilliss

Maribelle B. Leavitt

According to the ANA Social Policy Statement (American Nurses Association, 1980), clinical specialization occurs at the graduate level and includes supervised clinical practice in the area of specialization. Therefore, as has been argued by Gilliss (1991), graduate preparation in family nursing must include supervised clinical experiences in the care of families. Similarly Bell and Wright (1990) have called for the inclusion of advanced family nursing intervention skills, particularly in graduate nursing programs.

By tradition, psychomotor nursing skills have been taught by a supervisor who stands and observes the return demonstration of the learner. Two surveys of Canadian (Wright & Bell, 1989) and United States (Hanson & Bozett, 1987) nursing programs suggested that this has not been the case

AUTHORS' NOTE: Marlene Forde Casey, PhD, and Kay Tiblier, PhD, served as consultants to this educational project, which was greatly enriched by their thoughtful contributions. Janet Allen-Jacobsen, MA, and Byron Schneider, MA, assisted with manuscript production and preparation.

when teaching family intervention skills. Although students are provided opportunities to practice the nursing care of families, supervision associated with these experiences varies dramatically (Wright & Leahey, 1990). Methods most commonly used include clinical case conferences and process recordings. In an era of cost containment, these methods may be efficient for the faculty member; they are likely less effective for student learning (Wright & Leahey, 1990).

The purpose of this chapter is to describe (a) an approach-in-development for the live supervision of student clinical work with families and (b) the particular teaching opportunities afforded by the use of this method of live supervision.

Developing Family Clinical Skills: Educational Philosophy

Clinical skills are acquired through theoretical preparation, as well as through engaged clinical learning. Practice capabilities are advanced when learners are given the opportunity to work closely with experienced family nurses who can point out what is relevant in the family's presentation, what should be attended to and explored, and what may be passed over. Each family situation can be examined for its specific characteristics, for its capacity to illustrate family theoretical perspectives, and for its call for action on the part of the nurse. Although theory is not simply "applied" in practice, it sets up sensitizing perspectives from which each family can be viewed. Observing and participating in the whole treatment episode with families allow students to place into perspective both family problems and change initiated through treatment. Repeated experiences with multiple families coping with similar problems are optimal, so clear, qualitative distinctions in patterns of family response can be noted and grasped (Benner, 1985a; Benner, Tanner, & Chesla, 1992).

As a faculty we hope to transform our students' clinical perspective from one that focuses primarily on the individual client and considers the family as context to one that readily brings into focus the family as an interacting whole: to "think family." In addition we anticipate that students will become competent in recognizing basic family patterns of response to particular acute and chronic health conditions. Finally, we expect that students will demonstrate competent skills in convening and intervening with families experiencing health conditions. Recognizing that most of our students will be practicing in primary care settings that are structured to treat individuals, we realistically anticipate that our graduates infrequently may see or be able to treat families as a unit. We advise students, however, that a perspective on families and on ill members as embedded in their families and communities should enter and shape every treatment episode. In this we agree with Ransom (1988): "In family practice, family therapy is required only a small percentage of the time, although many of the skills and knowledge base of family therapy are relevant most of the time" (p. 293). We also hope that our students, because of their guided clinical preparation, actually may influence existing systems of care to incorporate the treatment of whole families.

Background

Family therapy and family therapy supervision have undergone substantial change and development in the past decade. Distinct schools of therapy, once led by the personal strength and charisma of the founding practitioners, have evolved and elaborated their own distinct theories and methods for treating families (Liddle, Breunlin, & Schwartz, 1988). In the wake of these developments, increasing attention has been paid to the knowledge and skills required to supervise students within particular schools. Supervisory philosophies and techniques have proliferated and frequently are as distinctive as the school of therapy that they are designed to further. Numerous authors note an isomorphism between the family therapy and the training structures for that therapy (Liddle et al., 1988; Liddle & Saba, 1985). Thus, although many schools of therapy use similar techniques, including live supervision of trainees, the intent, content, process, and tone of the supervisory experience are distinctly different.

A brief review of the nature and use of live supervision in two schools of family therapy—structural and systemic—are reviewed here. These two schools have been most influential in our development of a nursing service for training nurses in family work through use of live supervision. Three major aspects of training, including live supervision, will be described for these two schools: (a) the relationship between theory and practice, (b) the relationship between the teacher and the learner, and (c) the focus of the treatment/supervision team throughout the treatment sessions. This discussion draws from an excellent review by Liddle and colleagues (Liddle et al., 1988), and the reader is referred to this source for a more complete review of supervisory issues in seven contemporary schools of family therapy.

Structural family therapy focuses on family organization and functioning and attempts therapeutic change by helping the family restructure or make their current structure more fluid, flexible, and complex (Minuchin, 1974). Structural theorists and trainers make explicit their belief that conceptual development and development of therapeutic skills in the treatment room each must be given adequate space and time and optimally must occur simultaneously. Minuchin and Fishman (1981) advocated the "inductive" transmission of the skills of working therapeutically with families— an apprenticeship process in which the student learns the "small movements" of therapy. Direct observation of the session by the supervisor is necessary, along with a sufficient number of families, to provide a variety of therapeutic experiences for the student.

In structural family therapy, as in training, the relationships between the therapist and family and the trainer and trainee are hierarchical. Just as the therapist is expected to enter the family as a benevolent leader, so the trainer is expected to take a leadership and evaluative role with trainees throughout their training. Finally the focus of the team—including the trainer—during live family sessions, during pre- and postsession discussions, and in videotaped supervision is consistently the skill and adequacy of the trainee's interventions. During live sessions with families, calls or visits to the treatment room by the trainer are designed to help the trainee/therapist use him- or herself more effectively in the treatment of families. Similarly, in pre- and postsession discussions, the trainer will direct attention to the trainee's skills and deficits in managing the macro and micro processes throughout the session (Colapinto, 1988).

In *systemic family therapy,* a similar attitude is espoused about the relationship between theory and practice. Particularly in the writings of members of the Milan team (Pirrotta & Cecchin, 1988), the need to give students a deep grasp of family concepts alongside their technical and skills training is emphasized. Much of this team's focus throughout therapy is on attaining a deeper and richer grasp of the family's understandings and meanings that underlie behavior. The relation between therapist and family, as well as trainer and trainee, is nonhierarchical. Advocates of this therapy place great importance on encouraging and valuing the contributions of all members of the treatment team and argue that the joint product of unrestricted hypothesizing with the entire team produces more eloquent and effective questions than any one individual, no matter how skilled, might produce. Finally, the continuing focus of the team in systemic family therapy is the family process and the team's effectiveness in understanding and disturbing that process. The team is truly one, and thus the success and failure of the project rides with the entire team rather than on the skills or incapacities of the particular member who sits in front of the one-way mirror with the family (Pirrotta & Cecchin, 1988).

In our own work with students, where members of the faculty team have backgrounds in different schools of family therapy, we have incorporated aspects of both structural and systemic family therapy and supervision. As in both schools of thought, we provide conceptual and practical education simultaneously and attempt to integrate the theoretical with the practical in both the classroom and the supervised clinical practice. This concern matches the faculty's general educational philosophy and is reflected in the structuring of our curriculum. In our practice we primarily endorse systemic methods. Unlike the original systemic thinkers (Palazzoli, Boscolo, Cecchin, & Prata, 1980), however, we attend a great deal to the relationship established between the therapist and the family.

We draw on others, including nurses, who have extended the systemic model to attend explicitly to the relational aspect of therapy (Tomm, 1988; Family Nursing Unit, 1988). In addition, however, we attempt to incorporate some of Minuchin's eloquent writings and demonstrations of joining the family. Although we attempt to maintain a nonhierarchical relationship with students during the pre-, inter-, and postsession hypothesizing, we clearly take on a hierarchical relation during the regular family sessions; that is, the team behind the mirror primarily listens as the master therapist (a systemic therapist who serves as our consultant) guides interventions with the family via telephone contacts. Finally, our attention is focused primarily on family processes and the family and therapist as a therapeutic system rather than on the individual skills or learning needs of the particular trainee throughout the treatment episode. In this aspect of training, our methods are primarily systemic.

Evolution of the Educational Setting and Goals

As part of a graduate program for students becoming "specialists in the care of the family," a series of four courses on family care were developed and implemented. The second course, "Family Intervention," had no concurrent clinical laboratory in which to practice the new principles and skills discussed in the classroom. To remedy this deficiency, the faculty shortened the classroom time and added a seminar for the purpose of supervising students in making entrée and working with families accessed through acute and continuous health care settings in the community. Students took turns presenting the genograms and histories of family clients; some shared audiotapes of their work. The success of the seminar was dependent on individual students' comfort with approaching families and presenting their work with objectivity and openness, and this level of comfort and ability varied widely among students. Thus the faculty sought a teaching approach that offered more consistency and more structure for students trying to learn the complex communication skills of a family intervention.

A one-way mirror facility (two rooms separated by a one-way mirror, or "window," for viewing) in the School of Nursing was available to the faculty, who decided to add an optional family clinical laboratory to the course. A microphone, telephone, and video camera were installed in the room in which the families are interviewed.

The total time scheduled for each live supervision session is approximately 3 hours. The first half hour is used for a preconference in which the family case is presented by the student, tentative hypotheses and interview goals are identified, and at least a beginning approach for the interview is established. Faculty lead the discussion, which tends to have high energy due to pressures of time and the impending interview. The family interview lasts about 1.5 hours, including a short break, and a postconference discussion is scheduled for about 30 minutes but usually runs longer. All students in the class are encouraged to participate in the pre- and postconferences and learn through observation. The students tend to identify with both the student interviewer and the more objective supervising faculty, vicariously taking on the role and perspective of each at different times during the conferences and the interview.

After the preconference, the interviewing student exits to greet the family. The family are oriented to the room, mirror, telephone (and how it will be used), microphone, and video camera and are told of those present in the observation room.

We usually try to allow at least 5 minutes to elapse before the first telephone intervention. This interval allows the interviewer to establish some rapport with the family and to begin the assessment in his or her own way. The strategies and the thinking behind the supervisory movements are discussed during the postconference, including the student interviewer's responses to the suggestions. We have found the postconference discussion incorporating the supervisees' experience of the interview to be a lively arena to test conflicting hypotheses and to air individual impressions about what just happened. The notion that it is all right for any of those present to disagree with tactics or to express personal discomfort, as well as enthusiasm, about aspects of the interview is conducive to the grasp of practical skills and to the development of personal comfort in the work.

Curricular Goal

The curriculum directed toward practice incorporates the Calgary Family Assessment Model (CFAM), developed by Wright and Leahey (1984). Within this model, students are taught to examine systematically the structural, developmental, and functional aspects of the family. Intervention with families is guided by the theoretical and practice perspectives of Goodrich, Rampage, Ellman, and Halstead (1988); Luepnitz (1988); McDaniel, Campbell, and Seaburn (1990); Minuchin (1974); Minuchin and Fishman (1981); Palazolli et al. (1980); and Tomm (1984a, 1984b, 1987a, 1987b, 1988). The practice thus can be typified as primarily systemic and structural, and the team works very hard to incorporate feminist concerns throughout its practice.

Although several theories of family therapy are incorporated into the curriculum, we do not envision our graduates practicing as family therapists. Rather we educate nurses who can be primary care practitioners yet can demonstrate beginning to competent skills in both family assessment and intervention. We train our students to engage and treat relatively intact families who are experiencing simple to complex reactions to a change in health of a family member. Severely dysfunctional or disrupted families are considered to be too complex for the students' skills and are appropriately referred to family therapists for further evaluation and treatment.

As we conceptualize the practice of our students, it resides somewhere between the practice described by Wright and Leahey (1988) as family nursing and family therapy. Although we encourage our students to think of themselves as family nurses, Wright and Leahey's definition of *family nursing* is too restrictive; that is, they define family nurses as being educated at the undergraduate level, viewing family as context and having a capacity to complete family assessment and simple, probably educational, interventions. Our graduates view the family as focus and have specialized knowledge of the family. We are more in concert with the side in the debates in the Society for the Teachers of Family Medicine that uses the terminology "working with families" as opposed to "family therapy" to describe the practice capabilities of their graduates (Ransom, 1988). We believe that this language more appropriately represents the context and working relations that our graduates establish with families.

Unique Opportunities of Live Supervision

1. Creating an Identification With Clients.

As a rule, one of the earliest lessons to be learned by students who care for families is that all families are not like their families of origin. Moreover, although the purpose of education is not to provide therapy to students, increased self-awareness regarding the charged issues in one's family of origin cuts down on the tendency to project or reenact the scenes from the student's own family with clients. Therefore, as one aspect of live supervision of student work, we promote the examination of natural identifications and alliances and work to create some that seem less natural.

Several approaches are employed. In role playing, students are invited to participate as family members or as interveners in front of the mirror. Each family member is provided with a sketch of what concerns the family today and a brief history of the family. With this information they complete the characterizations and unfold a drama that is always truer than life. The student interveners are provided with typical intake information. In the act of role playing, each student employs what he or she knows to complete the character. This exercise often requires that the students become the nagging, protective mother that they cannot understand or the distant, unresponsive father that they cannot reach. In the roles of young children, they experience the fright of power afforded them by adults who are not able to provide leadership to the family. Meanwhile, behind the mirror, those observing quietly attach to particular characters in front of the mirror or are bothered and irritated by some others.

The postsession conference of the entire group invites those students to describe their feelings about their characters and others in the role-played family. Similarly student interveners and observers are asked whom they felt closest to and whom they "did not like." Through group discussion students share disparate perceptions of characters and begin to offer one another new information about understanding family characters. Students begin to explore personally why they feel as they do. They become more self-conscious about their issues and less sure about "truth."

2. Establishing a Unity
Between the Interviewer and the Team.

The experience of "working with" the faculty and students who are behind the mirror requires a shift in the thinking of most students. Historically students have been observed by faculty who evaluate them and interrupt them to correct errors. Thus when a telephone call interrupts the ongoing dialogue, the student assumes that a mistake has been made.

We encourage the student to view those behind the mirror as sharing in the responsibility for the client's care, thereby enlarging the responsibility for the intervention to the team. Calls then are not seen as corrections but communications from the team to the interviewer and sometimes to the family. Through this reframing, the telephone is viewed as a friend and resource to the student working in front of the mirror.

A related and important notion involves the use of praise. If we all are working together as an effective team, the performance of one individual should not stand out as good or bad or be evaluated separately from the team. Rather we comment about what is effective or not effective with regard to the results of our actions. Again this commenting represents a break with tradition, for as teachers we have become accustomed to praising behaviors that we wish to reinforce. In this instance praise and correctives must be provided by and applied to the entire team. The effectiveness of the interventions are weighed as the result of the entire team's efforts.

3. Coaching to Perform New Behaviors.

The most obvious and powerful advantage of live supervision lies in the ability to influence a student's behavior during a session with a family, to increase his or her repertoire of interventive tactics. Students can be coached to perform new interventions that they may have read about but never have tried. Immediate feedback is available as the student, with the help of those behind the mirror, can see the results in the new behavior. With the assistance of the team, events can be shaped as they unfold. Students can attempt these new strategies in the safety of a protecting environment.

4. The Use of Metaphor in Teaching.

Live supervision is not unique as an opportunity to employ metaphor. We have found, however, several metaphors particularly effective in live supervision. Already we have observed that "the phone is my friend." Students do take considerable comfort in this phrase; in fact some indicate that they miss the phone when it does not ring. In helping students join the team behind the mirror and feel the sense of shared responsibility for the family's care, we suggest that when they are in front of the mirror they "lie back and float down the river, trusting that the currents will carry you along."

5. Learning to See From Behind the Mirror.

Time spent behind the mirror is well spent in guiding students to develop their ability to see and feel what is happening without getting caught in the family's emotional system and rules for interaction. Although the telephone-linked supervising faculty member's attentions may be focused on the interviewing student, a second faculty member may point out certain family behaviors worth tracking as the interview progresses or may ask students to consider what else they might do in the given situation.

6. Decreasing Student Resistance to Live Supervision.

Despite their genuine excitement about seeing families with supervision, most students also are frightened that they will appear incompetent to those observing. (Obviously this stance is held by those who do not yet understand that we are a team.) Those who are ambivalent have innumerable ways to delay the progress of live supervision. Because our time with students is limited to a 10-week quarter, we have tried to anticipate obvious resist or delay tactics and to eliminate some of these.

Locating families is a major obstacle for most students. They have difficulty asking people to come to the laboratory, explaining what they will do there, and also may convey their own anxiety about being observed. Therefore faculty have become more directly involved in the recruitment of families for students. Faculty have established professional contacts with potential referral sources and have increased the visibility of the family supervision laboratory throughout the health science campus in which it exists by inviting referral sources to attend the labs.

Directions for Future Practice

The faculty presently are engaged in instituting a faculty practice of family nursing specializing in helping families respond to the demands of new and chronic health problems. Our primary goals are educational: (a) ensuring a flow of familiar clients for our students and (b) providing increased opportunity to model family work by experienced faculty. Two family therapist consultants and four doctorally prepared family nursing faculty who have experience working with families are the staff of the service. A brochure describes the service and how families or referring health professionals can reach us. A coordinating secretary takes inquiry calls and contacts one of the faculty on a rotating basis to return the intake call. We now are meeting with potential referral sources in acute care and community settings. Responses to our calls and visits to referral sources have been enthusiastic, as well as curious (What do we offer that social workers do not? Why a family-only approach?). These questions provide an opportunity to clarify and describe a service that is seen by most of the health or community agency professionals as unique, innovative, and needed. At this point, and largely because of its training focus, we have decided not to charge a fee for service. We are studying third-party reimbursement and university billing structures.

As an alternative to bringing the family into the laboratory for supervision, we also have encouraged students to videotape home visits to families and have purchased portable video cameras for their use. They have made use of the video cameras and have "brought in the family" in this manner. Faculty and students review the videotapes individually and in seminars. Although we do not believe that this is as powerful or effective as live supervision, a retrospective analysis of the visit nevertheless increases the student's clinical repertoire. Viewing the tapes helps the student see behavioral sequences and circular effects of interaction patterns and identify what works well and not so well, and why.

PART VI

Contemporary Issues

Catherine L. Gilliss, Editor

19

Cross-Cultural Family-Nurse Partnerships

Marta A. Browning

Jean H. Woods

The construction of effective cross-cultural partnerships to advance family nursing requires that the nursing community assume responsibility for developing and implementing appropriate health care services for families within minority populations that include ethnic peoples of color. Nursing should be concerned particularly about those who live in urban settings and who suffer from the effects of institutional racism and social class discrimination precipitated by poverty. This chapter will focus on four aspects of the nursing profession's responsibility: (a) identifying the existence of a problem, (b) identifying a probable locus for nursing intervention, (c) determining the role of nursing, and (d) overcoming resistance to change by trouble-shooting a "first step" activity.

Identifying the Existence of a Problem

As experts in community health and community mental health settings, we believe that the application of systems theory is useful in exploring the existence and extent of a problem. *Systems theory* emphasizes "studying and describing interrelationships rather than viewing units in isolation" (Ross & Cobb, 1988, p. 85). Two key concepts in systems theory are *negentropy,* which is energy that promotes order within systems, and *entropy,* which is energy resulting in disorganization and chaos. Functional systems can be described as maintaining a balance between negentropy and entropy. This balance is commonly referred to as a *system steady state.*

To identify the existence of a problem, nurses need to look at some alarming characteristics of three systems relevant to the practice of family nursing: (a) the United States health care system, (b) the dysfunctional family system, and (c) the local or interfacing health care system.

Some characteristics of these systems are shown in Table 19.1. These characteristics should alert nurses to the urgent need for reform.

System I: The United States Health Care System

The United States health care system appears to be blind to the needs of a significant percentage of the population. The facts illuminate alarming disparities in the health care provided to ethnic peoples of color when compared with their white contemporaries. Access and utilization threaten to worsen as the demography of the United States changes. For example, Hispanics will increase to 11.3%, Blacks to 13.1%, and other racial groups to 4.3% of the total U.S. population (U. S. Dept. of Health, 1990). The "minority" sector of the population is growing, and this growth will impact dramatically the character of the nation by the turn of the century. Unfortunately the politics of health care scarcity is lived out within culturally diverse families who are also poor. Thus it is apparent that the United States health care system is not functioning in a steady state but rather is a system tending toward a state of entropy.

System II: The Dysfunctional Family System

The term *dysfunctional* is used in its broadest sense to identify families, particularly those who are poor and have multiple problems, needing assistance in meeting their health care needs rather than those suffering from mental illness. Family systems having even a few of these characteristics, shown in Table 19.1, suffer a tendency toward entropy. Through professional practice in community health, home health, community mental health, and family therapy, we have observed that these families need most to have the following:

Table 19.1 Characteristics of Three Interacting Systems

System I: United States Health Care System	System II: Dysfunctional Family System	System III: Local or Interfacing Health Care System
31 million Americans uninsured[a]	Living at or near the poverty line	Fiscal constraint—it seeks to eliminate unprofitable clients from the system or to limit their use of the system.
Distribution of uninsured	Uninsured for health care	
18.6% white	Suffering the impact of institutional racism, which denies access to care	Time-limited interactions directly with health care professionals, typically lasting less than 30 minutes
29.8% black	Existing in a constant state of crisis	
41.4% Hispanic[b]	Inability to articulate health care needs due to inadequate verbal communication skills[g,h,i]	Focus on the individual as client, not the family group
Rationing of health care disproportionately affects blacks and Hispanics.[c]		Places a premium on verbal articulation of needs in standard English
Systematic institutionalized racial discrimination contributes to maldistribution.[d]		Applies assessment and treatment protocols based on standards developed by the study of white males
Black infant deaths are twice as high as white infant deaths.[e]		Staffing patterns that are made up predominately of majority group (white) professional caregivers
21% of U.S. children live in poverty.[f]		

NOTE: [a] (Davis, 1991)
[b] (Friedman, 1991, p. 2491)
[c] (Lundberg, 1991)
[d] (Freeman et al., 1990, pp. 313-315)
[e] (Clemen-Stone, Eigisti, & McGuire, 1991, p. 456)
[f] (Hoerlin, 1989)
[g] (Aleman, 1991)
[h] (Lash, 1991)
[i] (Martin & Henry, 1991)

Resources (food, clothing, shelter, transportation)

Time and attention of professional health and social service providers

Stability and consistency of helping professionals over extended periods of service

Culturally sensitive caregivers

24-hour availability of support services for crisis management

Training to acquire basic problem-solving skills

Long-term support in the incorporation and practice of behavior change

Services designed for individuals as representatives of a family group

Services provided to the total family in its natural setting—the home

In light of the specific intervention needs of dysfunctional, multiproblem poor families who are disproportionately represented in minority populations, it is important to examine the local or interfacing health care system.

System III: The Local or Interfacing Health Care System

The local or interfacing health care system is the first point of interaction between the client and the health care provider. The local health care system serves as an interface between the client and the macro level national health care system whose policies it manifests in the selection and implementation of specific services. In this system the theoretical assumptions of planners and policymakers are tested on human beings who either are able to obtain service or are rejected from service according to rules and criteria established in towns and boardrooms far from the scene of implementation. This local or interfacing health care facility is sought out by the family when crises precipitate a need for action. The characteristics of System III (see Table 19.1), however, appear antithetical to the actual needs of the dysfunctional family as discussed previously. System III is also a system out of balance when examined in relation to its ability to meet the needs of the dysfunctional family.

Results of System Interaction

The three systems discussed are like large beach balls that rebound off one another when thrown up into the air simultaneously. No mutual attraction binds the systems together in concerted action. Quite the opposite appears to be true. System I and System III, designed to meet the needs of System II, actually give evidence of repelling one another.

To improve the lives of poor, culturally diverse American families, these three systems must be reshaped. Targeted components of each system must be pushed and molded to resemble pieces of a jigsaw puzzle so that connections become interlocked in a dynamic exchange for mutual benefit.

Identifying a Probable Locus
for Nursing Intervention

We believe that nurses must direct their energies toward creating change in the local or interfacing health care system. Instigating change in System III can drive changes in Systems I and II as change in one system invariably brings about change in interlocking systems.

Designing "family-friendly" services specifically directed toward the needs of urban minority clients would include bilingual or multilingual nurses and multiple services for one-stop shopping (health care, dental care, etc.) and appointments on weekends or in the evenings. Additionally physical/ mental health assessment guidelines and client education services would be culturally relevant, while follow-up care would be home based and family centered. The presence of such services would indicate a desire on the part of health care providers to create an environment in which true collaborative partnerships could be established with ethnically different families. In the initiation of meaningful methods of service delivery for diverse clients, nurses can demonstrate objectively an openness to change. We are suggesting initial changes that are simple, born out of simple courtesy and a respect for the desire of clients to learn to care for themselves through access to instructions and treatments that they can understand and implement.

If nursing is able to create changes in System III, then change gradually will occur in System I. Small programs or service packages serve as models or demonstrations of the efficacy of family-centered services. These programs and service packages, once operationalized and refined, can be offered to the federal government as models of systems that work in family-centered urban health care delivery. A variety of unique local programs developed by nurses can offer federal policymakers an array of options for consideration.

Determining the Role of Nursing

Nurses are ideally suited to serve as the agents of systems change. They are acutely aware of the elements required for proper management of health care in the family system. Therefore nursing is the profession of choice to assume the role of "cultural brokerage" as described by Bulecheck and McClosky (Ross & Cobb, 1988, pp. 143-144). In this role the nurse must act as mediator between clients and the organized health care system. As culture broker the nurse performs the "act of translation in which messages, interactions and belief systems are manipulated and processed from one group to another" (Ross & Cobb, 1988, p. 143). It is this very act of translation, however, that poses a problem for nurses and thus leads to the fourth aspect of fulfilling nursing's responsibility for action.

Overcoming Resistance to Change by Trouble-Shooting a "First Step" Activity

To design health care systems for ethnically diverse families, cross-cultural collaboration and communication are essential. Systems that are culturally sensitive and culturally appropriate cannot be designed without input from members of the group that they are designed to serve.

Family nursing literature focuses heavily on the assessment of families, including the use of genograms and eco-maps (Miller & Winstead-Fry, 1982), and on intervention with individuals in the context of family (Wright & Leahey, 1987). Far less information is available on working with the family as a whole group, in one location, at one time or through time. This problem is compounded when the family's culture differs from that of the nurse. Transcultural nursing, while helpful, supplies answers to only a portion of this dilemma. Transcultural nursing literature stresses the importance of nurses learning about other cultures, and to that end the literature describes attributes of cultures, folkways, foodways, mores, and significant health-related practices of cultural groups (Boyle & Anderson, 1989; Giger & Davidhizer, 1991; Tripp-Reimer, Brink, & Saunders, 1984).

What the literature does not tell is how to take the problematic first step. We believe that establishing communication with clients may be more problematic, as flawed communication may occur among nurses themselves. If nurses' communication with one another is flawed, the systems designed by these professionals to serve families will also be flawed. As a first step, professional caregivers must learn effective ways of communicating across cultures in the professional relationship. By doing so they avail themselves of the rich opportunity for learning from and teaching one another the strategies of cross-cultural communication. These in turn can be transferred to the families served by nurses.

We have developed a paradigm to illustrate the barrier to action that can be posed by the first action step—establishing a meaningful dialogue. We are white and African American; our own cultures are used as examples for illustration purposes in the paradigm. The paradigm is in three parts (Browning & Woods, 1991).

Figure 19.1, "The Challenge," illustrates the impact of institutional racism on the provision of care and on the health care of African Americans. Institutional racism has resulted in a health care crisis for many people of color. The correction of its causes and the amelioration of its manifestations now pose a significant challenge to health care providers.

In initiating solutions to problems posed by "The Challenge," however, nurses confront "The Impasse" (Figure 19.2). Nurses from different cultures—in this case African American and white—meet together in the workplace to perform task-oriented job assignments, but they meet essentially as strangers. The vast majority of their lives have most likely been spent in segregated communities amidst social networks largely unknown and potentially misinterpreted by one another. These social networks provide definitions of one's self, one's own culture, and alien cultures by assigning designations as "us" versus "them." When drawn together on projects for joint planning to solve such critical problems as improving health care for underserved people, nursing professionals of differing ethnic backgrounds may come to the planning table knowing relatively little about how really to relate to one another. If issues to be discussed regarding client care tap sensitive areas in the lives of interacting professionals, they inadvertently may injure one another. Conversely, if issues are discussed with an overapplication of sensitivity, the professionals never may share enough to learn those things that they most need to learn from one another. A certain air of tension hovers around the initiation of the relationship. This tension can be traced to stereotypical views that have been developed from the "we" versus "they" definitions given to the individuals by their own cultures. These definitions have gone largely unchallenged and unrevised due to the lack of interaction with one another in the social spheres of their lives. Stereotypical views, in the case of the relationship between the African American and white nurses, can trigger black anger and white guilt. Thus feelings surrounding historical, institutional, or interpersonal racism can both overtly and covertly damage the ability of the two groups to relate truly and empathetically to each other. In their interaction they can become preoccupied with the anxiety engendered by their need to manage uncomfortable or unwanted guilt-producing thoughts and feelings. Depending on the level of anxiety stimulated by the interaction and the need to control that anxiety, denial of relevance of involvement

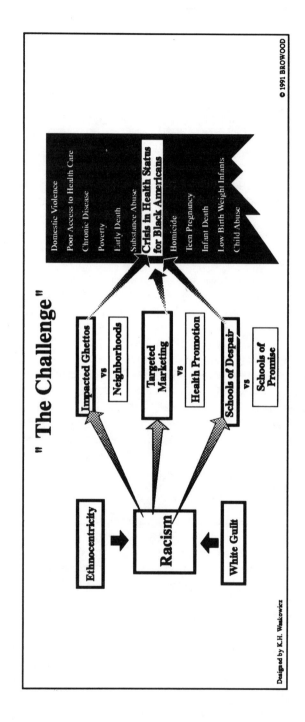

Figure 19.1. The Paradigm "Establishing a Meaningful Dialogue .:" The Challenge

184

(e.g., this problem is not mine; let "them" solve it) or actual flight from the working relationship may occur.

To prevent the fear, distrust, and defensiveness that lead to disengagement and flight from effective working relationships, the nursing profession must find ways to create situations in which empathetic cross-cultural relationships can occur. The profession must admit that problems exist in the area of race relations and must take steps to address them actively in the education of beginning practitioners and in the re-education of practicing professionals. This re-education can be accomplished when nurses can access those aspects of their colleagues' nonwork networks, the genesis of really knowing and feeling another's culture, and integrate that "knowing" into the workplace. In nonpsychiatric settings and in the development of professional human relationship skills, the profession largely has overlooked the experiential piece—walking a mile in another's shoes or the feeling-based portion of the educative process called empathy.

Empathy is defined as "an understanding of another . . . which must in some verbal or nonverbal manner, be communicated to another person" (Birkhead, 1989, p. 76). Williams (1990) stated that empathy is particularly applicable to nurses because it is congruent with the philosophy of nursing. According to Williams (1990) several components of empathy make the process of empathizing a complex one. These components are *emotional empathy,* which is the innate tendency to react emotionally to the emotions of others; *cognitive empathy,* which involves the individual's ability to detach the self from emotion and to use knowledge, experience, and theory; *communicative empathy,* which involves the ability to translate verbal and nonverbal language of others; and *relational empathy,* which describes the interpersonal experience itself (Williams, 1990).

As illustrated in Figure 19.3, nurses effectively using empathy would recognize that some feelings aroused during the initiation of a cross-cultural relationship would be uncomfortable and disquieting. In employing cognitive empathy, however, the colleagues would give internal acknowledgement to the presence of negative or frightening feelings arising from old stereotypes or historical emotional baggage but would resist the urge to act on these feelings in the old way. The tumultuous feelings would be accepted as human, as a new and risk-taking venture, and would be set aside gently through sublimation to create a neutral, nonvalue-laden zone in which new and functional communication and discovery could occur. The practitioners develop an awareness of each other and a readiness to actively listen to, interact with, and give feedback to each other on their respective ideas. As feedback is provided and shared, readiness to listen is increased (Woods & Browning, 1990).

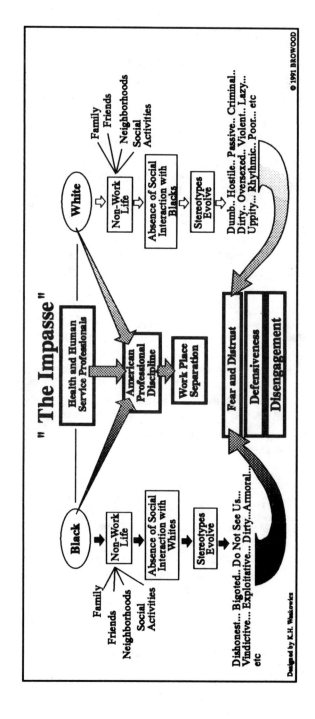

Figure 19.2. The Paradigm "Establishing a Meaningful Dialouge:" The Impasse

If the profession can assist its practitioners to operationalize empathy in all of its manifestations—cognitive, emotional, communicative, and relational (Williams, 1990)—nurses can override anxieties inherent in cross-cultural relationships and can create neutral playing fields for mutual problem solving (Figure 19.3). It is in this neutral zone where active empathy holds anxiety in check and prevents crippling disengagement. Problems and challenges are not divided into "yours" and "mine" but are remerged into "ours." Their solutions thus are derived as part of a collaborative process. When such collaborative relationships are formed, nurses can assume active roles in the process of cultural brokerage.

Nurses proficient in the role of culture broker will be able to translate what they have learned from establishing cross-cultural relationships with one another to the formation of working relationships with the families that they serve. Furthermore, after they have lived the experience of moving through alienation to collaboration, they will be more able to perform the role of culture broker. The culture broker is the bridge between the family systems that comprise the unit of service and the professional caregiving system that comprises the units of health care delivery.

We have followed this process of analysis as we struggled to establish our own cross-cultural relationship. We believe that our paradigm needs to be tested through research to explore its validity in other racial/ethnic relationships. It is our belief that our experience also indicates an urgent need for nurses to develop methodologies for creating environments in which cross-cultural empathy is generated and can flourish for both professional peers and the families served by the profession.

If nurses cannot yet relate effectively to professional colleagues whose culture differs from their own, how can they truly form partnerships with families from divergent cultural backgrounds? Until nursing takes this first step and transcends the initial barrier—establishing a meaningful dialogue—the profession cannot begin to address other critical issues necessary to create systems change.

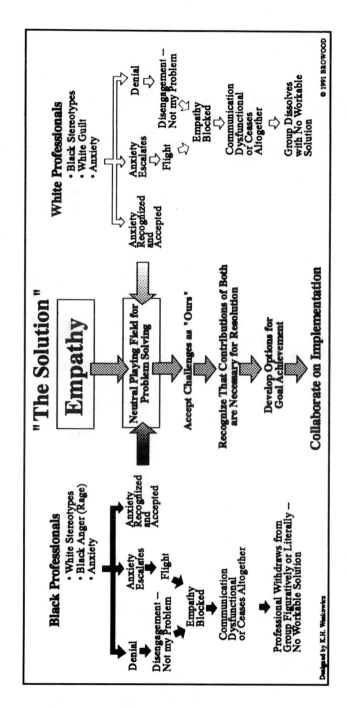

Black Professionals
- White Stereotypes
- Black Anger (Rage)
- Anxiety

Anxiety Recognized and Accepted

Anxiety Escalates → Flight

Denial

Disengagement — Not my Problem

Empathy Blocked

Communication Dysfunctional or Ceases Altogether

Professional Withdraws from Group Figuratively or Literally — No Workable Solution

Designed by K.H. Waskowicz

"The Solution"

Empathy

Neutral Playing Field for Problem Solving

Accept Challenges as "Ours"

Recognize That Contributions of Both are Necessary for Resolution

Develop Options for Goal Achievement

Collaborate on Implementation

White Professionals
- Black Stereotypes
- White Guilt
- Anxiety

Anxiety Recognized and Accepted

Anxiety Escalates → Flight

Denial

Disengagement — Not my Problem

Empathy Blocked

Communication Dysfunctional or Ceases Altogether

Group Dissolves with No Workable Solution

© 1991 BROWOOD

Figure 19.3. The Paradigm "Establishing a Meaningful Dialogue:" The Solution

188

20

The Black Box in Family Assessment: Cultural Diversity

Julie E. Sprott

Like the proverbial *black box,* a term that refers to a taken-for-granted entity of nebulous definition, cultural assessment in nursing, though considered essential, remains poorly specified. Rather than casting the assessment too broadly, it may be more useful to tailor cultural assessments of families to specific clinical settings. This chapter focuses on the health promotion context of care provided by nurse practitioners (NP) in clinic visits, because this specialty area of nursing continues to burgeon with ever-increasing numbers of NPs and because many of the extant guides for cultural assessment do not seem well suited for application to NP practice. Although the discussion is directed at the NP role, points made in this chapter relate as well to the state of the art of cultural assessment of families in contemporary nursing practice across a broad range of nursing roles and settings.

Three basic lessons from anthropology are presented to frame both content and process concerns in making culturological assessments and to provide a context for a critique of current assessment guides. Although time-worn, these lessons continue to have relevance to nursing theory and practice.

Lessons Offered by the Anthropological Perspective

Lesson 1. Culture is the blueprint and context for much of human behavior.
A culture or subculture must be understood on its own terms and via its own
system of meaning.

Fundamental to the discipline of anthropology, the *culture* concept purports
that persons are socialized from birth into one or more social groups that
provide a normative system for beliefs and behaviors, shaped conceptually
by symbols imbued in language. Characteristic of systems in general,
cultures are holistic and complex, formed of many parts or subsystems, in
which certain values are given greater emphasis over others (Kluckhohn,
1976).

Cultures are products of mental schemas bounded by value and normative demarcations. Membership in cultures and subcultures is not constrained by outward physical manifestations such as skin color but may
include classification, for example, by cohort (as in the postwar baby
boomers), religion (as in Mormon), or profession (nurses). *Ethnicity* is based
on "a consciousness of group belonging that is differentiated from others
by symbolic 'markers' (including cultural, biological, or territorial), and is
rooted in bonds of a shared past and perceived ethnic interests" (Burgess,
1978, p. 270). In the United States, socioeconomic level is confounded with
ethnicity to a large extent: The non-Anglo groups such as African-American,
Asian, and Hispanic subgroups also bear the burden of economic disadvantage and societal discrimination from the dominant culture (Children's
Defense Fund, 1989; Spencer, 1990).

The concept of *boundedness* of culture for minority ethnic groups within
a nation bears on a basic task in cultural assessment. The nurse (likely to
be a member of the dominant culture group) must appreciate the degree to
which the family or individual's cultural boundaries are either well defined
or indeterminate, as well as perceive divergent aspects of cultural norms in
relation to those of the dominant culture. A newly arrived immigrant or a
more traditionally oriented person would more likely exhibit contrasts in
beliefs and behaviors, compared with more acculturated groups/persons
who ascribe to part or most aspects of the dominant societal norms. It is
beyond the scope of this chapter to discuss theories of acculturation or variables used in its measurement. A brief list of such variables, however,
includes degree of exposure to formal schooling, urban settings, wage employment, and forms of the media, whether or not the individual has adopted
the language, religion, dress, and dietary habits of the dominant culture or
the degree to which the individual's social network reflects primarily ethnic,
mixed, or Anglo composition (Berry, Trimble, & Olmedo, 1986).

Despite the obvious implications of the culture concept for medical and nursing practice, little headway has been made in the incorporation of the concept into the education of health professionals, notwithstanding the consistent call to do so (Brink, 1982; Chrisman & Kleinman, 1983; Harwood, 1981; Henderson & Primeaux, 1981; Leininger, 1978; Spector, 1985). Nor is it clear how the practitioner should best conduct a culturological assessment.

For example, Leininger's sunrise model (1988) calls for a comprehensive assessment of individuals, families, groups, and institutions reminiscent of traditional structural/functionalism of ethnography. According to the model, parts of the system to be scrutinized entail education, economics, kinship and social structure, the political and legal system, religious and philosophical factors, and cultural values and lifeways. Implied is the idea that knowledge of the broad workings of a society is essential for understanding the client's motivations and choices related to health and illness experiences. Several nurse anthropologists have proffered assessment models similar to Leininger's in scope (Herberg, 1989; Orque, Block, & Monrroy, 1983).

Yet others question the practicality of comprehensive assessments for nursing practice and offer abbreviated guides (Friedman, 1990; Maheady, 1986; Tripp-Reimer, Brink, & Saunders, 1984). Maheady tapped six domains in her brief 14-question format for use by nurses who work on pediatric inpatient units: religion, diet, language usage, healing beliefs and practices, parenting practices, and family values. Tripp-Reimer et al. (1984) limited critical assessment areas to ethnic affiliation, religious preference, family patterns, food preferences, and ethnic health care practices. They advised that "nurses need to identify the major values, beliefs, and behaviors as they influence and relate to a particular clinical setting or health problem" (1984, p. 79). Friedman's (1990) outline for assessment is similar to that of Tripp-Reimer and colleagues, with the additional concern for the nature of the neighborhood and the degree of community prejudice encountered by the family.

Another model emphasizes use of racial/ethnic biophysical data for assessment of normal variations and deviations from normal between and within groups and group-specific susceptibility in terms of risks to health (Giger & Davidhizar, 1991). These authors implicitly borrowed from concepts in epidemiology in championing inclusion of macro-level, population-based data.

Although choice of any of these domains for assessment may be supportable, heeding the advice noted earlier of Tripp-Reimer and others (1984) that the choices be based empirically on specific needs of the nurse to know, it seems odd that little empirical research has addressed the question of how much information is enough and what constitutes critical data in cultural assessment. Until such studies are forthcoming, our choices for approach and content areas will continue to be based on custom, reasoned action, and trial and error.

An attractive, parsimonious alternative to the assessments discussed so far is the client-centered problem-oriented focus of Kleinman and colleagues (Chrisman & Kleinman, 1983; Kleinman, 1980). They suggested a short list of questions designed to reveal the subjective meanings (constructed via the cultural system in part) that clients imbue in the signs and symptoms of their illnesses. Their assessment also aimed to uncover meanings in terms of the broader "folk" system of healing. Tripp-Reimer et al. (1984) incorporated that idea as well as part of their two-phase model for cultural assessment and provided an additional list of questions following the nursing diagnosis to probe specifically for beliefs that would most affect nursing interventions.

Despite the importance of problem orientation in caring for clients with specific illness concerns, that focus ignores the health promotion aspect of primary care that often lacks a problem impetus, as for well baby care. An individual, problem-oriented approach also neglects the need for cultural normative information, group biophysical norms, and population-based health-risk data that could serve as important background from which to frame culturally relevant questions themselves; that is, the solely individual-oriented model lacks the community health perspective that "sensitizes" the nurse to probe relevant areas of concern specific to each ethnic/racial group. As a further critique of the individual-focus mode, it may be unwise, as suggested by Tripp-Reimer et al. (1984), that the nurse rely on the single client as representative of a culture group to provide information about specific cultural norms. If the practitioner has not been exposed to a range of families of that cultural group, she or he cannot judge the degree of "normalcy" of the client or the suitability of the individual or family as key informant for that culture. Thus a key dilemma in cultural assessment is the need to balance micro-specific (individual and family) with macro-level data and vice versa.

Lesson 2. No one cultural solution or manner of family structure or interaction is inherently better than another.

This lesson derives from the concept of *cultural relativity.* Simply stated, it means that no culture is intrinsically more worthwhile than any other. This lesson seems most difficult to apply, probably due to the tendency of bounded cultural entities to construct as part of their value system a high self-regard vis-à-vis other groups, a phenomenon called *ethnocentrism*. Although social groups are not necessarily conterminous with cultural ones, ethnocentrism is consistent with the idea in conflict theory that groups in positions of power attempt to maintain the status quo to maintain their advantage. The advantaged and more powerful group tends to impose its beliefs, practices, and values on the group in the inferior position (Leininger, 1978, p. 148). Such social forces may play a subtle role in the low recruitment of minorities into nursing despite vigorous efforts to increase their number by national nursing organizations in the last decade. Minorities comprised 6% of nurses in 1977 and only 7.6% in 1988 (Moses, 1990).

Manifestations of ethnocentrism are also apparent in research literature. Featured issues on minority children in the journals *Child Development* (April 1990) and *American Psychologist* (February 1989) point to the pervasive "deficit" model that has underpinned much of the research on non-Anglo populations. Children of African-American, Hispanic, or Native American subgroups, for example, often score less favorably than do Anglo children on tests that inherently have a construction bias toward the more socioeconomically advantaged Anglos. A "deficit" in the minority group is the presumed cause, with socialization patterns typically blamed as the root problem.

Similar biases are apparent in family assessment instruments. The middle-class Anglo image of healthy family cohesion underlies the circumplex model of family dynamics of Olson and colleagues (Olson, et al., 1989). Despite the authors' acknowledgment that many cultural groups emphasize family togetherness as "normal" (examples cited are Slovak Americans, Puerto Ricans, Italians, the Amish, and the Mormons; p. 67), an extreme score on the dimension of "cohesion" nevertheless falls into the category of "rigidly enmeshed." They conceded that such families are functioning well "as long as all family members are willing to go along with those expectations" (p. 67). Though seeming to illustrate flexibility in assessment of culturally diverse families, this evaluation serves to frame family interactional style in terms of a value system foreign to it. It results in the implication that there is no need for development or application of a more culturally relevant assessment. Furthermore it is insulting to attach a label to a family pattern that is considered to be aberrant in the dominant culture. In addition, the evaluator is left with no means to assess what would be considered an abnormal, unhealthy pattern in the nondominant culture group in terms of the culture's own value orientations.

Lesson 3. Cultures tend to perpetuate themselves unless massively assaulted or undermined by natural or human-generated causes.

Achebe's (1959) description of the detrimental effects on an Ibo African village of colonialism and the coming of missionaries echoes the experience of many other cultures during periods of European expansionism, and is a dominant/subordinate pattern of culture contact experienced by many indigenous peoples. Introduction of diseases at the time of contact with many of these populations decimated them in number and in cultural heritage: The physically weakest and most likely to succumb—the elderly— were typically the designated bearers of the oral traditions. Nevertheless it is believed that cultural groups as entities strive to survive despite heavy insult and injury.

In light of the tenacity of cultures to endure, it is not surprising that a melded uniform culture in the United States as imaged in the "melting pot" metaphor failed to come to fruition. Ethnic pride in one's unique heritage remains a viable force within American society; it is likely that cultural diversity will be even more salient as the "minorities" gain majority in number, estimated to occur in fewer than 100 years (Children's Defense Fund, 1989).

A paradox in asserting a fundamental tenacity of cultures is the fact that some cultural groups have disappeared, as in the poignant example of Ishi, the lone survivor of the Yahi Indians of California (Kroeber, 1964). Not uncommonly one finds in the literature a depiction of certain cultural groups as if on the verge of disintegration. As societal stressors and changes with negative impact maximally tax coping abilities of individuals and groups, it follows that groups would be increasingly unable to maintain boundaries, unique values, and cultural integrity.

This is not to imply that all socioeconomically deprived or otherwise stressed groups are culturally similar as suggested by Oscar Lewis's (1966) *culture of poverty* concept. Lewis proposed that the poor develop a unique subculture marked by the traits of alienation, noninvolvement, apathy, fear, and suspicion. Critics of Lewis's position have largely discounted it by pointing to (a) his failure to take into account the social structural constraints placed on the poor and (b) the circularity of his argument that essentially "blames the victim" (Valentine, 1968).

We can appreciate from Lewis's work, however, the point that poverty places an enormous strain on the family (Belle, 1982; Dohrenwend & Dohrenwend, 1974). As a result, families (and cultural systems) may fail to support the well-being of their members. In some situations the nurse must distinguish cultural traditions from effects of stress. For example, parental permissiveness and noninterference in child behavior have been traditional among many Native American groups (Driver, 1969, p. 380; Sprott, 1990). But as several Blackfeet Indian respondents indicated in a study on multicultural definitions for child harm and abuse, the assumption of noninterference was no longer a reliable one, as child neglect occurred under conditions of increasing alcohol and drug abuse on their reservation (Gray & Cosgrove, 1985).

Suggestions for Framing the Family Assessment in Ambulatory Care

The remainder of the chapter addresses issues of content and process to present cautions in the use of formal instruments and to offer strategies for interviewing, concurrently keeping in mind the three lessons gleaned from anthropology. In looking at the question of content, we first must ask what we want to know and why we need to know it. With systems theory as the framework and the focus on the family as the critical setting feature for the health of individuals, it follows that we need to know whether the family system is operating within an acceptable range of normalcy in the context of the cultural group of affiliation. We need to judge whether the family supports growth and development of each family member as each (as cognitively and developmentally able) evaluates it in his or her own system of meaning (adapting some of the proposed criteria for evaluating health by Pender, 1987, p. 27).

As suggested earlier, critical background information needed by the nurse practitioner in ambulatory care includes knowledge of ethnic group physical/biological normative differences, risks to optimal health that are associated with the targeted ethnic group, and skills in interventions for these particular areas. This means incorporating epidemiological data as a means to tailor the assessment to the family, a standard borrowed from role expectations of the public health nurse (Salmon, 1989).

Indicators of community/ethnic group health important to nursing of families must go beyond incidence and prevalence of disease to data on social and behavioral factors that impact health, such as educational attainment, housing conditions, and family composition. For example, the current research shows that for Alaska Natives risks to health are greatest in the area of violent death (including suicide) and preventable injuries (Mohatt, McDiarmid, & Montoya, 1988).

Multiple goals for assessment that include biophysical and psychosociocultural aspects of family health require interpretations of meaning for the family as central to the data-gathering process. The practitioner's success depends in part on the familiarity of the nurse with the cultural meanings and symbols specific to the client and the family, which may include knowledge of another language. A novice would do well to seek the advice of a culturally astute person in order to conduct a sound assessment.

In relation to the content of the *interview* of the client alone or with other family members present, the first task entails ascertaining the family structure itself: Who in fact is considered to be a family member? Inquiry about the family structure should extend beyond household members to those relatives who live nearby and to those with whom contact is frequent. Outward appearance of conformity to a life-style of the dominant culture does not necessarily exclude the presence of a nondominant culture family pattern, such as extended family support and interaction, as I found in a study with a sample of Alaska Native parents in Anchorage, who otherwise seemed highly acculturated (Sprott, in press). Other areas for inquiry involve questions typically asked in the health assessment interview (see Table 20.1).

Content issues related to *formal assessment instruments* for use in cross-cultural settings are too complex to treat in any depth here. One question, however, is deserving of comment because it is so frequently asked: Is it valid to assess an ethnic group on an instrument normed only on Anglo middle-class samples? As a general rule, if Lesson 1 of this chapter is taken seriously, a truly culturally context-free instrument is an impossibility. If certain precautions are taken, however, it is reasonable to employ an existing instrument with established reliability and validity. Those precautions include consideration of linguistic, functional, and conceptual equivalence (that words and the behavioral phenomena being compared have the same function and meaning in the societies being studied), as well as psychometric equivalence (a complex of issues that pertain to test construction itself; Irvine & Carroll, 1980; Poortinga, 1975).

Merely establishing in a pilot study that a sample of nondominant culture representatives can read English well enough to complete a standardized instrument does not constitute an adequate appraisal. In such instances respondents are unlikely to volunteer comments on difficulties that they may have in understanding the intent of questions, as few persons of any culture wish to appear ignorant. They even may elect to have fun by marking the most outrageous responses (Lonner & Berry, 1986).

Another issue related to content is the caution that practitioners become too preoccupied with knowledge of the "ideal" culture or normative descriptions of cultural groups via trait lists, only to fall into the trap of stereotyping families or clients (Sue & Zane, 1987; Tripp-Reimer & Fox, 1990). Sue and Zane (1987) wrote that "no knowledge of their [minority]

Table 20.1 Questions for Use in the Health Appraisal of Family Members for Culturally Relevant Assessments

1. What is the health status of each family member? What composes the family medical and social history, including recent major stress events, nutrition, individual recreation/ work patterns, habits, sleep patterns, participation in religion, and the quality of social contact and support?
2. What are the goals of the family as a unit and for individual members for health and well-being? What dreams do they hold for the future? What are the perceived barriers to accomplishing those goals? Do they work together or separately to reach these goals? In what way do they envision the health care practitioner as a resource to aid them in attaining their goals?
3. With what ethnic group (or groups) does the family as a whole or as individuals identify? Which ethnic traditions impact their health status? How does ethnic identity impact the decision-making processes of the family?
4. How do family members interact, and are they satisfied with those interactional patterns for recreation, mealtimes, chores, child care, and other family-oriented responsibilities?

culture is detrimental; however, even with this knowledge, its application and relevance cannot always be assumed because of individual differences among members of a particular ethnic group" (pp. 38-39). The advantage of bringing to the foreground the family interactional milieu as the critical context for assessment of family members' health and well-being means that culture trait lists and cultural normative data become relegated to the background, as necessary but not central in the assessment.

Bearing more on process concerns is the issue of the assumption underlying the literature on nursing of culturally diverse clients that the practitioner is "on her own" in the complex process of assessment and planning (other than in collaboration with the family itself). Being knowledgeable about a single culture other than one's own is a formidable enterprise; what greater task for those who work in large urban centers like San Francisco who may see clients of many different ethnic groups! And further, how "culturally competent" is the nurse to judge the client's behavior as adaptive, neutral, or harmful, a responsibility cited often as part of the intervention planning process (Tripp-Reimer et al., 1984)?

I believe that we should employ a different lens to view the efficacy of health or illness beliefs or behaviors of clients. Although devised to assess whether a child-rearing practice within an ethnic group constitutes harm, Korbin's (1977) schema to evaluate cultural "contextual factors" seems relevant to the evaluation of potential physical/psychological harm to family members of health practices in general. The behavior is not considered to be harmful if the following conditions are met: (a) The behavior in question actually reflects a sanctioned practice of that culture, (b) it falls within the limits of (behavior and) deviation acceptable in that culture, (c) the intent of the responsible caretaker is consistent with cultural "rules" governing the practice, (d) it is the perception of the child (person) that this is an appropriate practice in the situation, and (e) the practice is important in the development of the child (person) as a member of the culture (Korbin, 1977, p. 11).

We may benefit also from the advice of cross-cultural psychologists Sue and Zane (1987), who urged the hiring of bilingual/bicultural personnel in designated mental health facilities to provide culturally appropriate treatment with the aim of improving the documented dismal dropout rates of minority clients. They cited recommendations of the Special Populations Task Force of the President's Commission on Mental Health (1978) that "services to be provided for the special populations should be delivered, again with a view toward the best possible of worlds, by persons *who share the unique perspective, value system and beliefs of the group being served*" (p. 732).

Notwithstanding the belief that with specialized cross-cultural education in transcultural nursing nurses can attain high skill levels in provision of culturally sensitive care, few such specialty programs exist at the graduate level, and little emphasis is placed on cultural diversity at the undergraduate level in the majority of nursing schools. In a climate that reflects perhaps on our own ethnocentrism as a profession, we must think of alternative strategies. At the very least, could we not study the efficacy of forging a clinical partnership with key informants/cultural advocates as a transitional measure until more minorities are recruited into the profession?

Cultural advocates could be a valuable resource to disentangle the nuances of meaning of family behavior of their specific cultural group that might take years for the novice to appreciate. The NP/cultural advocate team periodically could tape and critique practitioner/family interactions at a clinic visit and exchange ideas to improve approaches and to clarify cultural miscommunication. Spinoffs of such a collaboration might include increased visibility of minorities as role models for others and increased interest in the pursuit of a career in nursing.

The *collaboration* concept is not meant to replace the hard work that it takes by the nurse to learn about and understand another culture in depth. For practitioners in relatively large institutions that provide services to clients from a myriad of cultural backgrounds, individual staff members could elect to concentrate on one of the majority groups, including learning the language of that culture. Working with the cultural advocate of that group, the nurse could act as the designated primary care provider for that group and could serve as a resource to other providers. Periodic in-service education on aspects of each culture could be presented by staff members to share experiences and expertise.

In summary this chapter presented three basic lessons from anthropology that provide a systems-based framework for the assessment of culturally diverse families. A critique of the extant approaches for cultural assessment was made to determine their suitability for the health promotion context of care provided by nurse practitioners in clinic visits. Alternative/reframed guidelines for content and process in interviewing were offered. A main thesis of the chapter was that focus on the family structure, function, and processes puts the level of analysis where the "action is" and places the biophysical/cultural norms and epidemiological data where they belong—in the background. Last, an alliance of the nurse practitioner with a translator/cultural advocate was suggested as a means to enhance exchange of cultural knowledge and to provide a more vital dialogue and meaningful assessment.

21

Family Nursing Research:
A Feminist Critique

Mary M. Cardwell

As nursing's interest in families and nursing's production of research have increased, the number of studies related to families also has increased (Gilliss, 1989a). Although the volume of research has increased, we have not seriously questioned our conceptualizations of or our assumptions about families. This chapter explores some of our thinking about families, presents an overview of feminist critique of research, analyzes some current family nursing research studies, and then discusses several issues raised by the research analysis.

Nursing and Families

In light of the history of the United States, many of the views of its inhabitants about families reflect historical influences from England. Stark (1979) described Victorian England as a country with an ideology that worshiped the woman in the home. Women were viewed only as wives and mothers. Husbands had total power over their wives—their money, their property, their children, and even their bodies. This was the society in which Florence Nightingale lived. A radical in her own time, Nightingale (1852/ 1979) rejected the family as stifling the individual. She strongly opposed the position that women were supposed to take in the family and society. Nightingale was a humanitarian interested in the needs of the poor and the deprived in society, but she was explicitly antifamily in some of her writings and also chose not to support women's issues (Woodham-Smith, 1951).

In spite of Nightingale's views on the family, nurses frequently have worked with and supported families since the early part of the century, when nurses did private care in homes and then worked in community health settings. The family as a focus for research by nurses did not really begin until the mid-1970s. Feetham wrote the first review of family research for the *Annual Review of Nursing Research* in 1984 (Feetham, 1984). Gilliss (1989a) completed a 4-year review of family nursing research in the 1980s, and Hayes has updated that work in this volume (Chapter 3). Both Feetham (1984) and Mercer (1989) have reviewed some of the most influential family frameworks used in nursing. These include symbolic interactionism, developmental perspectives, systems approaches, social exchange theory, structural-functionalism, and ecological frameworks. Most of these frameworks originated in sociology or psychology. The major, as well as the founding, theorists within all of these frameworks have been white Euro-pean and American males (Poster, 1978). Although nursing has been trying to move family conceptualizations and research into nursing theory-based research, nursing has not actually questioned basic assumptions of these theories about the family in society.

One exception to this lack of inquiry is Allen's (1985) analysis of introductory textbooks in nursing in which he found that many of the authors assumed that somehow a natural phenomenon called "the family" exists, that the family has essential functions, that the family needs fixing, and that the family is somehow adaptive or homeostatic. He used feminist criticism to challenge some of these beliefs about families.

Feminist criticism can be quite helpful in identifying issues and contradictions in our thinking about families. Thus a feminist-based critical analysis of some current family research was completed to explore basic assumptions about families that underpin our knowledge development in nursing.

Feminism and Feminist Critique

Harding (1987a) defined *feminism* as "a political movement for social change" (p. 182). "All feminists are united by a commitment to improving the situation of women," according to Jaggar and Rothenberg (1984, p. xiv). Feminist research is distinctive in that it not only generates its problems from the perspective of women's experiences but also uses women's experiences as a significant indicator against which hypotheses are tested (Harding, 1987b). Feminist critique is a critical analysis that looks at whether women's experiences have been taken into account.

Feminists have advocated various approaches to research in order to better understand the situation of women. Duffy and Hedin (1988) described feminist research as based in horizontal relationships and shared decision making among those involved in the research. They believed that feminism makes two major contributions to science. First, women are treated as human beings and are not studied only within the context of their maternal and reproductive roles; second, feminist science incorporates subjective, as well as empirical, knowledge. Thompson (1987) suggested the following creed for family researchers: "Feminists strive to generate emancipatory knowledge, use nonoppressive methodology, and take a critical stance toward prevailing approaches as well as their own work" (p. 2).

Harding (1987b), one of the most influential scholars regarding the issues of feminism and science, proposed that the following three questions be used to identify examples of feminist research:

1. Are women's experiences used as the test of adequacy of the problems, concepts, hypotheses, research design, collection, and interpretation of data?

2. Is the research project for women; that is, is it done with and for women and not to or on them as subjects?

3. Does the researcher or theorist place herself in the same class, race, culture, and gender-sensitive critical plane as the participants in the study?

Harding (1987b) also stressed that feminism rejects the concept of *relativism*—the position that both men and women have equal and valid views. This position exemplifies the belief that by supporting views that are currently dominant and oppressive, we legitimize the continuation of androcentrism and the centrality of men's views. The questions proposed by Harding were used in the critical analysis of the nursing studies included in this research analysis.

Analysis of Family Studies in Nursing

A convenience sample of the 91 articles published in *Nursing Research* and *Research in Nursing and Health* during the 1988 calendar year was used. All of the studies were read to determine eligibility for analysis as a family study. Gilliss's (1989a) criteria were used for inclusion. These included research reports that addressed the family as a unit, a dyad within the family, or a particular family role enacted by a family member. Studies that focused on prenatal maternal attachment to the infant were included, but those that measured pain during labor were not. One study that compared life cycle transitions of mothers to nonmothers was included as a role enactment study, and a study that investigated the perceptions and stereotypes of nursing students related to marital status during pregnancy was included because of the information it added about nursing students' values and expectations regarding family form or structure. A total of 23 studies met these minimal criteria to be included as family studies.

The studies are summarized by type of research (Table 21.1), by content of the studies (Table 21.2), and by social demographic information (Table 21.3). None of the studies analyzed could be said to address the family as a unit. Two research reports regarding the same sample mentioned intergenerational support as a factor in maternal and paternal fetal attachment for certain groups of participants; otherwise none of the studies mentioned family members other than those in the nuclear family.

Most studies reported marital status as a demographic variable, whether or not that variable was related to anything else in the research report. Several studies required that the parents be living together or be committed to living together if not married. Perinatal studies included only mothers by a ratio of 2:1 over studies including fathers; and of the four studies related to illness of a spouse, all included predominantly males as the ill spouse except for one study that focused on women with breast cancer.

Because of the variability in reporting income and socioeconomic status, categorizing this information was difficult. It was estimated that six of the studies did include predominantly lower-income persons. Several of the studies not reporting racial/ethnic mix did indicate, however, that participants had high income levels. Most of the studies seemed to include predominantly well-educated persons.

In summarizing the findings, one could say that (a) nursing research with families generally focuses on a dyad in the family or on the performance of a role within the family, (b) perinatal concerns are of primary importance, (c) the nuclear family based on a heterosexual relationship is considered to be the norm, and (d) white, well-educated, middle- to upper-income families are sampled most frequently. After completing her review of nursing research, Gilliss (1989a) concluded that very little has been published on nontraditional families or on families from nondominant cultures.

Table 21.1 Type of Study

	%*	n
Dyads	57	13
Role enactment	26	6
Response to event or illness	9	2
Attitudes	9	2
		23

NOTE: *% are rounded off.

Table 21.2 Content of Studies

	%*	n
Perinatal	57	13
Ill spouse	17	4
Response to death or illness	9	2
Single categories	16	4
		23

NOTE: *% are rounded off.

Table 21.3 Social Demographics

	%*	n
Predominantly white participants (up to 100% of participants)	61	14
Predominantly black participants	9	2
Mixed sample	4	1
Racial/Ethnic mix not identified	26	6
		23

NOTE: * % are rounded off.

Additionally interactions between family groups and the community generally have been overlooked.

None of the research reports indicated that the studies had been used to help emancipate women or that the researcher had participated in a gender/class/race/cultural-sensitive plane with participants. If this did occur as part of the studies, it was not indicated in the research reports. No reports indicated that participants had participated in the analysis of the data or had been informed of the results of the study. In all studies in which both males and females participated, the input of males and females was included equally or the results were homogenized. Thus *relativism,* or a maintenance of androcentrism, was permitted. None of the studies met the criteria for feminist research.

Issues for Discussion

Three major issues emerged from this analysis of family research in nursing: (a) the emphasis on the nuclear family, (b) women's reproductive and maternal roles, and (c) the low status of most women in society in relation to nursing research. Each of these will be discussed in relation to feminist literature.

The Nuclear Family

Nursing's endorsement of the traditional nuclear family as the "norm" is troubling from a feminist perspective. As was discussed earlier, most of our beliefs about families have evolved from the theories and practices of white European and American males. One of the contemporary insights in feminism is that the personal is political. Millett (1970) was one of the first contemporary feminists to make us aware that the activities in the bedroom and in the kitchen are related to the political activities in the society. Family life is no longer considered to be isolated from the beliefs and influences around it. Yet nursing research on families has viewed the family in an isolated way by focusing on the nuclear family or a family member without a context.

Many feminists have viewed the nuclear family as oppressive to women. The nuclear family is problematic for *liberal feminists* because women historically have been denied equal opportunity on the basis of traditional expectations for women in the family (Jaggar & Rothenberg, 1984). *Marxist feminists* have viewed women's oppression as located in the monogamous family because of the economic system that allows men to control the family's wealth. The Marxist view holds that the traditional nuclear family supports a capitalistic society (Jaggar & Rothenberg, 1984). *Radical feminists* see the heterosexual marriage as the primary institution through which men oppress women, while *socialist feminists* question the socialization of children in nuclear families. Some believe that exclusive female parenting in nuclear families perpetuates both capitalism and male dominance because of the sexually differentiated personality types that it produces. Women of color stress that families in various ethnic and class groups function differently from those of the mainstream in order for their

members to survive, and thus the traditional nuclear family is not representative of their experiences (Jaggar & Rothenberg, 1984). Regardless of their
philosophical position, most feminists agree that the nuclear family has
served to isolate women from other women, especially those from different
ethnic and class groups, and that it is through this isolation that male
dominance and control in society continue (Lipman-Blumen, 1984).

Both Barrett (1988) and Poster (1978) pointed out that the traditional
nuclear family is an ideology that has no cultural or biological basis. Multiple family forms have existed in many different places over time. Yet the
ideology of the modern nuclear family is so strong in our society that we
generally have assumed that what is good for the family is good for everyone in it (Goodrich, Rampage, Ellman, & Halstead, 1988).

Feminist criticism has identified several major issues that are ignored
when the focus of attention is on the nuclear family as a unit. Discussion
of two of these—denial of individual needs and changing family structures
follows.

Denial of Individual Needs

When the family unit is the focus of attention, individual needs become
secondary. A family focus usually assumes equality in the family, at least
equality between the spouses; yet women and children traditionally have
been oppressed in the modern family. Research on abuse indicates that in
the United States at least 1.8 million women are assaulted severely by their
partners and 6.9 million children are assaulted severely in their families
each year (Straus & Gelles, 1990). Abuse is so common that the typical
American woman is many times more likely to be assaulted in her own
home than anywhere else (Straus & Gelles, 1990).

In addition to the high risk of physical injury experienced by women and
children in families, marriage itself has been shown by some authors to be
detrimental to the mental health of women. Bernard (1982) concluded that
the psychological costs of marriage are considerably greater, and the benefits
considerably less, for wives than for their husbands. Through analyzing a
number of studies, she described the emotional and mental health of wives
as being dismal, "like a low-grade infection that shows itself in a number
of scattered symptoms" (Bernard, 1982, p. 37). Women "dwindle" into
being wives, redefining the self and actively reshaping the personality
to conform to the wishes or needs or demands of husbands (Bernard, 1982,
p. 39). Additionally Ross (1991) recently reported that, after adjusting for
differences in income, married women have the lowest sense of personal

control of any group among married and unmarried women and men, with unmarried women having the highest sense of control.

Yet although women report more marital stress than their husbands, they also report more overall marital satisfaction (Bernard, 1982). This seeming incongruity may be reflective of the intense pressure within our society for women to conform to expectations that one should get married (Bernard, 1982). Many women may judge themselves to be happy by definition; that is, being married is the ultimate ideal for women. Additionally women may evaluate themselves as having adjusted well to the demands of marriage, thus interpreting their adjustments as happiness (Bernard, 1982). For Ross (1991) marriage is a trade-off for women. Marriage increases household income, indirectly increasing a sense of control, while at the same time also decreasing women's sense of personal control, probably because of subordination, dependence, and lack of autonomy.

When we fail to question the belief that the nuclear family is the ideal family, we risk equating conformity with health. We frequently overlook the obvious and subtle power imbalances that often exist in these families. We ignore the effects of current family arrangements on individual family members, and we also overlook the growing number of families who no longer resemble the ideal nuclear family.

Changing Family Structures

A second major area of feminist criticism of the modern nuclear family is that it is used as a standard by which all other family forms are evaluated. The term *alternative* families means different from some accepted norm. Thus single-parent, lesbian, gay, multigenerational, or communal-type families all are considered to be different from "normal" families. Yet only 57% of all households in the United States are of the married-couple type (Rix, 1990). Using one ideology of the family as a standard sets up a hierarchy in which some are valued more than others.

The structure of the modern nuclear family has tended to focus the family inward toward self-reliance, stressing a strong bond between the husband and wife. Thus heterosexual bonding has been the primary force in these families. Although this has been thought of as a "natural" arrangement, Stacey (1986) has suggested that "one could argue that the breakdown of the conventional nuclear family has the capacity to generate communitarian behaviors and oppositional attitudes" (p. 223). Some are predicting that family forms currently labeled as "alternative" may be more functional than traditional nuclear families in the future (Gerber, Wolff, Klores, & Brown, 1989; Rapping, 1990).

Perhaps one reason the ideology of the nuclear family has remained so strong is that we still believe that our needs for intimacy and affection are met within the nuclear family. "Concern about the future of the family is often concern about the fate of care giving and nurturance, about values and needs denied and undermined by the fragmentation and impersonality fostered by capitalism" (Thorne, 1982, p. 19). If we were to focus on the diversity of ways in which persons can be supported and nurtured within the family, as well as outside the family, rather than assuming that certain family forms are better than others, we could begin to create a society in which everyone could benefit.

Women's Reproductive and Maternal Roles

A second issue identified in the critical analysis of family nursing research was the focus on women's reproductive and maternal roles. An interesting finding of this study was that 20% of the total sample of 91 research reports reviewed in this analysis focused on perinatal issues involving women—pregnancy, childbirth, and the immediate postpartal period. This percentage does not include studies that focused exclusively on infants. In addition, 57% of the family studies focused on the perinatal period. Gilliss (1989a) also found in her review that 55% of family studies focused on infants and their parents or the family during birth, with most of the studies addressing the mother-infant relationship. It is intriguing that although the perinatal period is such a relatively short period in women's lives, it is a major focus in nursing research.

In her review of women's health research in nursing, Woods (1988) found that only 3% of the studies dealt with older women, while 15% dealt with middle-aged women, and 69% dealt with young adult women. The other studies focused on women from several age groups, primarily young and middle-aged adults. The articles selected for review were from journals published in the United States.

Interestingly, Moody et al.'s (1988) analysis of published nursing research found that *Nursing Research,* a journal based in the United States, had the highest percentage of maternal-infant studies (19.2%), whereas the *Journal of Advanced Nursing,* a British journal, and the *International Journal of Nursing Studies* had the highest percentages of gerontology studies, 25% and 21% respectively. Thus cultural values may influence not only whether we study women but also may influence what it is that we study about women.

Nursing's focus on women's reproduction and maternal-infant attachment reinforces and may reflect an underlying belief in society that women are somehow closer to nature than are men. Reproduction and nurturing are natural for women but not for men. Ortner (1974) pointed out that in every culture women's physiology is seen as closer to nature than men's. How could this be when men are also part of the species? As a result of this view of women's physiology, women's social roles have become the traditional domestic ones, imposed on them by the men who have assumed control of the cultural processes. Ortner pointed out that even in cultures in which some of the deities have been women, women still have been controlled by men by use of taboos about what women are and are not allowed to do. Many of these taboos are related to menstruation, pregnancy, and lactation. "Nature" has been seen as something threatening and as something needing to be controlled. One need only look at the tremendous energy we as a society spend on reproductive issues to recognize that the control of women's bodies is still a major issue.

Nursing's continued high level of interest in and focus on that short period of time in women's lives when they become pregnant and bear an infant reinforces the belief in biological determinism, still a dominant view in our society. *Biological determinists,* or conservatives in regard to the family, take the traditional family as biologically given and attempt to defend on biological grounds the traditional divisions of labor between the sexes in which the woman's responsibility is domestic work and child care. The man's task is to protect his family from the outside world and to teach his offspring how to meet the world successfully. The biological determinists believe that a strong mother-child bond must be established right at the beginning of an infant's life (or even before birth, as the nursing literature now suggests?) and must be maintained for a child to have healthy mental development. Biological determinists have not explained why it is that men are biologically incapable of entering into primary bonds with children (Jaggar & Rothenberg, 1984). Is nursing as a profession reinforcing the status quo of women in our society through the research we do? Have we critically asked ourselves what our research means?

Low Status of Most Women in Society

"While families maintained by women today account for 16 percent of all families, they account for 48% of all poor families. Nearly 40% of the American poor are children, and over half of them live in female-headed families. Moreover, the poverty statistics for families headed by black and Hispanic women are even more bleak" (Sidel, 1986, p. xvi).

Nursing's acceptance of married, white, young, well-educated women as representative for advancing knowledge within the profession is racist, sexist, ageist, classist, and out of touch with the realities of most women's lives. Sidel (1986) has emphasized that while the economic conditions have improved for some women in our society, increasing numbers of women continue to slip into poverty and to survive at the barest levels. Well-educated nurses are among the privileged women in society. As a predominantly female discipline, nursing could lead the way in conducting research to improve the situation of women, and through them, entire families. So far we have not chosen to do so.

Conclusion

The purpose of this chapter was not to advocate that nursing abandon the care of families or the conduct of family research. Rather the intent has been to critically examine predominant assumptions within nursing related to families. This feminist-based critical analysis of family research has indicated that our research is reflective of views about women that help maintain the status quo rather than advocate for improvements in the situation of women.

Thompson (1987) proposed what she calls a more radical research agenda for generating emancipatory knowledge in social science. Components of this agenda include the following:

1. Feminists can help women comprehend their everyday lives and experiences and how their experiences are embedded in larger social, political, historical, and economic processes.
2. Feminists can chronicle women's active struggle and resistance, as well as their subordination and oppression.
3. Feminists can transform the knowledge in their discipline by rethinking basic concepts, theoretical frameworks, and orienting assumptions.
4. Feminists can provide a vision of the future by exploring sexual equality as a possible and desirable alternative to current arrangements (Thompson, 1987, p. 13).

What an exciting research agenda this could be for nursing!

22

Caregiver Stress in Families of Persons With HIV/AIDS

Marie Annette Brown

AIDS can devastate an individual's ability to care for him- or herself. To help the ill person remain at home and avoid institutionalization, family members are the key component for care and support of their loved one during the course of HIV disease. Families provide the foundation for society's response to the AIDS epidemic; they are called on to provide a wide range of assistance, from management of the ill person's finances to daily personal hygiene.

Literature on the family suggests that families are affected significantly by the health problem of an ill member (Gilliss, 1989c; Leahey & Wright, 1987a; Lewis, 1985). Even more profoundly affected is the person who assumes the primary caregiver role for a sick family member (Biegel, Sales, & Schulz, 1991; Gruetzner, 1988; Miller & Montgomery, 1990; Rabins, Fetting, Eastham, & Fetting, 1990; Sommers & Shields, 1987). Although negligible research has been conducted to date about the particular challenges

AUTHOR'S NOTE: This study was funded in part by a Biomedical Research Support Grant from the University of Washington School of Nursing and the Psi Chapter of Sigma Theta Tau. I gratefully acknowledge the generous contribution of time from the study participants, as well as from Gail Powell-Cope, in the conduct of the study.

for families of a loved one with HIV infection/AIDS, we may assume that the impact of HIV disease is equally significant. Certainly consumer-oriented books by family members of persons with AIDS dramatically attest to their suffering (Haque, 1989; Moffatt, 1986; Monette, 1988).

Although HIV infection currently is considered to be a life-threatening illness with an average life expectancy of approximately 2 years from time of Class IV (AIDS) diagnosis, more effective drug therapy has increased the expectation that HIV will become more like a chronic illness (Arno & Shenson, 1990; Miller, Turner, & Moses, 1990). Popular literature reflects, however, that Americans tend to view HIV as a "fatal illness" (Shilts, 1987). Therefore it is not surprising that consumer and clinical literature highlights the distress faced by families and significant others from the very beginning—at the time of their loved one's initial diagnosis (Eidson, 1988; Flaskerud, 1989). Some families become aware of the HIV infection diagnosis when the individual is healthy and asymptomatic. Many, however, must face the shock of the diagnosis concurrent with the reality of the patient's severe health crisis. It is not unusual for family members to be thrust into the caregiving role during an acute opportunistic infection when the person with AIDS (PWA) is very ill and needs emotional support, as well as concrete assistance in managing his or her care (Horowitz, 1985; Wilson, 1989).

The challenges for family caregivers have been well documented with frail elderly, Alzheimer's, and cancer patients. Although these difficulties usually are described as *caregiver burden* (Harper & Lund, 1990; Pruchno & Resch, 1989) or *caregiver strain* (Cantor, 1983; Nygaard, 1988), a variety of concepts and aspects of this phenomenon is used in the literature to elaborate the distress of family caregiving: caregiving stress (Baillie, Norbeck, & Barnes, 1988; Stephens & Kenny, 1989); stress effects (Bunting, 1989; Noelker & Poulshock, 1982); caregiving demands (Stetz, 1987, 1989); caregiving consequences (Horowitz, 1985); personal strains and negative feeling (Cicirelli, 1980); caregiving impact (Lawton, Kleban, Moss, Rovine, & Glieksman, 1989; Poulshock & Deimling, 1984); and caregiving burnout (Cline, 1990). Despite a lack of consensus of terminology in the family caregiving literature, this phenomenon of the stresses associated with the primary caregiving role includes the following important elements: emotional responses to the caregiver role, impact of caregiving on various life spheres, and difficulties performing caregiving tasks. Horowitz's (1985) review of literature on family caregivers of the frail elderly noted that the emotional strain of this role arises most often from families' concerns about the ill person's health and safety and subsequent changes in the relationship. Adverse effects (such as role alterations) in the various spheres of personal or family life from the impact of caregiving were noted as the second most common area of concern. Other potentially problematic areas identified in this literature review included financial concerns, difficulties encountered in performing the various caregiving tasks, compromises in caregiver health, and strains in the caregiver/care receiver relationship (Horowitz, 1985).

Literature about family caregivers of other populations of ill persons suggests various components of the emotional stress involved in providing care to a family member. Depression has been noted as a major problem among caregivers (Cohen & Eisdorfer, 1988; Moritz, Kasl, & Berkman, 1989). In addition many families experience anger (Yaffe, 1988), anxiety (Jones & Vetter, 1984), uncertainty (Stetz, 1989), and burnout (Maj, 1991). Cantor (1983) noted that the overriding problem for caregivers of the frail elderly was the emotional strain of dealing with the progressive deterioration of the patient. Hinds's (1985) study of caregivers of cancer patients noted that one-third of the families were coping poorly with providing care to their ill relatives because of the caregivers' unmet needs. Significant psychological concerns were identified in the areas of personal discomfort resulting from patient suffering, uncertainty about the disease, insecurity in providing physical care, and dealing with patient depression.

Families caring for loved ones with AIDS are often subjected to a kind of "guilt by association," as well as stigma, rejection, and/or harassment (Powell-Cope & Brown, 1992). Dealing with AIDS phobia and stigma simultaneously with the tremendous demands of caregiving may become overwhelming for family members (Moffatt, 1986). In addition, family members, as well as the PWA, are affected by the challenges of life-threatening illness and accompanying issues of death and loss, which can cause existential crisis, anxiety, and depression for both ill persons and caregivers alike (Flaskerud, 1989; Govoni, 1988). Extensive literature on psychosocial stresses of the PWA has documented common symptoms of fear, anxiety, and depression, as well as guilt, fear, anger, and suspicion (Christ & Wiener, 1985; Cohen & Weisman, 1986; Wolcott et al., 1986). Living with a person who has AIDS therefore often requires that lovers, spouses, and other family members respond to the PWA's emotional reactions, as well as deal with the psychological and social effects of family caregiving (Govoni, 1988; Tibler, 1987). In AIDS family caregiving, issues of communicability; the unpredictable illness trajectory of HIV infection; AIDS phobia and stigma; alternative, stigmatized life-styles; and multiple and premature losses can coalesce to place even more significant demands on families (Maj, 1991; Meisenhelder & LaCharite, 1989; Pearlin, Semple, & Turner, 1988).

This chapter describes the demands of family caregiving in the instance of HIV infection/AIDS. In this study *family* is defined broadly to acknowledge a variety of current family forms, to honor the commitments made in nontraditional relationships, and to include family of origin and family of choice. "Family" members may be related biologically (parent, sibling), by legally sanctioned marriage, by nonlegally sanctioned marriage (partner, significant other), or as a friend who performs primary caregiver functions.

Methods

Grounded theory (Glaser & Strauss, 1967; Strauss, 1987) provided the methodological basis for qualitative data generation and analysis and is described in more detail elsewhere (Brown & Powell-Cope, 1991). Theoretical sampling and constant comparative analysis were used to guide data collection and analysis. Interviews were tape-recorded and were transcribed verbatim. Validity and reliability of the data were addressed systematically through use of the criteria outlined by Sandelowski (1986) and Lincoln and Guba (1985): (a) truth value, (b) applicability, (c) consistency, and (d) neutrality. Member checks, debriefing by peers, triangulation, prolonged engagement with the data, persistent observation, and reflective journals were techniques used to ensure validity and reliability. During the final phases of analysis, focus groups of study alumni, family caregivers who did not participate in the study, and professionals and community volunteers working in the area of AIDS family caregiving were solicited for feedback.

Procedures

Participants were recruited from a variety of AIDS community sources, including clinics, support groups, a caregiver course, volunteer organizations, and a community newspaper. After consent was obtained, participants were asked: "What has it been like for you living with and taking care of someone with AIDS?" Relevant probes were used to gain further insight into issues raised. In addition an interview guide was used to ensure consistency of topics across interviews. Interviews were conducted in either one or two sessions, lasted a mean of 4.5 hours, and yielded over 200 hours of interview data. Confidentiality was maintained.

Sample

The sample consisted of 53 family caregivers of people with symptomatic HIV infection or AIDS. Approximately one-third (32%) were partners or lovers in gay relationships, 6% were partners or spouses in heterosexual relationships, 43% were friends (9% were former lovers), 13% were parents, 4% were siblings, and 4% were other family of origin. The parents included those of both adult and minor children with HIV/AIDS. Seventy-seven percent lived in the same household with the PWA, and 60% of the households also included other individuals such as the caregiver's partner, child, or housemate. Approximately two-thirds (64%) of the family caregivers were male, 36% female. Approximately two-thirds (68%) were gay or bisexual, 32% heterosexual. The sample ranged in age from 22-65, with a mean of 36. Fifty-seven percent had less than a college degree, and 92% were white. Fifty percent of the caregivers were employed full-time, 19% part-time outside the home. Family incomes (which supported an average of 1.9 persons) were low, with 18% reporting under $10,000, 41% between $10,000-20,000, 16% from $20,000-30,000, 16% from $30,000-40,000, and 9% over $40,000. In almost half (47%) of the families, the PWA had been diagnosed within the past 12 months. Eighty-four percent of the caregivers knew the PWA prior to the diagnosis of AIDS. The sample contained few ethnic minorities and a large number of caregivers of gay PWAs, thus reflecting the demographics of AIDS in the geographical area where the study was conducted (DSHS & Seattle-King County Health Department, 1990). Compared with family caregivers of people who had other health problems, this sample was younger and with a greater proportion of men, fewer spouses, and fewer members from families of origin.

Results

The data for this analysis are included in the category "Managing and Being Managed by the Illness," one aspect of the grounded theory study of AIDS family caregiving (Brown & Powell-Cope, 1991). *Managing and being managed by the illness* is defined as vigilantly monitoring the mercurial illness of HIV/AIDS and constantly responding to the demands and uncertainties associated with caregiving tasks. The experience of being managed by the illness reflected the part of this category that included caregivers' responses to the demands and challenges associated with their caregiving role.

Study findings suggested that the demands of caregiving seemed so pervasive that caregivers felt as if they were "being managed by AIDS." Caregivers reported multiple stresses in the course of caregiving for persons with AIDS. As a young man in his 20s who was caring for his partner reflected:

> This [caregiving] is the hardest thing I have ever done in my life. Nothing even prepared me for this. Sometimes I wonder if I'll ever recover.

Although study participants considered it their "job" as caregivers to keep the illness (AIDS) in a manageable state and to treat each symptom that the ill person experienced, they felt that they were not always the one in command. Sometimes it was as if the tables were turned and the illness had taken complete control of the caregiver's life. One family member talked about this perception:

> I didn't feel like I was in control. I felt like times and events were controlling my life instead of my being able to manipulate my life. I was being manipulated. Sort of like a puppet, a marionette. Yeah, I've been bombarded with this over the last 2½ years, and it's painful.

For most families, taking care of their loved ones with AIDS was not simply an important aspect of their lives, it became their lives. One family member related his realization that AIDS had essentially taken over his life:

> Recently I went out for the first time in a very, very long time and I had a flash: "Oh, I haven't thought about AIDS for an hour and a half now." And that's a long time not to think about AIDS . . . I dream about AIDS.

Overall, the caregiver's perception of "being managed by the illness" provided a foundation on which the stresses of AIDS family caregiving were built.

Emotional Responses to the Caregiver Role

Although the extent to which the family caregiver felt managed by the illness depended on the style of the caregiver, as well as on the needs of the PWA, most individuals experienced considerable emotional strain from the demands of caregiving. Some participants described this demand in general terms such as "difficult," "hard," or "stressful," while others detailed specific emotions. One family member summarized her struggle:

I'm spinning up on top, but I'm barely holding on and so that scares me. But it's just that it's so incredibly demanding.

Despite caregivers' enormous amount of work to manage the illness, as the months progressed and the demands of caregiving increased, many family members found that the relentlessness of the demands became an increasing source of strain. One middle-aged businessman who eventually quit his job to take care of his ill partner explained the all-consuming nature of this role:

Other people who are in a caregiving setting in a hospital, they can shut it off after 8 hours. I can't ever shut it off; I have no way of ever shutting it off. I'm not sure I'd wish to if I could, but I have to live with it 24 hours a day, 7 days a week. If there were only some way of getting other folks to be able to cross that threshold and see what it's like—that there is no easy way of doing this.

Caregivers reported that sometimes the feeling of "never being able to do enough" contributed to their perception of being managed by the illness. Many family members, like this man caring for his life partner, viewed this disease as complex and exhausting, making constant demands on their strength:

It [caring for a person with AIDS] has its ups and downs, and it's really hard. Especially when they really never get better. If it's not one thing, it's something else and you're in and out of the hospital and you almost lost him one time and then they're back and if it isn't, you know, diarrhea, it's skin infection, if it isn't that his kidney stops working, if it isn't that it's this. I mean, it's always something.

This source of stress is intensified when, despite the caregivers' best efforts, they were unable to obtain positive results. One mother talked about her discouragement:

But if it's in the situation where he's not getting better and there's nothing you can do and he feels bad all the time, then that's what's so very hard.

Sometimes the frustration of being unsuccessful about "making a difference" in the PWA's health was coupled with anger and disappointment with the ill person's response to the caregiving activities. One woman, whose brother had moved in with her after he could no longer live alone, spoke of her frustration:

I work very hard on something and it doesn't taste good to him and I'm just angry at the situation . . . you try to give him some good information or something the doctor has said and they don't want to hear it. You're trying to do the right thing for them and sometimes nothing is right. It's frustrating.

This helplessness and frustration often escalated into anger, a reaction especially difficult for caregivers to accept and manage. Caregivers directed this anger toward a variety of different targets: other family members, friends, health care providers, "the system," and so forth. One common target, particularly with caregivers in the gay community, was the government's ineffectual response to the AIDS epidemic, which most caregivers attributed to homophobia. The health care system's and health care providers' lack of knowledge and uninformed approach to patient care was also a significant target for caregivers' anger, as this middle-aged teacher noted:

I'm furious at the federal government and the basic failure to deal with the drug possibilities . . . and there are other drugs . . . and another one of the things I am angry about is that not enough health care professionals know about this.

Another caregiver agreed:

It makes me angry at this disease, and it makes me angry that so far in all the massive research nothing has come about to alleviate it in any real tangible light.

Depression was the most commonly reported emotional reaction among family members. Even caregivers who did not report current depression had no difficulty recalling episodes of depression. One mother reported how the depression brought on by caregiving had affected her life:

Well, in terms of my emotional stability, of course it [caring for a PWA] has affected it. I had several bouts of deep depression, and when I get depressed I'm one of these people that sleep—my escape.

Another man talked about his partner getting sicker, his escalating caregiving demands, and his increasing depression:

This whole thing is a mess. . . . It [caregiving] does certainly take the edge off a kind of joy, I mean I have been very depressed and it's getting worse.

Anticipatory grief was also apparent as caregivers acknowledged the eventual death of their loved ones. The sources of caregivers' depression was not only death of the PWA but also the potential horrors associated with dying of AIDS. A middle-aged professor expressed his emotional response about the fear and depression associated with the impending death of his lover:

> No matter how well he does, we're dancing on the edge. We're on that edge and it's very scary. While I've always known that, I haven't realized that my system was also knowing that at a very deep level and it was basically making me very depressed.

Many caregivers, however, had difficulty contemplating the future, which they viewed pessimistically. One father reflected on his concern and uncertainty about the future of his young adult son:

> Truly I don't know how he's going to do and . . . I do worry about that and it is a burden, a psychological burden that we're never free of.

In addition the life-style changes and other losses experienced by caregivers also were associated with sadness and depression. Another father discussed his feelings about his 9-year-old son's illness and how it had affected their entire family and had devastated them financially:

> I call it going out and feeling sorry for myself and it sounds really self-centered, but yeah, there are a lot of things in my life that are not very good right now. You know, involved with his illness, and it bothers the heck out of me. It makes me very sad and makes me very angry.

Study participants reported depression, sadness, and isolation, which came together to form a particular kind of loneliness. Families affected by AIDS usually felt very isolated, in part due to the secrecy and selective disclosure that often surrounded the AIDS diagnosis. Some families simply felt the uniqueness of their situation as compared with others in their social network. A mother caring for her young adult son stated:

> I get resentful and a little envious of friends whose kids are all healthy. Nobody else was going through this but us, you know. Everybody else is just going on with their lives. Why doesn't everything just stop because my son is sick? And there's nothing I can do.

Even when friends were aware of the situation, AIDS family caregivers reported that others simply did not "understand" the incredible difficulty of their situation. For one partner caregiver, the comments of a co-worker and friend pointed out to him other people's lack of empathy:

> Somebody said something to me the other day which really hurt me. I said to her, "It's amazing how stressed out I have been over Mike's illness, and when he's been away for this past week, how stressless I have been." And she said to me, "Well, you only bring it upon yourself. The stress you bring out is because you're just so involved." And it hurt me, because she doesn't know what it's like to live with somebody who's got a terminal illness. She has no idea.

Impact of Caregiving on Various Life Spheres

For most study participants, virtually all spheres of their lives were affected. Employed caregivers reported less energy for work, as well as strain associated with balancing caregiving with the demands of a job. A 30-year-old man struggled to maintain his work as a bank teller while being "on duty" day and night to help his lover:

> He went into hysterics and I couldn't calm him down, and I finally made the decision that we were going to the hospital, and I stayed with him for 12 whole hours in the emergency room while they decided what they were going to do with him. Then they didn't have a bed available, so I took him back home and waited 24 hours and they finally had a space for him so I brought him back. That 48 hours was probably the worst I've spent yet, and I told him I wouldn't leave him, and in fact at one point I had to call work because I hadn't had any sleep and I was gonna try to get about 2 hours and then go back into work.

Caregivers reported that the additional tasks and time demands associated with caregiving narrowed daily activities to only the most essential. Hobbies, recreation, relaxation, and other "quality of life" activities significantly diminished or disappeared. One caregiver, whose lifeblood had been politics and social action, replaced those activities with evenings at home watching television to provide companionship for his ill partner. He talked about the toll that this compromise had taken on him:

> It's difficult. It's a drag. I mean, I have a lot of zest for life and there are a lot of things I want to do, a lot of passion for life . . . It's difficult to have to devote so much time and energy to something that's actually so negative.

Difficulties Performing Various Caregiving Tasks

The requirements of providing care for someone with AIDS, a disease with complex, often frightening, confusing, or overwhelming symptoms, could push caregivers to their limits. Often the pressures on caregivers centered on how the large amount of day-to-day caregiving activities could take a toll on individuals. A middle-aged woman described the constant demands of providing care for her husband:

> He's tired all the time, he can't make his own food half the time, and he gets sick like that, and when he does, whether he's in the hospital or not, it takes constant brainpower. You're constantly thinking and worrying about him, and having to bring him things, and help him speak with the doctors, and just work everything out.

Managing the PWA's dementia was particularly stressful for most caregivers. One man talked about feeling overwhelmed by new symptoms of dementia that took away his partner's ability to communicate normally:

> He woke up one morning and I realized he was not relating the way he had, all he could do was repeat back to me what I had said . . . and I sort of lost it and I called a friend up in a terrible panic and he came over. I basically couldn't deal with the situation. . . . I think I was too close and it was too upsetting.

Another symptom that was particularly difficult for caregivers to manage was the PWA's depression. Study participants noted that living with someone who was depressed frequently was stressful and tended to potentiate any depression that the caregiver might be feeling. One brother faced the challenge of keeping the PWA's depression from negatively affecting his own health:

> It's very hard to deal with a person who's very depressed constantly in terms of getting them motivated to do things for themselves or whatever. I've had major hassles about things like are they gonna take drugs or how to deal with extended states of depression and how it affects other kinds of functioning.

Finding ways to help the PWA deal with his or her depression could be difficult. Caregivers usually realized, however, how potentially destructive depression was for the PWA's physical health and ability to continue self-care. Some study participants encouraged the PWA and his or her physician to consider antidepressive medications, while others tried various "cheer up" activities to motivate the PWA to engage in life more actively.

In some situations the stresses associated with caregiving, whether that was managing the PWA's way of dealing with his or her illness or the tasks of caregiving, became more than the caregiver could tolerate. One study participant, who assumed the role of family caregiver for an ill neighbor whose family of origin had abandoned him, said that the stress became so great that he eventually withdrew from caregiving:

> This was dangerous to my health. It was frustrating. Because of the stress and obviously as a recovering alcoholic I can't be involved with people that are abusing drugs or alcohol. His life-style, his untruthfulness and things like that caused me to become extremely stressed. In fact, it caused a relapse in my recovery. I feel guilty [about leaving him]. He's a lonely man, and he's a sick lonely man. But, I also know I have to take care of myself and with my health status [HIV positive], I can't deal with stress. I mean I shouldn't have to deal with stress . . . so I feel I've made the right decision.

Discussion

Study findings lend support to current conceptualizations of challenges faced by families as they care for ill or disabled members suffering from a variety of health problems. These qualitative data highlight the particular demands surrounding caring for family members with HIV infection as a devastating, life-threatening illness. These demands were extensive and pervaded all aspects of caregivers' lives, leading them to feel as if they were "being managed by AIDS." The sources of these demands included (a) the pain of loss, (b) the pressures of an altered relationship between the caregiver and the care receiver, and (c) the stigma and potential danger of HIV joined with all the mental, physical, and emotional work of managing the sick person's illness on a daily basis. An in-depth analysis of these sources of demands is presented elsewhere (Brown & Powell-Cope, 1991, 1992; Powell-Cope & Brown, 1992). This chapter focused on the caregiver's experience of the emotional stress associated with these demands.

Study findings parallel caregiver responses noted in predominantly quantitative research on family caregivers of other populations. The intensity of the emotional responses reported by these families was particularly striking. Although emotions ran the entire gamut of possibilities, depression, frustration/anger, and sadness were the most common emotions reported by study participants. The relentless nature of these stresses intensified the families' perceived strain of their caregiving work. Stress arose from three major areas previously identified in Horowitz's (1985) review of family caregivers for the elderly: (a) emotional response to the caregiving role, (b) impact of caregiving on various life spheres, and (c) difficulties performing various caregiver tasks. One example of a difficulty in caregiver tasks surrounded the PWA's depression and the caregiver's attempts to minimize its deleterious and often "contagious" effects on the family.

Coping with the extensive demands of AIDS family caregiving required considerable energy, time, and commitment that often go unrecognized and unsupported. Family members are not commonly included as a primary target for nursing intervention for PWAs. These data reflect a significant need for clinical therapeutics designed to provide direct support to AIDS family caregivers to enable them to better cope with the stresses of their role and to continue to provide urgently needed home care for persons with HIV/AIDS.

23

The Health of Homeless Mothers and Their Children

Edna M. Menke

Janet D. Wagner

Homelessness is a national social problem affecting many families. Some children are born into homeless families; other children experience homelessness as a result of a change in their family of origin. The largest growing group is children living with their mothers, who comprise over 30% of the homeless; however, little research has focused on these families (Bassuk & Rubin, 1987; Institute of Medicine, 1988; Natapoff & Essoka, 1990; Rosenman & Stein, 1990). Homeless mothers and children in a nation of affluence and opportunity have become a politicized issue that has received a great deal of media attention. Myths that the homeless are different from the rest of the population have obscured the paucity of facts as homeless families continue to be shrouded in mystery (Bachrach, 1987; Kozol, 1988; Wagner & Menke, 1991).

A homeless family often is headed by a woman who has at least two children to support (Bassuk & Rubin, 1987; Institute of Medicine, 1988).

AUTHORS' NOTE: This study was funded by Ohio Department of Mental Health Grant Number 89.1019.

Such mothers are likely to be African American or from another ethnic minority group (Rossi, 1989). Eviction for nonpayment of rent, overcrowding, and interpersonal conflict are the most commonly cited precipitating reasons for their homelessness (Bassuk, Rubin, & Lauriat, 1986). Homeless families that include two parents are more likely to be white and to live in rural areas (Institute of Medicine, 1988). Homeless families usually are isolated and have impoverished social support networks (Institute of Medicine, 1988; Wagner & Menke, 1991). Few researchers have studied homeless families. Some researchers have included homeless women as subjects (Merves, 1986; Roper & Boyer, 1987; Roth, Bean, Lust, & Saveanu, 1985), but children, the mother-child dyad, or homeless families have been virtually ignored (Gewirtzman & Fodor, 1987; Kozol, 1988). Only three studies have reported on the health status of homeless children and their mothers staying in shelters (Bassuk & Rosenberg, 1988; Bassuk & Rubin, 1987; Boxill & Beaty, 1990).

The homeless are at greater risk for physical illness, mental health problems, and social incompetence by virtue of the added stress of street life (Hopper & Hamberg, 1984). Few researchers have focused on the health status of the homeless. Most studies have used primarily homeless males as subjects and have included only small numbers of homeless females. An exception to this is a national study by Wright (1987), in which approximately 30% of the subjects were women and children; 15% of the children had chronic health problems. Other studies have found similar incidence of chronic health problems in homeless children (Bassuk et al., 1986; Hu, Covell, Morgan, & Arcia, 1989; Wagner & Menke, 1988). No consensus exists regarding the incidence of psychopathology in the homeless (Wright & Weber, 1987). Even though the mental health status of homeless women has been studied less than that of men, their psychiatric problems are thought to be more severe and complex (Crystal, 1984).

Most of the information concerning homeless children and their families has been generated by anecdotal impressions rather than by systematic empirical observation. Information about homeless families has been inferred from research on groups who have suffered components of the homeless experience, for example, those who have migrated, moved, or lost their homes (Gewirtzman & Fodor, 1987). The application of these findings to homeless children is questionable.

In only one study was the mental health of homeless children living in shelters considered (Bassuk et al., 1986). In another study of families living in shelters or in temporary housing, mothers linked aggressiveness, anxiety, and sadness to their children's immediate responses to homelessness;

however, the mothers believed that the homeless experience would not have any permanent ill effects on their children (Wagner & Menke, 1988).

Purpose

The purpose of this study was to examine the health of homeless children and their mothers. The research objectives were as follows:

1. To determine the developmental status of homeless children
2. To determine the mental health of homeless children and their mothers
3. To ascertain the health status and health care practices of homeless children and their mothers

Framework for the Study

The ecological model of the family interacting with the environment guided the study (Andrews, Bubolz, & Paolucci, 1980; Feetham, 1991a). The emphasis was on ascertaining the health of the individual homeless family members, because if one family member experiences a health problem, the entire family system is affected. This perspective is congruent with the model developed by Berne, Dato, Mason, and Rafferty (1990) to address the health needs of homeless families. Their model was derived from Pesznecker's (1984) adaptational model of poverty, in which the individuals/family develop health-promoting or health-damaging behaviors in response to the stressors associated with poverty.

Methods

A descriptive cross-sectional research design was used to study homeless children and their mothers. Human subject approval was obtained from the institutional Behavioral and Social Sciences Human Subjects Review Committee. A *family* was defined as a mother who had at least one child staying with her. Additional children and the child's father or another male father figure could be with the homeless mother. The rationale for limiting the definition to a mother and at least one child was that many homeless families are female headed (Sidel, 1986).

Sample/Procedure

A power analysis indicated that a sample of at least 250 children would be needed for an effect size of .50 with power of .80 (Cohen, 1989). A family was considered homeless if they were living on the streets; in automobiles, abandoned buildings, shelters or missions, or cheap hotels; or staying with family, friends, or other individuals or in another situation where the intended stay was 45 days or less (Roth et al., 1985). The child had to be under 12 years of age and living with the mother. No more than two children from one family could participate. If more than two children met the criteria, the investigators randomly selected which children would participate.

Homeless families were recruited from seven agencies that provide shelter and services to the homeless, two soup kitchens, and a community settlement house in a large Midwest metropolitan city. In addition the investigators walked the streets and parks in the downtown area in an attempt to locate homeless families who might not use soup kitchens or agencies that help the homeless. Contact was made with potential subjects to ascertain whether the woman and any of her children met the study criteria. If they met the study criteria, the study was explained to the mother and her child(ren). When the mother and her child(ren) were willing to participate, the mother was asked to sign a consent form, and her children over 7 years of age were asked to give assent.

Instrumentation

Data were obtained from both the mother and her child(ren). The mother participated in a tape-recorded interview and completed some standardized questionnaires regarding herself and the child(ren) who were subjects. For subjects under 6 years of age, the Denver Developmental Screening Test was administered. For subjects over 2 years of age, the mother completed the Child Behavior Checklist. Each child over 7 years of age completed the Children's Depression Inventory.

The *Homeless Children Interview Schedule-Mother's Version* was developed by the investigators (Wagner & Menke, 1988). It consists of 90 questions regarding the family and the family's experience of being homeless. The interview schedule was reviewed by several experts on homelessness to establish content validity and was pretested with several homeless mothers prior to being used in this study.

The *Denver Developmental Screening Test* was used to measure developmental status in children under the age of 6 years (Frankenburg, Dick,

& Carland, 1975). This is the most widely used test in pediatric practice that has been shown to have predictive validity in terms of later school problems (Sturner, Green, & Funk,1985).

The *Child Behavior Checklist* was used to assess the mental status of children over the age of 2 years. The tool has reported reliabilities ranging from .74-.92 and has been associated with treatment outcomes (Achenbach & Edelbrock, 1983; Achenbach, Edelbrock, & Howard, 1987).

The *Children's Depression Inventory* was used to assess depression in children over the age of 7 years. Test-retest reliability coefficients have ranged from .50-.84 (Kovacs, 1985). In this study the Cronbach alpha coefficient was .83.

The *SCL-90-R* was used to obtain data regarding the mental health status of the mother (Derogatis, 1983). The reported reliabilities have ranged from .77-.90 for the subscales and a Cronbach alpha of .95 for the total scale (Derogatis, 1983). In this study the Cronbach alpha coefficient for the total scale was .98, and the Cronbach alpha coefficients for the subscales ranged from .74-.89.

Data Analysis

Data from the tape-recorded interviews were transcribed by using *Ethnograph* software. The investigators and research associate analyzed the transcriptions separately until interrater reliability had been established prior to analyzing all of the tapes. The data from the interviews were quantified in regard to mental health, physical health, and health care practices. Descriptive and inferential statistics were used to analyze the data. An alpha level of .05 was used to ascertain any statistically significant results.

Results

The sample consisted of 160 mothers with 251 children. Ninety-seven (66.9%) of the families had been homeless less than 3 months, and only 20 (12.5%) of the families had been homeless longer than a year. The mothers attributed being homeless to a variety of reasons, including being evicted, loss of shared housing, deciding to leave the situation, and loss of employment. Sixty-three (39.4%) of the families were staying in shelters, 41 (25.6%) were in cheap hotels, 20 (12.5%) were staying with relatives or another family, 19 (11.9%) were in agency apartments, and 14 (68.6%) were staying in churches overnight. Only 2 (1.4%) families reported living on the streets.

Thirty-five (21.8%) of the families had a relative who was or had been homeless.

The number of individuals in the family ranged from 2-12, with the mean being 3.94 (sd = 1.48) members. The number of children in the family ranged from 1-11, with the mean being 2.47 (sd = 1.47) children. The mothers ranged in age from 16-43 years of age, with a mean of 27.43 years (sd = 4.92). In regard to ethnicity, almost two-thirds (n = 102, 63.8%) of the families were African American, 46 (28.8%) were white, and 12 (7.4%) were biracial, Asian, or Hispanic. Seventy (43.8%) families had a father figure who was the biological father, stepfather, or a male cohabiting with the mother and children. In 90 (50.3%) of the families, the mother did not report an adult male as part of the family structure.

The 251 child subjects ranged in age from 2 weeks to 12 years, with a mean age of 4.51 years (sd = 3.63). The sample was almost equally divided between females (n = 121, 48.2%) and males (n = 130, 51.8%). The majority (n = 157, 62.5%) of the child subjects were African American. Fewer than half (n = 106, 42.7%) of the children had a father figure living with them. Only five (4%) of the school-aged children did not attend school.

Children's Developmental Status

Data from the Denver Developmental Screening Test (DDST) were used to ascertain the children's developmental status. Table 23.1 presents the children's DDST results. A subject must pass all four categories in order to bypass additional assessment for a development lag. Seventy (45%) of the 157 children, who were under 6 years of age, had scores on the DDST that indicated the need for additional screening to ascertain the presence of a developmental lag. The Chi-square statistic was used to ascertain any statistically significant differences for the children's scores on the DDST and some variables. These variables were the child's ethnic background, the child's gender, the child's age, the length of time homeless, where the family was staying, the mental health status of the mother, and the presence of a father figure in the family structure. No statistically significant differences were found for the Denver Developmental Screening Test scores and any of the variables.

Mental Health

Data from the interviews with the mothers, the Child Behavior Checklist, the Children's Depression Inventory, and the SCL-90-R were used to ascertain the children's and mothers' mental health status. Mothers reported

Table 23.1 Homeless Children's Denver Developmental Screening Test Results

Category	Pass		Not Pass	
	Number	Percentage	Number	Percentage
Personal/Social	138	88	19	12
Fine motor	110	70	47	30
Language	121	77	36	23
Gross motor	132	84	25	16
Total test	87	55	70	45

that eight (4%) of the children had a diagnosed mental health problem and that four of these children had been hospitalized for a mental health problem.

Data from the Child Behavior Checklist and the Children's Depression Inventory indicated that some of the children might have mental health problems. The mean scores for the 143 children ages 2-12 years on the Child Behavior Checklist were within the normal limits (Table 23.2). A mean T score over 70 on the Child Behavior Checklist and/or a mean T score under 30 on the Social Competencies scales is indicative of possible behavioral problems requiring further evaluation (Achenbach & Edelbrock, 1983). Thirty-eight (27%) of the children had scores indicating that they should have additional evaluation for behavioral problems. Data from the Children's Depression Inventory were available for 76 of the children over 7 years of age. The mean score for these children was 10.73 ($sd = 7.57$). A score over 9 indicates that a child should have additional evaluation for depression (Kovacs, 1985). Thirty-five (46%) of the children had scores indicating that they were depressed or might be at risk for depression.

Analysis of variance and t-test statistics were used to ascertain any statistically significant differences for the children's scores on the Child Behavior Checklist and the Children's Depression Inventory. The variables used were the child's ethnic background, the child's gender, the child's age, the length of time homeless, where the family was staying, the mental health status of the mother, and the presence of a father figure in the family structure. No statistically significant differences were found for the total scores on the instruments and these variables. In addition, no relationship was found between the children's scores on the Children's Depression Inventory and the scores on the depression subscale of the Child Behavior Checklist ($r = .15, p = .24$) that the mother had completed about the child.

Sixteen (10%) of the mothers reported having mental health problems. Thirteen (8%) had been hospitalized for a mental health problem. The major-

Table 23.2 Homeless Children's Child Behavior Checklist Scores

Scale	Number	Mean T Score	Standard Deviation
Child Behavior Problems			
Total score	143	56.70	13.21
Internalizing	143	55.30	11.87
Externalizing	143	55.58	11.83
Aggressive	143	60.35	7.06
Somatic	143	59.54	7.68
Depression	143	59.91	8.17
Withdrawal	143	60.35	7.06
Social Competencies			
Total Score	105	38.19	11.50
Activities	105	42.63	9.90
Social	104	39.08	10.09
School	74	43.50	10.04

ity ($n = 106$) of the mothers' scores on the SCL-90-R scale indicated that they needed additional psychiatric evaluation. Twenty-seven (17%) of the mothers had sought help for drug abuse at some time in their lives.

Health Status and Health Practices

Data from the interviews with the mothers were used to ascertain the health status and health care practices of the homeless children and their mothers. Fifty-five (22%) of the children were perceived by their mothers as having a major health problem. The health problem that the largest number of children had was allergies ($n = 32$). Other health problems that were reported for over 5% of the children were asthma, bronchitis, and headaches. Seventy percent ($n = 175$) of the children had no health problems, 21% ($n = 54$) had one health problem, 4% ($n = 11$) had two health problems, 2.5% ($n = 5$) had three or four health problems, and data were unavailable for the other children ($n = 5$). Sixty-nine percent ($n = 173$) of the children had been to a physician or health clinic within the last 3 months.

Sixty-two (39%) of the mothers had a major health problem. Over 20% of the mothers had allergies, anemia, gynecological problems, and/or kidney problems. The average number of health problems for the mothers was 2.27 ($sd = 1.07$). Twenty percent ($n = 32$) of the mothers did not report having any health problems. Fifty-six percent ($n = 90$) of the mothers had one to three health problems, and 24% ($n = 38$) had four to eight health problems. One hundred (64%) of the mothers had been to a physician or a health clinic within the last 3 months. Eighty-two (51%) of the mothers reported drinking alcohol, and 114 (72%) reported smoking cigarettes.

Eighteen percent (*n* = 29) of the mothers were pregnant at the time they participated in the study. Sixty-two percent (*n* = 18) of the pregnant women were receiving prenatal care. Twelve of the pregnant women received prenatal care beginning in the first trimester, four in the second trimester, and nine were not receiving any prenatal care. Eleven of these women were drinking alcohol, and 20 were smoking during their pregnancy.

The mothers were asked whether they perceived a change in the health of their children and themselves since becoming homeless. Twenty-three percent (*n* = 37) of the mothers thought that their children's health had changed, and 41% (*n* = 66) perceived that their own health had changed. The kinds of changes were acute respiratory infections, anorexia, diarrhea, constipation, weight loss, and insomnia.

Discussion

The average number of children was 2.64 per homeless family, a figure similar to findings of other studies (Alperstein & Arnstein, 1988; Bassuk & Rubin, 1987). Fifty-six percent of the sample were female-headed families; this is suggestive of the feminization of poverty (Sidel, 1986). The ethnic breakdown of the families indicates that a majority of them were African American; this is different from the findings of other studies, which had a higher percentage of white families (Bassuk & Rubin, 1987; First, Toomey, & Rife, 1991). The length of time that the families had been homeless is similar to the findings of First, Toomey, and Rife (1991), who have studied the rural homeless in Ohio. A subgroup of their sample was 247 homeless families with children. In the urban study, a higher percentage were staying in shelters or temporary housing; in the rural study, a higher percentage (60% vs. 12.5%) were doubled up with another family.

The findings for the Denver Developmental Screening Test and the Children's Depression Inventory results are similar to those of Bassuk et al. (1986) for homeless children in the Boston area. The scores for the children on the Child Behavior Checklist differ from those of the Boston study, in which a higher percentage of children needed additional psychiatric evaluation. The incidence of health problems of children and their mothers are similar to the findings of a national study of the health of the homeless (Wright, 1987). A limitation of the study was that data were not obtained regarding when the health problem initially had been diagnosed. The fact that the majority of the families had been homeless for fewer than 3 months suggests that most of the major health problems existed prior to becoming homeless. Future research needs to document the onset of health problems to ascertain whether they occur prior to or after becoming homeless. Twenty-three percent ($n = 37$) of the mothers thought that their children's health had changed, and 42% ($n = 66$) perceived that their own health had changed. On the basis of these perceptions, many of the families are experiencing health changes since becoming homeless. The seriousness of these health changes needs to be assessed.

Data need to be obtained about what happens to the health of families after they become homeless. The empirical data have documented primarily acute episodes of illness where mothers have sought assistance in emergency rooms or clinics. Future research needs to follow children and their families after they become homeless to ascertain what occurs to their health. This research could be accomplished by tracking these families in clinics that provide services to the homeless.

Sixty-seven percent ($n = 106$) of the mothers had SCL-90-R scores indicating the need for additional psychiatric evaluation. In contrast 90% of the women in the Boston study had psychiatric problems (Bassuk & Rubin, 1987). Past investigators have indicated that a large number of homeless persons have chronic mental health problems and have not received treatment (Pittman, 1989). Even though the SCL-90-R scores indicated the need for case referral for additional evaluation, most of the subjects denied past treatment for emotional or mental problems, and all denied present involvement with the mental health system.

The findings indicate the need for further evaluation of the mental health status of homeless children and their families. The children should be evaluated for mental health problems that require intervention. In addition the mothers should be evaluated for mental health problems, including assessment for addictions. Access to services for the evaluation and treatment of health problems of homeless children and families needs to be available; for instance, providing health care at shelters, in the buildings where soup kitchens are located, or in the neighborhoods where the homeless congregate. Some model programs for the provision of care to the homeless have been developed by nurses and could be adapted to providing health care to homeless children and their families (Lindsey, 1989; Rafferty, 1989).

The school-age children's scores on the Children's Depression Inventory did not correlate with their depression scores on the Child Behavior Checklist completed by the mothers. This finding supports the need to obtain primary data from school-age children. School-agers are capable of expressing their thoughts and feelings about their experiences. Adults can make inferences about children's behaviors, but they need to be validated by the children. The findings also supports the need to obtain data from more than one family member when studying family phenomena.

The findings of this study suggest that homeless families are indeed suffering from mental and physical health problems that need evaluation and follow-up. Nurses, with their strategic placement in health care delivery systems, are in a unique position to work effectively with this vulnerable population. Nurses can be advocates for changes in health care policy that would provide more comprehensive health care for homeless families.

24

Mothering in the Midst of Danger

Lee SmithBattle

Since the 1970s, teenage mothers have become an increasingly visible part of the social landscape in the United States. They are the subject of newspaper stories and television talk shows; they figure prominently in discussions of welfare policies and costs; and the entire subject engenders heated debates among policymakers and researchers (Furstenberg, 1991, 1992; Geronimus, 1991, 1992). The prevailing perception of teenage parenting emphasizes individual failures, misconceived choices, truncated lives, deficits, and deviance from norms. For all the visibility of teenage mothers, their personal and family stories go largely unrecorded.

This chapter offers one example of interpretive family research that draws on Heideggerian phenomenology (Benner, 1985, 1991; Benner & Wrubel, 1989; Dreyfus, 1991; Leonard, 1989; Packer, 1985). The goal in this interpretive study of teenage mothering is not to uncover universals or laws but to explicate context and world (Rabinow & Sullivan, 1987) in

AUTHOR'S NOTE: I gratefully acknowledge the financial support provided by the Fahs-Beck Fund for Research and Experimentation; the Century Club Fund, School of Nursing and the Graduate Division of the University of California, San Francisco; the Alpha Eta Chapter of Sigma Theta Tau; and the National Center for Nursing Research for a National Research Service Award (NR1F31NR06266). Names and identifying information have been changed to maintain confidentiality.

order to show how mothering for teenagers is constituted and organized by personal concerns, family practices, and the wider social world. This study departs from scientific normalizing procedures, which easily capture the deficits and failures of young mothers based on formal decontextualized criteria. In contrast this study favors an interpretive approach in which the goal of understanding participants' lives in their own terms captures short-comings, suffering, and constraints, as well as the strengths and possibili-ties of young mothers as socially enacted within the traditions, practices, and resources of particular families and communities. The aim of under-standing is furthered through the power and validity of narratives for re-vealing participants' understanding of their lives and concrete circumstances.

I have chosen to tell one family's story from among the 16 participating families; 10 families were white and 6 of were African American. Data were collected from multiple joint and separate interviews with each young mother and at least one grandparent over a 3-month period beginning when the teenager's infant was 8-10 months of age. Interviews of family routines, history, and coping elicited narrative accounts of the difficulties and re-wards of being a mother or grandparent and the changes in family relation-ships and routines. Narrative accounts were fixed by verbatim transcription of interviews that provided the basis for textual analysis and presentation of findings. Four patterns of family care have been identified; the following story illustrates the pattern of adversarial care as lived out in the midst of danger and begins with the words of Josie, a 37-year-old African-American grandmother whose daughter Tamika gave birth at age 15 to a baby daughter named Angel.

> Gm: Me and my sisters, we could have got turned out on drugs because it's coming at us every which way, you know, but we just chose another route. We didn't do nothin' with our lives, but we also chose not to get off into drugs, you see . . . them the only two choices you have. . . . I started going to Bingo when I was 17 years old because that's where it stopped dead. I started going to Bingo and that has been my life. Bingo.

Josie's words begin to tell a story that points to a world of limited pos-sibilities, of constricted time, of pervasive danger, a world that is back-ground to the family's set of practices, habits, relationships, emotions, and concerns. To grasp the possibilities and constraints available in their world, I first describe the community where they live, because in the words of Mair (1988), "We are, each of us, locations where the stories of our place and time become partially tellable" (p. 127).

The Community Story

New City was originally a white farming community. During the 1950s, however, the widening of the interstate freeway system forced white-owned businesses in its path to relocate. With the increased migration of Southern blacks to the area, white families began leaving in ever-increasing numbers so that by the 1970s the majority of residents were people of color. Encouraged by their numbers and strengthened by the civil rights movement, blacks began exerting political pressure to incorporate the city. In spite of bitter opposition by white absentee landlords, they finally succeeded in 1983.

In spite of political successes, the daily lives of city residents have not improved dramatically. Infant mortality and the number of low birth weight infants is twice that of the county at large. Unemployment and underemployment is high; the likelihood of graduating from high school is low. New City is the most economically depressed city and has the highest crime rate in the county. The pervasiveness of drugs, crime, and poverty shows itself in boarded-up buildings, impenetrable-looking fences surrounding some homes, and empty playgrounds that have been the site of drug deals and gang warfare. Prominently displayed hand-painted signs declaring "Sum- mer is for chilling; Not for killing" are testimony to the danger of living in a virtual war zone.

Despite the pervasive violence and impoverishment of many families, neighborhood life is by no means destitute. People know one another from having long-established ties to their homes, churches, and neighborhoods. These connections have made it incumbent on some residents to take heroic stands to report drug deals or to get crack houses condemned. As Josie's narrative of survival makes clear, the most impoverished families contend with the harshest realities of providing for and safeguarding the children.

Josie's Story

Josie is an engaging storyteller who weighs no more than 86 pounds and looks younger than her 37 years. Her almost fragile appearance is quite at odds with her forceful presence. In lively conversation and with earnest candor, she describes her life as a mother and grandmother. I am sometimes surprised by her candor, although as she explains, she enjoys telling the story of her life to someone who does not already know about her problems. Part of her flair for storytelling comes from her survival-honed language and her unique way of punctuating dramatic moments with the phrase "you see what I'm saying?" She prides herself on her quick and caustic tongue as a deliberate means of surviving in the midst of danger. She is adept at intimidating "without using my fists. Because I can take a word that somebody say to me and reverse it." She is not averse to fighting with her fists, however, as becomes apparent below.

Josie and Tamika are members of a large extended family consisting of four households. The household where Josie lives includes her three youngest children, her grandchild, her mother, and her sister's family, for a total of four women and six children. Family obligations and patterns of cooperation bind all four households together in a domestic web much like Stack (1974) describes in *All Our Kin*. The domestic web shows itself in shared child care, living arrangements, and patterns of daily visiting when kin gather to learn about last night's Bingo, to watch TV, or to learn the latest community news. It was here during my visits that I would hear story after story of indiscriminate shootings, rapes, gang warfare, or fights of teenage girls and of women waged over men.

As a single mother, Josie has supported her children either on welfare or by working on low-paying assembly lines. Either way, it has been a constant struggle to make ends meet. Even if she is fortunate enough to pay her bills, unanticipated expenses result from scams or theft. Josie's seeming nonchalance about money reflects the brutal fact that she is always penniless by the end of the month:

> Gm: Money ain't going to make me, and it ain't going to break me, you know. I can't die with no money, so it ain't no big thing to have it. Cause once I have it, it's gone anyway.

Her words bespeak the stark reality that there is never enough cash to cover basic expenses or any surplus to deal with emergencies, thefts, or late welfare checks. Only patterns of obligation and reciprocity dispersed over several households fill in the breach by continuously redistributing resources among members of the domestic network (Stack, 1974).

The mother of four children, Josie's oldest two have presented difficult challenges. Her first-born son, now 20 years old, is mentally handicapped; he became involved in drugs 2 years ago. Tamika, her oldest daughter, was not hers to raise for her first 4 years. Prized for being "light-skinned," Tamika's paternal grandparents fought for and were awarded legal guardianship in court proceedings that Josie could not afford to contest. Although Josie eventually regained custody of Tamika, she concedes that her relationship to her daughter has been tenuous "because I didn't raise her." Tamika became pregnant at age 14 and continues to run the streets. Because of the street-related activities of her two oldest children, Josie declares in a grim yet unembittered fashion that they are "lost, that they won't survive."

> Gm: There's no chance. They lost. They gone. . . . It's just no remorse, it's no feeling, it's just, you know—you know they're lost. There's nothing that can be done about it.

Josie places greater hope for her younger children, but only if she is able to move her children out of New City:

> Gm: I want to raise my two little ones [in a northwestern city] because I believe that I see potential in them. I see something that—they can accomplish something, you see what I'm saying? Which they can't do it here because it's too many stumbles and too many obstacles for them to go around.

Her dreams for her children are shaped by the standards and possibilities available in her social world:

> Gm: I want [my son and daughter] to grow up to be better kids. I mean, I don't want them to become just your average black kid, you see what I'm saying? This city hasn't produced anything. Not nothing. You don't have no basketball players come from here, you don't have no football player, no nothing has been produced [here] to benefit anything. If it is, it's maybe a quiet airline stewardess. It's like uh, you hear most parents say, I'll move heaven and hell to get my kids out of here.

Survival: "Only the Strong Survive"

Josie and her children must reckon daily with the adversity and violence that permeate their lives. In a world where making ends meet is capricious, where manipulation and intimidation dominate social interactions, where relationships can turn exploitive, survival becomes a focal concern and a coherent way of understanding her life. Josie's self-understanding as a tenacious survivor is apparent in many of her stories. She relates one incident in which she was stranded with her children without money or food in a northwestern city. This story serves as a marker of her tenacity and reinforces the importance of teaching her children to survive:

> Gm: Because once you been there, you say, "God that was really frightful cause I didn't know how I survived. I don't know how I let my kids go through it." But once they go through it, they'll say theyself, "God, we had

some hard times back in that city. Sometime my mama didn't even have cigarette money. . . . " It's hard on you and it's hard on them, but it teaches them. It teaches them that they have to survive. We have to be strong to survive out there.

Josie's self-understanding as a tenacious survivor offers her a coherent way of coping with misfortune, a set of practices to avoid or confront the poverty and violence that surround her, and a way of judging her own and others' moral worth according to one's ability to survive. An ethos of survival organizes how she conducts herself in social settings and how she appraises situations as threatening or nonthreatening. Where intimidation and manipulation are taken for granted, Josie may beguile or intimidate others in order to avoid a fight. But when the situation demands it, Josie is ready to fight.

Gm: My boyfriend, I busted him with another girl, and I mean, I was pissed and this girl is huge, and I called her all kind of names and tried to hit her and ran after her, and chased her down the stairs and kicked the door in—I mean, just an example, you know.

In fact, fighting is a family tradition in which sisters call on one another to back each other up:

Gm: It's nothing but females in our family, and all of us is, we're real tight and we all believe in fighting, you know, one go down, all go down.

Fighting is so pervasive that even babies are understood to be (and praised for being) fighters. Josie proudly tells me that Angel has all the signs of being a good fighter because of the way she flails her arms and legs:

Gm: I mean anybody can fight. (laughter) . . . I mean even a baby. You know, you try to do something against a baby against their will, they're going to fight you. You see what I'm saying? To let you know that that's not what they want. Cause Angel, we play with her a lot of times and I say, "Fight, fight!" And she get to throwing her hands up, you know, and that's just, that's part of the instinct. . . . That's survival.

A media campaign to prevent violence by reframing fighting as a way to leave the community strikes a chord with Josie:

Gm: Like they try to tell you to fight to get out of here. You know, to improve yourself. But in order for you to get to do that, you have to fight somebody.

It was so much fighting down here before that they got on the TV and said, "If you're going to fight, fight to get out. Fight to improve," and all this stuff.

When I reveal to her that I have never personally fought, she is politely dubious and advises me: "You'd better learn. That's all."

Fighting is both a community norm among some groups and a family tradition. The metaphor that reframes fighting as a way to improve one's circumstances is a powerful one precisely because it resonates with long-standing norms and practices. In the following sections, survival shapes temporality and the imperatives of mothering.

Temporality and a Prayer for Deliverance

When survival becomes the prevailing end, personal time does not cohere into an ongoing past, present, and future. Rather, time seems to have stopped, as Josie makes clear:

> Gm: I can't see myself going forward. I can't see myself going backward. I'm just at a standstill. I'm not moving. I'm not doing anything. I don't know where I'm going, but I know where I been.

While the past is all too real for Josie, the future is obliterated by the real possibility of untimely death. When I ask, "What do you hope for tomorrow?" she replies:

> Gm: I can't. . . . I never plan for tomorrow cause I don't know if I'm going to be alive or not. . . . I could die in my sleep and get killed walking outside, go to the store, get shot, get stabbed, get robbed. Whatever. So I just don't plan.

When possibilities available in *this* life are so narrowed and circumstances seem so immutable, prospects for a better world are imagined only in the afterlife. The despair of living without a future becomes painfully palpable when she reads me her favorite passage from Revelations:

> Gm: With that I hear a loud voice from the throne saying, "Look, the tent of God is with mankind, and he will reside with them. They will be his people, and God himself shall be with them. And he will wipe out every tear from their eyes, and there will be no more. Neither will mourning nor outcries nor pain be anymore." That's my favorite one. Meaning that one day it's gonna be a new world. It's not gonna be no crime. It's not gonna

be no drugs. It's gonna be a much, much better place for everybody to live in. And sometime I just can't wait for that one to come. Cause I'm tired of this one. I don't like this one.

The new world she imagines is not of this earth. But until death releases her, Josie's care for her children gives her life purpose and makes her persevere. It is with her young children and grandchild that she experiences commonplace joys and ways of relating that are all but obliterated in the harshness and exploitation of the wider social world, a world that requires her to teach her children to survive.

Tamika's Story: "A Wild Person"

Tamika described herself as wanting to have a baby from the time she was 10 or 11. She was happy when her first pregnancy was confirmed at age 14, believing that it would keep her and her boyfriend together. After their relationship ended, she still looked forward to having a baby because all her peers were mothers. As an expected rite of passage among her peer group, having a baby bestows the positive status of becoming a woman where other routes to adulthood are severely constricted by the lack of economic and educational opportunities (Jones et al., 1985; Ladner, 1971; Sandven & Resnick, 1990).

In the first interview, Tamika wept briefly when she described herself as a "wild person, always hanging out, running here, running there. Drinkin." Being "a wild person" reflects a relational history of severed relationships and unstable connections that have left her existentially without a place, unknown and wild. She experiences caring for Angel as an impediment to "runnin' the streets." Of all the teenagers in the study, she shows the least pleasure in being a mother. Most of her interaction with Angel is negative, brusque, and often geared to get her to be less demanding. For example, during one interview Tamika held Angel on her lap, facing her chest. In response to almost any movement or sound made by Angel, Tamika hushed her in an irritated voice and ordered her not to move. Her flagrant disregard for Angel's welfare is especially conspicuous in her street-related activities. In one story related by Josie, a girl pulled a knife on Tamika with Angel in her arms. When Tamika told me of the same incident later, her main concern was for how mad her mother was going to be for having the baby with her on the streets.

Conflict between Josie and Tamika intensified with Angel's birth. Until Angel was 3 months of age, Josie cared almost exclusively for Angel because Tamika "slept all the time." Tamika's early lack of engagement may have been due in part to symptoms of lupus, diagnosed several months later. In any case, when Angel was 3 months old, Josie insisted that Tamika care for Angel, hoping that it would "put some stability in Tamika's life and make her responsible." Josie's demands, however, had no claim on Tamika because her mother's involvement and authority felt arbitrary, hostile, constant, and contemptuous. As Tamika explained, the hardest thing about being a mother is "my mom always jumping in and tell me what to do."

> M: She always jumps in, every day, all day, about every little thing. Do this, don't do that. Angel need to do this, she need to do that. Like she is MY baby.
>
> I: So what do you do?
>
> M: Just get my baby and leave. So I don't have to cuss her out because I will end up telling her somethin' real bad.

The protracted struggle that ensues over the care of Angel literally pushes Tamika into those activities on the street with her peers that Josie rails against and further undermines Tamika's relationship to Angel. Other studies of child care practices among impoverished African-American families reveal the legitimate authority of grandmothers in the lives of their grandchildren (Burton, 1990; Ladner, 1971; Stack, 1974). In some families the first child simply is raised by the grandmother or other family kin. The twist in this particular family story is that Tamika can neither fully relinquish her role as mother nor act as a mother so long as her relationship to Angel feels coerced by Josie. In the absence of a strong mother-daughter bond, Angel has become the battleground for mother-daughter conflict, failure, and disconnectedness.

As this research project seeks to demonstrate through interpretation of family narratives, mothering practices are shaped by family practices and social arrangements. In this particular family, personal and family histories, life circumstances, and the lack of alternative stories in their identity-forming community coalesce to derail the young mother's care of her child. With little room in her world to act as a mother, caring for Angel has become an external demand imposed by her mother rather than a project directed by the moral claim of the baby. Experienced as an external demand rather than an internally driven good, being a mother for Tamika conflicts with "runnin' the streets:"

> I: What do you like most about being a mother?

M: Spending time with my baby.

I: And what do you like least?

M: (pause) The way she came and changed my life. . . . Not being able to do the things that I want to do, the things I used to do.

The tragedy of Tamika's story is that there is so little room in her social world to become the good mother that stays home with her baby (her terms for a good mother), given the strong but contradictory situational press for being a "wild person" in the social landscape of violence. Tamika realizes that being "a wild person" is incompatible with being a mother and concedes that she is:

M: . . . always going back to it (the way she led her life before the baby was born). Yeah. Like I used to tell my mom, I'll go a certain place—well, I meant to go to that certain place and then I wouldn't come back for the next day and then my mom would be mad. "You got a baby, you can't be staying out all night."

Other authors (Musick, 1987) explain the deficits of adolescent mothers in individualistic terms—where perceptions, actions, feelings, and thoughts are located strictly in the self. This position, which underpins empirical-rational research, fails to recognize that who we are and who we might become are always situated and dependent on the stories and practices available in one's family and identity-forming communities (Bruner, 1987; MacIntyre, 1984; Taylor, 1989). For Tamika, mothering is not a practice that sets up meaning, identity, story, connection, or future. Like many other aspects of her life, mothering is another disappointment, another burden. The pervasive situational constraints offer few possibilities and sources for elaborating an alternative set of practices consistent with becoming the mother who stays home with her baby. Who then will care for Angel? Who will know her and care for her before she too must be risked to, and learn to survive in, the wider world? Josie offers these last discomforting words:

Gm: Like I told Tamika, Angel will get raised. Even if she got to raise herself. She will get raised. . . If I'm not around, she will raise herself because with me being here, I stays on Tamika to raise her. But Angel's smart and she see that Tamika's not paying her no attention whatsoever. . . . (I)n the future you just wait, you contact them 5 years later, and you see who's raising who. So Angel will be raising herself.

Commentary

The phenomenological underpinnings for this study contend that human beings and their activities are neither predestined nor necessary or open to unlimited possibility. Rather possibilities always are situated within the set of available practices and stories of a given historical time and a given place. In this family portrait, the ethic of survival is perpetuated by bureaucratic policies that segregate, regulate, and blame the poor (Kotlowitz, 1991; Piven & Cloward, 1971; Ryan, 1971/1976) and at the same time are intrusive, inflexible, and unresponsive to family needs and community conditions (Bush, 1988; Dill, Feld, Martin, Beukema, & Belle, 1980). The poor are suspended thereby in a web of entanglements, while those outside the situation with the power to define the problem and to frame its solution are caught in a language of pathology and bureaucratic management that disregards the extent to which maternal practices are socially embedded.

Tamika lacks many concrete possibilities. She is a child-woman of her time and place. She is a child of violence and danger, of despondency and despair, consigned to living in a savage world where becoming a wild person is itself an attempt to cope with and survive the chaos. She is an African-American child prized and seized for her light brown skin color in a world where skin color pervades and corrupts familial and social relations. She came as a stranger at 4 years of age to a distracted mother already preoccupied with coping with a disabled son without the benefit of community resources and constantly besieged without resources or partner to make anything but a tortuous way for her children. No luxury, no slack, no comfort. The family legacy of hopelessness and survival has become Tamika's future.

Tamika's story of "a wild person" and Josie's practices of surviving in the midst of danger are related, shaped, and constrained by the wider social world. In the end, after years of growing up with violence and having been failed by schools, social welfare, health care, and political institutions, many children inevitably succumb, are lost. Langston Hughes's poem "Dream Deferred" (1951) captures what it means to live on the outside, without hope, without possibility:

> What happens to a dream deferred?
>
> Does it dry up
> like a raisin in the sun?
> Or fester like a sore—
> And then run?
> Does it stink like rotten meat?

Or crust and sugar over—
like a syrupy sweet?

Maybe it just sags
like a heavy load.

Or does it explode?

This family narrative exemplifies adversarial care that severely constrains possibilities for becoming a mother. In interpreting other family stories, there are much less constraining ways for mothering to be taken up by teenagers. For some families mothering becomes a shared project where the capacities, skills, and voice of the teenager are nurtured by the grandparent. In these family narratives and practices, a different world—where care is generous for the baby and for the teenager—gets elaborated.

This particular family story points to how our current cultural narrative of mothering misunderstands mothering and family life as an individual, private affair rather than as a collective responsibility. That there are no safe parks and no pencils in schools points to the larger social context where quality child care, good education, and health care are all severely limited for impoverished children. In the absence of a collective resolve to care for children, individual mothers and their families are left to fend as best they can. What this family story demands of us is the courage and vision to create those social arrangements, based on an ethic of responsiveness and citizenship, that pursues the creation of the good in caring for children. Such a vision is sighted on deepening conditions of possibility, opportunity, dignity, integrity, worth, and care of teenage parents and their children.

25

Assessment of Rural Family Hardiness: A Foundation for Intervention

Jeri W. Dunkin

Colleen Holzwarth

Terry Stratton

Introduction

The purpose of this study is to describe the ways that rural families cope with hardships, using family strengths to buffer the negative impact of un-expected life events. The Family Hardiness Index (McCubbin & Thompson, 1987) was used to measure the family's patterned approach to life's hard-ships and its typical pattern of appraising the impact of life events and changes on family functioning.

Hardiness, the personality characteristic composed of control, commit-ment, and challenge, has been viewed as an inherent health-promoting factor (Lambert & Lambert, 1987). It is the personality characteristic that

AUTHORS' NOTE: This research is supported in part by funding from the Office of Rural Health Policy in the HERSA, U. S. DHHS (HA-R-000004-02). The work of Katherine Maidenberg on this project is greatly appreciated.

enables individuals to remain healthy even when confronted with stressful life events or a stressful environment. The hardy person recognizes that life requires use of judgment to make good decisions (control), becomes actively involved with others in various activities of life (commitment), and perceives change as ultimately beneficial to personal development (challenge) (Lambert & Lambert, 1987; Lee, 1983; Pollock, 1989).

Commitment implies a curiosity about life and a sense of the meaningfulness of life; *control* encompasses the belief that one can influence the course of events (e.g., similar to an internal vs. external locus of control); and *challenge* reflects the belief that it is normal for life to change and that change brings about stimulation and growth rather than a threat to security. These beliefs combine with *behavior,* which moves the hardy individual to take decisive action to find out more about life changes, transform events in order to learn from them, and incorporate them into ongoing life plans (Kobasa, Maddi, Puccetti, & Zola, 1985). Persons low in hardiness tend to feel alienated, powerless in the face of stressors, and tend to be more vegetative than vigorous in their approach to the change events in their lives.

Nursing has defined its major concern as human responses to actual and potential health problems. The concept of hardiness has particular significance to nursing in the quest to understand these responses. It reflects a positive, health-promoting approach to understanding human stress responses (Bigbee, 1991). The relationship between hardiness and stress as it affects individual reactions to illness has been studied extensively (Adeyanju & Creswell, 1987; Daniel, 1987; Johnson & Hall, 1988; Kobasa et al., 1985; Pollock, Christian, & Sands, 1990). For example, persons with high stress and low hardiness had more illness than persons with higher hardiness levels. Support has been found for the stress-buffering effects of hardiness (Nowak, 1986; Weibe & McCallum, 1986).

Another way to view hardiness is as a learned personality style based on the interaction between persons and their interpersonal environments. This personality style is most often learned within the context of the family and is part of family development (McCubbin & Figley, 1983). The family is the group in which learning develops (Kravitz & Frey, 1989).

Family hardiness is an extension of individual hardiness. It is the family's internal strengths and durability. It is characterized by an internal sense of control of life events and life's hardships, a sense of meaningfulness in life, involvement in activities, and commitment to learn and to explore new and challenging experiences. It is the strength that families have to manage the impact of family stressors and strains and to recover from a family crisis (McCubbin & Thompson, 1987).

Family hardiness is a broader concept than individual hardiness in that it adds the dimension of *confidence* to interrelated components of co-oriented commitment, challenge, and control. *Co-oriented commitment* is the ability of the family to work together to manage difficulties. *Confidence* is the ability of the family to handle problems. *Challenge* is the ability of the family to seek new life experience. *Control* is the family's sense of internal control rather than being a victim of circumstances (Figley & McCubbin, 1983).

The Family Hardiness Index (FHI) (McCubbin & Thompson, 1987) was developed to measure the characteristic of hardiness as a stress resistance and adaptation resource. Family hardiness functions as a buffer in mitigating the effects of stressors and demands and as a facilitator of family adjustment. The FHI was used initially in an investigation of family traditions, celebrations, and routines in 304 nonclinical families as part of the ongoing research of the Family Stress, Coping, and Health Project at the University of Wisconsin-Madison (McCubbin & Thompson, 1987).

Hardiness seems to fit well with rural culture, which emphasizes independence, self-reliance, and self-care (Bigbee, 1991). The expectation is that rural people will solve their own problems rather than seek outside help (Bushy, 1990). In fact there is a real reticence to trust outsiders (Long & Weinert, 1989). With the depressed economy and subsequent changes in rural communities, individual family members may have multiple role expectations, and an individual's goals may be subjugated for the family's well-being (Bushy, 1990). Families in sparsely populated areas employ different coping mechanisms for contending with life transitions (Bigbee, 1991; Bushy, 1990). Rural families rely on social support from within the extended family and informal organizations such as church groups and homemaker clubs. It is for these reasons that family hardiness of rural populations is of particular interest.

Methodology

Data Collection

This study utilized a convenience sample. The sample came from persons attending a meeting at the Farm Union in a rural Midwest community, a 1990 county fair, screening at local businesses, and those persons using the community-based primary care clinic from February 1990 to March 1991. All data were collected in the same rural Midwest county. The information was gathered as part of Health Risk Appraisal (HRA) screening. Two hundred ninety-eight persons participated in the screening. Of these, 206 usable questionnaires were obtained. Only questionnaires with the demographic data, health-risk appraisal information, and the hardiness questionnaire completed were used.

Instrument

The Family Hardiness Index is a 20-item instrument consisting of four subscales (Co-oriented Commitment, Confidence, Challenge, and Control), which calls for the respondents to assess the degree (False, Mostly False, Mostly True, True) to which each statement describes their current family situation. The Co-oriented Commitment subscale measures the family's sense of internal strengths, dependability, and ability to work together. The Confidence subscale measures the family's sense of being able to plan ahead, being appreciated for efforts, their ability to endure hardships, and to experience life with interest and meaningfulness. The Challenge subscale measures the family's efforts to be innovative, to experience new things, and to learn. The Control subscale measures the family's sense of being in control of family life rather than being shaped by outside events and circumstances.

Reliability

The internal reliability using Cronbach's alpha for the FHI in McCubbin's work was .82. The Cronbach's alpha for this study was .80.

Results

Of the 206 respondents, approximately 75% were women ($n = 151$). The mean age of the study group was 45 years, with a range of 16-77 ($sd = 13.94$). Eighty-five percent were married ($n = 175$), and 54% resided in communities of 2,500 or less. Over 89% had completed high school, with 33% of these having completed college or above (see Table 25.1).

The occupation most frequently checked by the respondents was homemaker (26.5%), followed by manager/educator/professional (15.5%). Ten percent selected farmer/rancher as their occupation. The most frequently reported occupation of the spouse was farmer/rancher, followed by manager/educator/professional.

Table 25.1 Respondent Characteristics

Characteristic	Number	Valid Percent
Sex		
Male	49	24.5
Female	151	75.5
Marital status		
Single	16	8.0
Married	175	85.0
Divorced	9	4.5
Widowed	3	1.5
Family type		
Not Married	27	14.0
Couples	29	15.0
Pre & School	43	22.0
Adolescent/Launch	56	28.5
Empty Nest/Retire	41	20.5
Level of education		
Less than high school	16	7.9
High school	59	29.5
Some college	55	27.5
College	50	25.0
Graduate school/Professional	20	7.8
Rural/Nonrural residence		
2,500 or less	105	53.6
Over 2,500	91	46.4

NOTE: $N = 196$

Questions were asked about distances to health services. The average distance to a doctor/clinic was 10.70 miles (range = 0-55 miles, $sd = 12.66$). The mean distance to the nearest hospital was 13.20 miles (range = 0-55 miles, $sd = 14.09$). This is in line with the recently reported study of health services availability to rural residents (U.S. Congress, 1990). It was an average of 101 miles, however, to the nearest town of 50,000 or greater.

Family Type

Because family hardiness is a function of family development (McCubbin & Thompson, 1987), we felt that we should consider the stage of family development in relation to hardiness. The family typology used was the system described by McCubbin and Thompson (1987). It defines the five family types as single, couple, pre & school-aged children, adolescent &

Table 25.2 Analysis of Variance: Hardiness and Components by Respondent's
Characteristics

Source	df	SS	MS	F
Control				
Spouse's occupation	9	54.48	6.05	2.17[*]
Error	158	441.49	2.79	
Total	167	495.98		
Hardiness				
Rural/Nonrural	1	193.02	193.02	4.22[*]
Error	189	8,640.48	45.72	
Total	190	8,833.50		
Control				
Rural/Nonrural	1	20.09	20.09	6.34[*]
Error	189	599.34	3.17	
Total	190	619.43		

NOTE: [*]$p < .05$

launching of children, and empty nest & retired. These levels were determined by the respondent's age and the age of the oldest child (see Table 25.1).

Hardiness

The scores on Hardiness, as well as the subscales of Control, Challenge,
Co-oriented Commitment, and Confidence, were distributed in a normal
curve. Control was the weakest subscale, at 1.93; Challenge was next, with
2.11; Hardiness was third, with 2.28; Commitment was next to the highest,
with 2.41; and Confidence was the highest, with 2.46. The scales were rated
on a 0-3 ($x = 1.5$). This means that generally speaking the respondents'
family hardiness was fairly high, with all scales above the numerical
average.

Differences on Hardiness
for Demographic Variables

Analysis of variance was used to determine group differences on Hardiness. No significant difference was found between family type and Hardiness (or any subscale). Likewise no significant differences were found for
age of respondent, gender of respondent, or respondent's occupation. Significant differences were found, however, on Hardiness for several other
demographic variables. Control was significant at the .05 level for spouse's

occupation (see Table 25.2). The greatest Control was demonstrated for those spouses who were retired.

Community of residence (rural/nonrural) was examined to find that Hardiness and the subscale of Control were significantly different at the .05 level for the rural and nonrural groups (2,500 or less and over 2,500) (see Table 25.2). The more urban groups were hardier.

Discussion

Although this study used a convenience sample, the demographics were very similar to population statistics for the state. The percentage of married respondents was somewhat higher (85% vs. 61%) than the general population. It is not likely that this selection bias significantly affected the data outcome.

The level of education of our sample was representative of the state. Analysis did not detect any significant effect of education level on Hardiness. Nor did marital status make a difference. In fact, spouse's occupation, while it demonstrated significance, should be interpreted cautiously. Indeed, rurality appears to be the only demographic characteristic associated with family hardiness. It is somewhat surprising to note that the more rural families are less hardy. On reflection, however, one might conclude that those persons involved in a less rural life-style may feel that they have more ability to withstand stressful life situations. They are not as remote and are not dependent on such things as rainfall for income. In addition they probably are employed in a less hazardous occupation than the more rural respondents. These and other potential factors will be explored as we delve further into this data set.

McCubbin and Thompson, in their presentation of the Family Hardiness Index (1987), discussed the patterns of family hardiness over the life cycle. The patterns found in this study were different from those found by McCubbin. The biggest differences are during the couple and pre/school family stages. The two studies found very similar patterns during the single and adolescent/launch stages (see Figure 25.1).

The families in the current study then were divided into rural ($n = 105$) and nonrural ($n = 91$) families. The patterns of these two subgroups were somewhat different from the combined group, which indicates some relationship between family hardiness and place of residence. The rural and nonrural patterns were more similar to the total group in this study than what McCubbin and Thompson (1987) reported (see Figure 25.1). The stages of greatest similarity and differences remained the same, however.

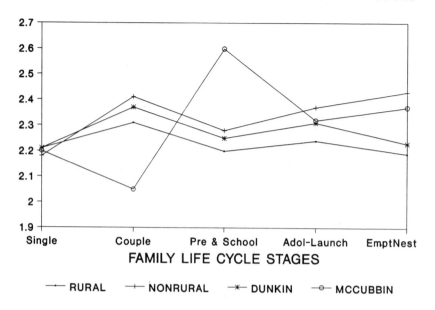

Figure 25.1. Family Hardiness Over the Life Cycle

Implications for Practice

The significance of this study and the theory surrounding family hardiness is geographically more inclusive than for rural America alone. Much of the world's population is rural, and the literature reveals that rural populations, wherever they are found, share similar problems (Bushy, 1990).

Rural populations are at greater risk for both acute and chronic illnesses, accidents and disabilities, depression, alcohol abuse, and isolation of the elderly. The strengths that rural families possess to cope with these and other similar problems have yet to be explored in the literature (U.S. Congress, 1990).

Significant interactions may occur between family hardiness and the success of primary health care in many countries of the world. A major determinant of health is life-style (Bushy, 1990; Nelson & Simmons, 1983), and life-style is a function of culture. Part of that culture is how families respond to life's stresses (Bushy, 1990). Therefore the assessment of family hardiness is essential in meeting the primary health goal of health promotion and disease prevention. Indeed, the assessment of family hardiness in a target population is an important foundation for planning interventions for rural families. If the patterns of rural families for handling problems were better known, interventions to strengthen the family's hardiness could be implemented.

PART VII

Does Family Intervention Make a Difference?

Catherine L. Gilliss, Editor

26

Does Family Intervention Make a Difference? An Integrative Review and Meta-Analysis

Catherine L. Gilliss

Linda L. Davis

The reciprocal relationship between health problems and family functioning is well known to clinicians and theoreticians and is well documented throughout this volume. Health problems influence family perceptions and behaviors; likewise family perceptions and behaviors influence health outcomes. Thus family-focused health care interventions are of considerable interest. Despite the interest in family health care research, the evaluation of these studies remains seriously handicapped for the lack of integrative research on the completed work in the field. The work collected in this book assumes and sometimes claims that family intervention makes a difference, but do we know that?

The purpose of this final chapter is to present results from an ongoing integrative review and meta-analysis of family health intervention studies similar to those described herein.

AUTHORS' NOTE: We acknowledge the statistical assistance of Dr. Malcolm Turner, Professor, Department of Biostatistics and Biomathematics, UAB.

Background

Family health research is widely acknowledged as complex, and studies are often severely flawed (Feetham, 1984; Gilliss, 1983; Gilliss & Davis, 1992). Among the problems commonly identified are the use of conceptual frameworks/theories that do not articulate with the concepts measured, the data gathering or analytic methods, or the conclusions and vice versa.

Published research reports of interventions with families combine the complexities seen in family research with the intricacies of intervention research, often the randomized clinical trial. Thus the literature on family health interventions is difficult to critique and integrate in a meaningful way. Yet a growing number of authors have described a process for undertaking such a review, the criteria to be employed to establish clarity and rigor in such reviews (Ganong, 1987), and the analytic techniques for integrating the findings from such reviews (Cooper, 1989; Light & Pillemer, 1984; Smith & Stullenbarger, 1989; Wolf, 1986).

A number of well-known meta-analytic reviews have addressed psychotherapy and family therapy outcomes. Smith and Glass (1977) coded and statistically integrated nearly 400 controlled reports of psychotherapy, providing evidence that the treated psychotherapy client was better off than 75% of the untreated comparisons. Hazelrigg, Cooper, and Borduin (1987) compared outcomes (family interaction and behavioral ratings) from family therapy—no treatment and alternative treatment—to determine that family therapy resulted in more positive effects, sustained, though diminishing, over time. Shadish and Sweeney (1991) explicated an elaborate model in which the mediators and moderators of psychotherapy outcomes were analyzed. Their work offers one example in which the subtle patterns, often overlooked, might be better detected through meta-analytic techniques.

Though the psychotherapy and family literatures have been integrated through meta-analysis, the family health intervention research (family interventions that are not rendered by a mental health specialist as family therapy but are more typical of family education or family primary health care) has not been so integrated. Therefore, believing that family health intervention differs from family therapy in intensity, length of treatment, substantive content, and appropriate client selection, we sought to undertake a review of interventions more commonly employed by health practitioners in primary care of the family (physicians, nurses, dietitians, health educators).

Integrative Review

Our examination began with a review of biomedical and biobehavioral science research from the period 1985-1989, with the goal of describing those reports. Specifically we wanted to know what kind of interventions were being reported and which family members were the target(s) of the intervention. We deliberately attempted to locate published papers across health disciplines. Computer searches using the key words *family* and *intervention,* augmented by hand searches, identified 59 English-language citations for this period. Of these, 19 papers were classified as conceptual in nature, 5 were methodological, and 35 were descriptions of family research studies. Of the 35, 6 were descriptive reports of family characteristics or patterns, 4 were interventions carried out by mental health specialists (psychotherapy), and 25 were reports of interventions that might be carried out by non-mental-health specialists across a variety of health disciplines.

We then examined these 25 reports for two dimensions: the level of involvement with the family and the type of intervention. The level of involvement was characterized according to Bozett's (1987) schema, in which he described three levels. Level 1 interventions are focused on an individual within the family; Level 2 interventions address a select subset of family members (often mother-child); and Level 3 interventions involve the total family. To characterize the type of intervention employed, we used Wright and Leahey's (1984) classification of interventions as cognitive, affective, behavioral, or a combination of these.

The 25 categorized studies are organized by these dimensions and displayed in Table 26.1. The majority of reports described use of a combined intervention method ($n = 13$), followed by the cognitive approach ($n = 11$). Interventions were most often Level 1 (individual member) or 2 (subset of family member). Only 6 studies were characterized as Level 3 (family) interventions. Individual family members most often received cognitive interventions; subsets of family members received a combination of intervention types; and family groups also received a combination of intervention types.

An attempt to integrate the statistical findings from these interventions failed, as the data of the identified studies proved inadequate. Thus we began the second phase of our work, in which we planned a statistical integration of findings, using meta-analysis.

Although limited by sample size and time period covered, the first phase of our work highlighted some of the problems that we could expect in

Table 26.1 Intervention Studies (1985-1989): Type of Intervention by Level of Involvement

| | Type of Intervention | | | | |
	Cognitive	*Affective*	*Behavioral*	*Combination*	*Totals*
Level of involvement					
1 (Individual)	7	0	0	2	(9)
2 (Subset)	3	0	0	7	(10)
3 (Family)	1	1	0	4	(6)
Totals	(11)	(1)	(0)	(13)	(25)

sampling for a meta-analysis. Among these were clarity regarding the level of the intervention and what unit(s) of analysis and concepts were used for the outcome measure. Because the type (cognitive, affective, behavioral) of interventions did not vary substantially, this variable was coded but no longer was treated as a primary interest for the meta-analysis. Finally the data set was enlarged to include controlled studies in which adequate statistical data were reported so as to be usable in the meta-analysis.

Meta-Analysis

Studies published between 1986-1990 were included if they reported outcome results of a controlled study of family health intervention (intervention aimed at family members, subsets, or groups provided by a health professional who was not a mental health specialist). Reports that compared two forms of family intervention were excluded from the analysis because they did not address the question guiding this analysis.

Methods

The researchers developed two instruments for coding selected characteristics of family intervention studies: the Family Intervention Report Coding Form (FIR) and the Family Study Quality Rating Scale (FSQR) (both available from the authors). The FIR is a codebook used to record information on 12 different study characteristics, such as the type and level of family intervention used (the independent variables), the population/sample, setting, data collection instruments/methods, and outcome measures reported. The FSQR assesses the methodological quality of the written report and includes an assessment of such factors as reliability and validity of the instruments used and the control threats to internal validity. Interrater reliability for applying the FSQR to a subset of family studies was acceptable ($r = .80$).

A computer search was undertaken to identify studies for the period 1986-1990 to include in addition to the earlier identified studies published between 1985-1989.

Findings

A comprehensive search of published literature for the 5-year period 1986-1990 yielded 69 data-based reports, of which 22 were excluded because they did not meet the sampling criteria. Of the 47 remaining studies, all were coded; with respect to outcome, 31 measured patient outcomes, 23 measured family member outcomes, and 20 measured family outcomes. (The total exceeds 47, as most studies employed more than one outcome measure).

Among the 20 reports of family outcomes, which were the focus of our interest, only 5 contained adequate data, collected with a standardized instrument, and reported an outcome with enough conceptual commonality to justify integration. Therefore the meta-analysis was conducted on 5 studies, representing a total sample of 567 subjects. The studies included appear in Table 26.2.

Abramowitz & Coursey (1989) ($n = 48$) employed a nonequivalent control design to measure the effect of a program of family education and support on their ability to manage a chronically mentally ill member. A stress and coping framework was used; the caregiver's report of family stress was measured as outcome.

Chiverton & Caine (1989) randomly assigned 40 spouses who were caring for persons with Alzheimer's disease to educational groups or to no treatment and measured the effect of these on the caregiver's Health Specific Family Coping Index.

Evans, Matlock, Bishop, Stranahan, and Pederson (1988) employed a randomized clinical trial to test the effect of education and support to 188 families of stroke patients. The primary caregiver's report of family functioning was obtained by using the McMaster Family Assessment Device.

Gilliss, Neuhaus, and Hauck (1990) used a randomized clinical trial design to evaluate the effectiveness of a nursing education and support service offered in a hospital and by telephone to 67 pairs of patients and caregivers after cardiac surgery. Family functioning was measured with the Family APGAR.

Table 26.2 Meta-Analysis (1986-1990): Combined Probabilities: Family Functioning Studies

Study	Precise p	$-2 \ln p$
Abramowitz & Coursey (1989)	.0059	10.2656
Chiverton & Caine (1989)	.0052	10.5182
Evans et al. (1988)	.0000001	16.1181
Gilliss et al. (1990)	.43	1.6879
Parkerson et al. (1989)	.37	1.9885
		40.5783 ($2 \times 5 = 10$ df)
		$p < .001$

Parkerson et al. (1989) also employed the telephone to conduct a randomized clinical trial of supportive intervention to families identified as having high stress levels. Controls ($n = 108$), who received no treatment, were compared to 116 high-stress families. The Duke University Family Social Support and Stress Scale was administered to patients in this study.

Table 26.2 indicates that the precise p, calculated for each study, was significant for the Abramowitz and Coursey (1989), Chiverton and Caine (1989), and Evans and colleagues (1988) studies. Gilliss and colleagues (1990) and Parkerson et al. (1989) reported nonsignificant results for the outcome variables included in this analysis. In the final column appears the log linear transformation of these p values. (Added together, these equal a $\chi^2 = 40.5783$, with $2 \times 5 = 10$ df, $p < .001$.) Using Fisher's method, as cited in Hedges and Olkin (1985), we were able to reject the null hypothesis that there is no effect on family functioning when non-mental-health family interventions were used. (In other words the results demonstrated a positive effect of family health intervention on family outcomes.) As a conservative strategy, the study with the single most significant results was omitted, and we recomputed the χ^2. The combined result for the remaining four studies was still significant at the $p < .01$ level.

Discussion

This single meta-analysis of a small number of family intervention studies provides partial support for the value of family-focused health care. We do not claim, however, that this is the definitive meta-analysis on family intervention research. Our work is ongoing, and of particular concern is enlarging the sample. Two specific activities are now underway: (a) identifying nonpublished reports and (b) searching back to include the period 1980-1985.

A second area of concern is the conceptual overlap between outcome measures. Because of our interest in the effects of the intervention on the family, we hope to continue to measure family variables; however, note that in each of the five included papers, the outcome data were sourced from a single family member. Although this may be the state of the science of family health care, these outcome measures are imperfect proxies for family functioning.

As our data set enlarges, we hope to explore the dimensions that influence the outcomes of family health interventions. Which outcomes are we best able to influence? What types of interventions are most effective for what types of families? What types of interventions are most effective for what types of clinical problems?

In spite of the limitations of this work, we are encouraged to continue our examination. Reports of family health interventions clearly make a difference. Our beginning integration of these reports suggests that they do make a statistically significant difference in measures of family health. Thus may the readers of this volume be encouraged to continue their work, enlightened by the topics covered in the chapters that have preceded.

References

Aboitiz, F. (1985). A critique of the modern concept of localization. *Journal of Social and Biological Structure, 8,* 307-312.

Abramowitz, I. A., & Coursey, R. D. (1989). Impact of an educational support group on family participants who take care of their schizophrenic relatives. *Journal of Consulting and Clinical Psychology, 57*(2), 232-236.

Achebe, C. (1959). *Things fall apart.* Greenwich, CT: Fawcett.

Achenbach, T. M., & Edelbrock, C. (1983). *Manual for the Child Behavior Checklist and Revised Child Behavior Profile.* Burlington: University of Vermont.

Achenbach, T. M., Edelbrock, C., & Howard, C. T. (1987). Empirically based assessment of the behavioral/emotional problems of 2- and 3-year-old children. *Journal of Abnormal Child Psychology, 15,* 629-650.

Acton, G. J., Irvin, B. L., & Hopkins, B. A. (1991). Theory-testing research: Building the science. *Advances in Nursing Science, 14*(1), 52-61.

Adeyanju, M., & Creswell, W. H., Jr. (1987). The relationship among attitudes, behaviors, and biomedical measures of adolescents "at risk" for cardiovascular disease. *Journal of School Health, 57*(8), 326-331.

Affleck, G., Tennen, H., Pfeiffer, C., Fifield, J., & Rowe, J. (1987). Downward comparison and coping with serious medical problems. *American Journal of Orthopsychiatry, 57*(4), 570-578.

Aleman, A. R. (1991). Nursing care with the multiproblem poor family. In B. W. Spradley (Ed.), *Readings in community health nursing* (pp. 388-395). Philadelphia: J. B. Lippincott.

Alexander, S. (1991, June 21) Families turn to school nurse for health care. *Wall Street Journal,* pp. B1, B4.

Algase, D. (1990). Links between nursing science and nursing practice. In K. Berger & M. Williams (Eds.), *Collaborating for optimal health* (pp. 1628-1657). Norwalk, CT: Appleton & Lange.

Allen, D. G. (1987). Critical social theory as a model for analyzing ethical issues in family and community health. *Family and Community Health, 10*(1), 63-72.

Allen, D. G. (1985). Nursing and oppression: "The family" in nursing texts. *Feminist Teacher, 2*(1), 15-20.

Alperstein, G., & Arnstein, E. (1988). Homeless children: A challenge for pediatricians. *Pediatric Clinics of North America, 35,* 1413-1425.

Alwin, D. F. (1977). Making errors in surveys. *Sociological Methods and Research, 6*(2), 131-150.

Anderson, J. M. (1981). The social construction of the illness experience: Families with a chronically ill child. *Journal of Advanced Nursing, 6,* 427-434.

Anderson, J. M. (1986). Ethnicity and illness experience: Ideological structure and the health care delivery system. *Social Science and Medicine, 22,* 1277-1283.

Anderson, J. M. (1990). Home care management in chronic illness and the self-care movement: An analysis of ideologies and economic processes influencing policy decisions. *Advances in Nursing Science, 12*(2), 71-83.

Anderson, J. M., & Chung, J. (1982a). The differential construction of social reality in chronically ill children: An interpretive perspective. *Human Organization, 41,* 259-262.

Anderson, J. M., & Chung, J. (1982b). Culture and illness: Parents' perceptions of their child's long-term illness. *Nursing Papers, 14*(4), 40-52.

Anderson, J. M., & Elfert, H. (1989). Managing chronic illness in the family: Women as caretakers. *Journal of Advanced Nursing, 14,* 735-743.

Anderson, J. M., Elfert, H., & Lai, M. (1989). Ideology in the clinical context: Chronic illness, ethnicity, and the discourse on normalization. *Sociology of Health and Illness, 11,* 253-278.

Andrews, M., Bubolz, M., & Paolucci, B. (1980). Ecological approach to study of the family. *Marriage and Family Review, 32,* 29-49.

Aradine, C. E. (1980). Home care for young children with long-term tracheostomies. *MCN: American Journal of Maternal/Child Nursing, 5,* 121-125.

Arno, P. S., & Shenson, D. (1990). From AIDS to HIV disease: Transformation of an epidemic. *AHCPR Conference Proceeding,* 97-104.

Austin, J. (1988). Childhood epilepsy: Child adaptation and family resources. *Journal of Child and Adolescent Psychiatric Mental Health Nursing, 1,* 18-24.

Austin, J. K. (1990). Assessment of coping mechanisms used by parents and children with chronic illness. *American Journal of Maternal/Child Nursing, 15,* 98-105.

Bachrach, L. (1987). Homeless women: A context for health planning. *Milbank Quarterly, 65,* 371-396.

Bailey, D. B., & Simeonsson, R. J. (1988). *Family assessment in early intervention.* Columbus, OH: Charles E. Merrill.

Baillie, V., Norbeck, J. S., & Barnes, L. E. A. (1988, July/August). Stress, social support, and psychological distress of family caregivers of the elderly. *Nursing Research, 37*(4), 217-222.

Ball, D., McKenry, P. C., & Price-Bonham, S. (1983). Use of repeated-measures designs in family research. *Journal of Marriage and the Family, 80,* 885-896.

Bane, M. J., & Ellwood, D. T. (1989). One fifth of the nation's children: Why are they poor? *Science, 2245,* 1047-1053.

Banks, M. J. (1977). A family's overconcern about a child in the first two years of life. *Maternal-Child Nursing Journal, 6,* 187-194.

Barhyte, D. (1987). Levels of practice and retention of staff nurses. *Nursing Management, 18*(3), 70-72.

Barnard, K. E. (1978a). Nursing Child Assessment Feeding Scale. *Nursing Child Assessment Satellite Training Program manual.* N.C.A.S.T. Program, University of Washington, Seattle, WA 98195.

Barnard, K. E. (1978b). Nursing Child Assessment Teaching Scale. *Nursing Child Assessment Satellite Training Program manual.* N.C.A.S.T. Program, University of Washington, Seattle, WA 98195.

Barnard, K. E. (1979). Nursing Child Assessment Sleep/Activity Record. *Nursing Child Assessment Satellite Training Program manual.* N.C.A.S.T. Program, University of Washington, Seattle, WA 98195.

Barnard, K. E. (1980). Knowledge for practice: Directions for the future. *Nursing Research, 29,* 208-212.

Barnard, K. E. (1984). The family as a unit of measurement. *American Journal of Maternal/Child Nursing, 8,* 21.

Barnard, K. E. (1988a). Community Life Skills Scale. *Community Life Skills Scale manual.* N.C.A.S.T. Program, University of Washington, Seattle, WA 98195.

Barnard, K. E. (1988b). Difficult Life Circumstances Scale. *Difficult Life Circumstances Scale manual.* N.C.A.S.T. Program, University of Washington, Seattle, WA 98195.

Barnard, K. E. (1990, June 20). *Pediatric nursing in the 21st century: The child, the parent, and the nurse—revisited.* Keynote address at Taking Pediatric Nursing Into the Next Decade. Sponsored by the University of Wisconsin-Madison School of Nursing and the University of Wisconsin Children's Hospital.

Barnes, C. M. (1985). Training nurses to care for chronically ill children. In N. Hobbs, J. M. Perrin, & H. T. Ireys (Eds.), *Chronically ill children and their families* (pp. 498-513). San Francisco: Jossey-Bass.

Barnsteiner, J., & Gillis-Donavan, J. (1990). Being related and separate: A standard for therapeutic relationships. *MCN, 14,* 223-228.

Barrett, M. (1988). *Women's oppression today: The Marxist/feminist encounter* (rev. ed.). New York: Verso.

Bassuk, E., & Rubin, L. (1987). Homeless children: A neglected population. *American Journal of Orthopsychiatry, 57,* 279-286.

Bassuk, E. L., & Rosenberg, L. (1988). Why does family homelessness occur? A case-control study. *American Journal of Public Health, 78,* 783-788.

Bassuk, E. L., Rubin, L., & Lauriat, A. S. (1986). Characteristics of sheltered homeless families. *American Journal of Public Health, 76,* 1097-1101.

Beardslee, C. (1975). A mother's reactions to the surgery of her adopted son. *Maternal-Child Nursing Journal, 4,* 183-196.

Beckingham, A. C., & Baumann, A. (1990). The aging family in crisis: Assessment and decision-making models. *Journal of Advanced Nursing, 15,* 782-787.

Bell, J., & Wright, L. (1990, June). Flaws in family nursing education. *Canadian Nurse, 86*(6), 28-30.

Belle, D. (Ed.). (1982). *Lives in stress.* Beverly Hills, CA: Sage.

Benner, P. (1984). *From novice to expert.* Menlo Park, CA: Addison-Wesley.

Benner, P. (1985). Quality of life: A phenomenological perspective on explanation, prediction, and understanding in nursing science. *Advances in Nursing Science, 8*(1), 1-14.

Benner, P. (1991). The role of experience, narrative, and community in skilled ethical comportment. *Advances in Nursing Science, 14*(2), 1-21.

Benner, P., Tanner, C., & Chesla, C. (1992). From beginner to expert: Gaining a differentiated clinical world in critical care nursing. *Advances in Nursing Science, 14*(3), 13-28.

Benner, P., & Wrubel, J. (1989). *The primacy of caring: Stress and coping in health and illness.* Menlo Park, CA: Addison-Wesley.

Benoliel, J. Q. (1970). The developing diabetic identity: A study of family influence. In M. V. Batey (Ed.), *Communicating nursing research: Methodological issues in research* (Vol. 3, pp. 14-32). Boulder, CO: Western Interstate Commission of Higher Education.

Berman, W., & Turk, D. (1981). Adaptation to divorce: Problems and coping strategies. *Journal of Marriage and the Family, 43,* 179-189.

Bernard, J. (1982). *The future of marriage* (2nd ed.). New Haven, CT: Yale University Press.

Berne, A. S., Dato, C., Mason, D. J., & Rafferty, M. (1990). A nursing model for addressing the health needs of homeless families. *Image: Journal of Nursing Scholarship, 22,* 8-13.

Berry, J. W., Trimble, J. E., & Olmedo, E. L. (1986). Assessment of acculturation. In W. J. Lonner & J. W. Berry (Eds.), *Field methods in cross-cultural research* (pp. 291-324). Beverly Hills, CA: Sage.

Beutler, I., Burr, W., Bahr, K., & Herrin, D. (1989). The family realm: Theoretical contributions for understanding its uniqueness. *Journal of Marriage and the Family, 51,* 805-816.

Biegel, D. E., Sales, E., & Schulz, R. (1991). *Family caregiving in chronic illness.* Newbury Park, CA: Sage.

Bigbee, J. L. (1991). The concept of hardiness as applied to rural nursing. In A. Bushy (Ed.), *Rural nursing* (Vol. 1, pp. 39-58). Newbury Park, CA: Sage.

Birenbaum, L. K. (1987). *Description of family communication about chronic illness in children with cancer.* Unpublished doctoral dissertation, University of Washington, Seattle.

Birkhead, L. W. (1989). *Psychiatric mental health nursing: The therapeutic use of self.* Philadelphia: J. P. Lippincott.

Blecke, J. (1991, May). *Variation in children's self-care health behavior within differing family contexts.* Poster presented at the Second International Family Nursing Conference, Portland, OR.

Bomar, P. J. (1990). Perspectives on family health promotion. *Family and Community Health, 12*(4), 1-11.

Boss, P. G. (1987). The role of intuition in family research: Three issues of ethics. *Contemporary Family Therapy, 9*(1-2), 92-100.

Both, D. R., & Garduque, L. (Eds.). (1989). *Social policy for children and families.* (Report of the Steering Group of the National Forum on the Future of Children and Families). Washington, DC: National Academy Press.

Bowen, M. (1978). *Family therapy in clinical practice.* New York: Jason Aronson.

Bowers, B. J. (1987). Intergenerational caregiving: Adult caregivers and their aging parents. *Advances in Nursing Science, 9*(2), 20-31.

Bowmar, P. J. (1990). Perspectives on family health promotion. *Family and Community Health, 12*(4), 1-11.

Boxill, N., & Beaty, A. (1990). An exploration of mother-child interaction among homeless women and their children in a public night shelter in Atlanta, Georgia. In N. Boxill & A. Beaty, *The waiters and the watchers: American homeless children* (pp. 49-64). New York: Hawthorne.

Boyle, J. S., & Andrews, M. M. (1989). *Transcultural concepts in nursing care*. Glenview, IL: Scott, Foresman.

Bozett, F. (1987). Family nursing and life-threatening illness. In M. Leahey & L. Wright (Eds.), *Families and life-threatening illness* (pp. 2-25). Springhouse, PA: Springhouse.

Bradburn, N. M. (1983). Response effects. In P. H. Rossi, J. D. Wright, & A. B. Anderson (Eds.), *Handbook of survey research* (pp. 289-328). New York: Academic Press.

Bradburn, N. M., & Sudman, S. (1988). *Polls and surveys*. San Francisco: Jossey-Bass.

Bradt, J. O. (1980). The family with young children. In E. A. Carter & M. McGoldrick (Eds.), *The family life cycle* (pp. 121-146). New York: Gardener.

Brink, P. (1982). An anthropological perspective on parenting. In J. A. Horowitz, C. B. Hughes, & B. J. Perdue (Eds.), *Parenting reassessed* (pp. 66-85). Englewood Cliffs, NJ: Prentice-Hall.

Bronfenbrenner, U. (1979). *The ecology of human development: Experiments by nature and design*. Cambridge, MA: Harvard University Press.

Brooten, D., Brown, L. P., Munro, B. H., York, R., Cohen, S. B., Roncoli, M., & Hollingsworth, A. (1988). Early discharge and specialist transitional care. *Image: Journal of Nursing Scholarship, 20*(2), 64-68.

Brown, J., & Ritchie, J. A. (1990). Nurses' perceptions of parent and nurse roles in caring for hospitalized children. *Children's Health Care, 19,* 28-36.

Brown, J. S., Tanner, C. A., & Padrick, K. P. (1984). Nursing's search for scientific knowledge. *Nursing Research, 33,* 26-32.

Brown, L. P., Brooten, D., Kumar, S., Butts, P., Finkler, S., Bakewell-Sachs, S., Gibbons, A., & Delivoria-Papadapoulos, M. (1989). A sociodemographic profile of low birth weight infants. *Western Journal of Nursing Research, 11,* 520-528.

Brown, M. A., & Powell-Cope, G. (1991). AIDS family caregiving: Transitions through uncertainty. *Nursing Research, 40*(6), 338-345.

Brown, M. A., & Powell-Cope, G. (1992). *Caring for a loved one with AIDS: Experiences of families, lovers, and friends*. Seattle: University Press.

Browning, M., & Woods, J. H. (1991). *Cross-cultural communication of caregivers*. Poster presented at the 68th Annual Meeting of the American Orthopsychiatric Association, Toronto, Canada.

Bruner, J. (1987). Life as narrative. *Social Research, 54,* 11-32.

Bunting, S. M. (1989). Stress on caregivers of the elderly. *Advances in Nursing Science, 11*(2), 63-73.

Burgess, M. E. (1978). The resurgence of ethnicity: Myth or reality? *Ethnic and Racial Studies, 1*(3), 265-285.

Burke, M. L. (1989). *Chronic sorrow in mothers of school-age children with a myelomeningocele disability*. Unpublished doctoral dissertation, Boston University, Boston.

Burke, S. O., Costello, E. A., & Handley-Derry, M. H. (1989). Maternal stress and repeated hospitalizations of children who are physically disabled. *Children's Health Care, 18*(2), 82-90.

Burke, S. O., Kauffman, E., Costello, E. A., & Dillon, C. (1991). Hazardous secrets and reluctantly taking charge: Parenting a child with repeated hospitalizations. *Image: Journal of Nursing Scholarship, 23,* 39-46.

Burr, W. (1973). Families under stress. In W. Burr (Ed.), *Theory construction and the sociology of the family* (pp. 199-217). New York: John Wiley.

Burr, W., Herrin, D., Day, R., Beutler, I., & Leigh, G. (1988). Epistemologies that lead to primary explanations in family science. *Family Science Review, 1,* 185-210.

Burton, L. M. (1990). Teenage childbearing as an alternative life-course strategy in multigeneration black families. *Human Nature, 1,* 123-143.

Bush, M. (1988). *Families in distress: Public, private, and civic responses.* Berkeley: University of California Press.

Bushy, A. (1990). Rural determinants in family health: Considerations for community nurses. *Family and Community Health, 12*(4), 29-38.

Caldwell, B. M., & Bradley, R. H. (1978). *Manual for the home observation for measurement of the environment.* Child Development Research Unit, University of Arkansas at Little Rock, 33rd and University Avenue, Little Rock, AR 77204.

Canam, C. (1986). Talking about cystic fibrosis within the family—What parents need to know. *Issues in Comprehensive Pediatric Nursing, 9,* 167-178.

Canam, C. (1987). Coping with feelings: Chronically ill children and their families. *Nursing Papers, 19*(3), 9-21.

Cantor, M. (1983). Strain among caregivers: A study of experience in the United States. *Gerontologist, 23*(6), 597-604.

Caplan, G. (1960). Patterns of parental responses to crisis of premature birth. *Psychiatry, 23,* 365-373.

Carey, P., Oberst, M., McCubbin, M., & Hughes, S. (1991). Correlates of caregiving demand and distress in family members caring for patients receiving chemotherapy. *Oncology Nursing Forum, 18,* 1341-1348.

Carnes, P. (1987). *Counseling sexual abusers.* Minneapolis: CompCare.

Carpenito, L. J. (1991). *Handbook of nursing diagnosis* (4th ed.). Philadelphia: J. B. Lippincott.

Carroll-Johnson, R. M. (Ed.). (1989). *Classification of nursing diagnoses: Proceedings of the Eighth Conference, North American Nursing Diagnosis Association.* Philadelphia: J. B. Lippincott.

Caty, S., Ritchie, J. A., & Ellerton, M. L. (1989). Mothers' perceptions of coping behaviors in hospitalized preschool children. *Journal of Pediatric Nursing, 4,* 403-410.

Cautley, P. (1980). Family stress and the effect of in-house treatment. *Family Relations, 29,* 575-583.

Children's Defense Fund. (1989). *A vision for America's future.* Washington, DC: Author.

Childs, R. E. (1985). Maternal psychological conflicts associated with the birth of a retarded child. *Maternal-Child Nursing Journal, 14,* 15-18.

Chiverton, P., & Caine, E. D. (1989). Education to assist spouses in coping with Alzheimer's disease: A controlled trial. *Journal of the American Geriatrics Society, 37,* 593-598.

Chodoff, P., Friedman, S. B., & Hamburg, D. A. (1964). Stress, defenses, and coping behavior: Observations in parents of children with malignant diseases. *American Journal of Psychiatry, 120,* 743-749.

Chrisman, N. J., & Kleinman, A. (1983). Popular health care, social networks, and cultural meanings: The orientation of medical anthropology. In D. Mechanic (Ed.), *Handbook of health, health care, and the health professions* (pp. 569-590). New York: Free Press.

Christ, G. H., & Weiner, L. S. (1985). Psychosocial issues in AIDS. In V. T. DeVita, Jr. (Ed.), *AIDS: Etiology, diagnosis, treatment, and prevention* (pp. 275-297). Philadelphia: J. B. Lippincott.

Cicirelli, V. G. (1980). *Personal strains and negative feelings in adult children's relationships with elderly parents.* Paper presented at the 33rd Annual Scientific Meeting of the Gerontological Society of America, San Diego, CA.

Clarke, H. F. (1989). Developing consensus on Canadian family health needs: A step toward policy development. *Canadian Journal of Nursing Research, 21*(4), 21-33.

Clarke, J. (1984). *The family types of schizophrenics, neurotics, and normals.* Unpublished doctoral dissertation, University of Minnesota, St. Paul.

Clemen-Stone, S., Eigsti, D., & McGuire, S. L. (1991). *Comprehensive family and community health nursing.* St. Louis: C. V. Mosby.

Clements, D. B., Copeland, L. G., & Loftus, L. G. (1990). Critical times for families with a chronically ill child. *Pediatric Nursing, 16,* 157-161.

Cline, D. J. (1990). The psychosocial impact of HIV infection: What clinicians can do to help. *Journal of the American Academy of Dermatology, 22*(6, pt. 2), 299-302.

Coddington, M. N. (1976). A mother struggles to cope with her child's deteriorating illness. *Maternal-Child Nursing Journal, 5,* 39-44.

Cohen, D., & Eisdorfer, C. (1988). Depression in family members caring for a relative with Alzheimer's disease. *Journal of the American Geriatric Society, 36*(10), 885-889.

Cohen, J. (1989). *Statistical power analysis for the behavioral sciences* (2nd ed.). New York: Academic Press.

Cohen, M. A., & Weisman, H. W. (1986). A biopsychosocial approach to AIDS. *Psychosomatics, 27*(4), 245-249.

Cohen, M. H., & Martinson, I. (1988). Chronic uncertainty: Its effect on parental appraisal of a child's health. *Journal of Pediatric Nursing, 3,* 89-96.

Colapinto, J. (1988). Teaching the structural way. In H. A. Liddle, D. C. Breunlin, & R. C. Schwartz (Eds.), *Handbook of family therapy training and supervision* (pp. 17-37). New York: Guilford.

Comeau, J. (1985). *Family stressors, resources, and perceptions: Impact on the health status of the chronically ill child.* Unpublished doctoral dissertation, University of Minnesota, St. Paul.

Cooper, H. (1989). *Integrating research: A guide for literature reviews* (2nd ed.). Newbury Park, CA: Sage.

Cotroneo, M., DeFeudis, R., Moriarty, H., & Natale, S. (1992). *Family processes in intrafamilial abuse: A cross-cultural study of Italian families and American families.* Unpublished manuscript.

Cotroneo, M., Hibbs, B., & Moriarty, H. J. (1992). Uses and implications of the contextual approach to child custody decisions. *Journal of Child and Adolescent Psychiatric and Mental Health Nursing, 5*(3), 13-26.

Cotroneo, M., Moriarty, H. J., & Smith, E. (1992). Managing family loyalty conflicts in child custody disputes. *Journal of Family Psychotherapy, 3*(2), 19-37.

Council on Scientific Affairs. (1991). Hispanic health in the United States. *Journal of the American Medical Association, 265*(2), 248-252.

Crnic, K. A., & Greenberg, M. T. (1989). *Parenting Daily Hassles Scale.* Available from K. A. Crnic, Department of Psychology, 612 Moore Blvd., Pennslyvania State University, University Park, PA 16802.

Cromwell, R. E., & Olson, D. H. (1975). *Power in families.* Beverly Hills, CA: Sage.

Crummette, B. (1979). The maternal care of asthmatic children. *Maternal-Child Nursing Journal, 8,* 23-27.

Crystal, S. (1984). Homeless men and homeless women: The gender gap. *Urban and Social Change Review, 17,* 2-6.

Dailey, C. P. (1985). Teaching parents and children preventive health behaviors. *Family and Community Health, 7*(4), 34-43.

Damrosch, S. P., Lenz, E. R., & Perry, L. A. (1985). Use of parental advisors in the development of a Parental Coping Scale. *Maternal-Child Nursing Journal, 14,* 103-109.

Dance, F. E. X. (1979). Acoustic trigger to conceptualization. *Health Communication Informatics, 5,* 203-213.

Daniel, E. (1987). The relationship of hardiness and health behaviors: A corporate study. *Health Values, 2*(5), 7-13.

Daniels, E., Davis, B., & Sloan, P. (1991). *African-American family resources for coping (Study I); African-American family interactions (Study II); and Elderly African-American family coping behavior (Study III).* Bethesda, MD.: National Institutes of Mental Health.

D'Antonio, I. J. (1976). Mother's responses to the functioning and behavior of cardiac children in child-rearing situations. *Maternal-Child Nursing Journal, 5,* 207-264.

Davidson, G. (1990, October). *When a child dies.* Presentation at Lutheran General Hospital, Park Ridge, IL.

Davies, B. (1987). Family responses to the death of a child: The meaning of memories. *Journal of Palliative Care, 3*(1), 9-15.

Davis, K. (1991). Expanding Medicare and employer plans to achieve universal health insurance. *Journal of the American Medical Association, 265*(19), 2525-2528.

Dean, P. G. (1986). Monitoring an apneic infant: Impact on the infant's mother. *Maternal-Child Nursing Journal, 15,* 65-76.

Deatrick, J., & Knafl, K. (1988). Developing programs for hospitalized children: Clinical significance of qualitative research. *Journal of Pediatric Nursing, 3*(2), 123-126.

Deatrick, J., & Knafl, K. (1990). Management behaviors: Day-to-day adjustments to childhood chronic conditions. *Journal of Pediatric Nursing, 5*(1), 15-22.

Deatrick, J., Knafl, K., & Walsh, M. (1988). The process of parenting a child with a disability: Normalization through accommodations. *Journal of Advanced Nursing, 13,* 15-21.

Deatrick, J., Mason, K., & Davidson, R. (1990). *Collaborative assessment and management of selected orthopaedic problems.* Philadelphia: University of Pennsylvania and The Children's Hospital of Philadelphia.

Deatrick, J., Stull, M., Dixon, D., Puczynksi, S., & Jackson, S. (1986). Measuring parental participation: Part II. *Issues in Comprehensive Pediatric Nursing, 9,* 239-246.

Deatrick, J. A. (1990). Developing self-regulation in adolescents with chronic conditions. *Holistic Nursing Practice, 5*(1), 17-24.

Deatrick, J. A., & Faux, S. A. (1991). Conducting qualitative studies with children and adolescents. In J. M. Morse (Ed.), *Qualitative nursing research: A contemporary dialogue* (pp. 203-223). Newbury Park, CA: Sage.

Denyes, M. J. (1980). Development of an instrument to measure self-care agency in adolescents. *Dissertation Abstracts International, 4,* 1716-B. (University Microfilms No. 8025672).

Denzin, N. (1970). *The research act: A theoretical introduction to sociological methods.* Chicago: Aldine.

Derogatis, L., Abeloff, M., & Melisaratos, N. (1979). Psychological coping mechanisms and survival time in metastatic breast cancer. *Journal of the American Medical Association, 242*(14), 1504-1508.

Derogatis, L. R. (1983). *SCL-90-R: Administration, scoring, and procedures manual. II* (rev. ed.). Townson, MD: Clinical Psychometric Research.

Derogatis, L. R., & Melisaratos, N. (1983). The brief symptom inventory: An introductory report. *Psychological Medicine, 13,* 595-605.

Diers, D. (1985). Preparation of practitioners, clinical specialists, and clinicians. *Journal of Professional Nursing, 1,* 41-47.

Dill, D., Feld, E., Martin, J., Beukema, S., & Belle, B. (1980). The impact of the environment on the coping efforts of low-income mothers. *Family Relations, 29,* 503-509.

Dimaggio, C. T., & Sheetz, A. H. (1983). The concerns of mothers caring for an infant on an apnea monitor. *MCN: American Journal of Maternal/Child Nursing, 8,* 294-298.

Dobson, S. M. (1989). Conceptualizing for transcultural health visiting: The concept of transcultural reciprocity. *The Journal of Advanced Nursing, 14,* 97-102.

Doherty, W., & Baird, M. (1986). Developmental levels in family-centered medical care. *Family Medicine, 18*(3), 153-156.

Doherty, W. J., & McCubbin, H. I. (1985). Families and health care: An emerging arena of theory, research, and clinical intervention. *Family Relations, 34,* 5-11.

Dohrenwend, B. S., & Dohrenwend, B. P. (Eds.). (1974). *Stressful life events: Their nature and effects.* New York: John Wiley.

Dominica, M. F. (1987). Guest editorial: A message from Mother Frances Dominica, Founder of Helen House Hospice for Children. *Journal of Advanced Nursing, 12,* 149-150.

Donahue, M. P. (1985). *Nursing: The finest art* (p. 469). St. Louis, MO: C. V. Mosby.

Donaldson, S. K., & Crowley, D. M. (1978). The discipline of nursing. *Nursing Outlook, 26,* 113-120.

Donnelly, E. (1990). Health promotion, families, and the diagnostic process. *Family and Community Health, 12*(4), 12-20.

Dowd, E., & Vlastuin, L. (1990). In M. Craft & J. Denehy (Eds.), *Nursing interventions for infants and children* (pp. 240-256). Philadelphia: W. B. Saunders.

Dracopoulos, D. T., & Weatherly, J. B. (1983). Chronic renal failure: The effects on the entire family. *Issues in Comprehensive Pediatric Nursing, 6,* 141-146.

Draper, T. W., & Marcos, A. C. (Eds.). (1990). *Family variables: Conceptualization, measurement, and use.* Newbury Park, CA: Sage.

Dreyfus, H. L. (1991). *Being-in-the-world: A commentary on Heidegger's being and time, division I.* Cambridge, MA: MIT Press.

Driver, H. E. (1969). *Indians of North America* (2nd rev. ed.). Chicago: University of Chicago Press.

DSHS & Seattle-King County Health Department. (1990). *Washington St./Seattle-King County HIV/AIDS epidemiology report* (4th quarter). Seattle: Author.

Duffy, M., & Hedin, B. A. (1988). New directions for nursing research. In N. F. Woods & M. Catanzaro (Eds.), *Nursing research: Theory and practice* (pp. 530-539). St. Louis: C. V. Mosby.

Duffy, M. E. (1987). Strategies for change: The one-parent family. *Family and Community Health, 10*(2), 11-21.

Duffy, M. E. (1988). Health promotion in the family: Current findings and directives for nursing research. *Journal of Advanced Nursing, 13,* 109-117.

Dufour, D. F. (1989). Home or hospital care for the child with end-stage cancer: Effects on the family. *Issues in Comprehensive Pediatric Nursing, 12,* 371-383.

Dulock, H. L., & Holzemer, W. L. (1991). Substruction: Improving the linkage from theory to method. *Nursing Science Quarterly, 4*(2), 83-87.

Dunst, C. J., Cooper, C. S., Weeldreyer, J. C., Snyder, K. D., & Chase, J. H. (1988). Family Needs Scale. In C. J. Dunst, C. M. Trivette, & A. G. Deal (Eds.), *Enabling and empowering families: Principle and guidelines for practice* (pp. 149-151). Cambridge, MA: Brookline.

Dunst, C. J., Trivette, C. M., & Deal, A. G. (Eds.). (1988). Family Resource Scale. *Enabling and empowering families: Principle and guidelines for practice* (pp. 139-141). Cambridge, MA: Brookline.

Dunst, C. J., Trivette, C. M., & Jenkins, V. (1988). Family Support Scale. In C. J. Dunst, C. M. Trivette, & A. G. Deal (Eds.), *Enabling and empowering families: Principle and guidelines for practice* (pp. 155-157). Cambridge, MA: Brookline.

Dzik, M. A. (1979). Maternal comforting of the distressed infant. *Maternal-Child Nursing Journal, 8,* 163-171.

Edelman, M. W. (1987). *Families in peril: An agenda for social change.* Cambridge, MA: Harvard University Press.

Eidson, T. (1988). *AIDS caregiver's handbook.* New York: St. Martin's.

Elfert, H., Anderson, J. M., & Lai, M. (1991). Parents' perceptions of children with chronic illness: A study of immigrant Chinese families. *Journal of Pediatric Nursing, 6,* 114-120.

Ellwood, D. T. (1988) *Poor support: Poverty in the American family.* New York: Basic Books.

Erickson, J. R. (1988). *Coping with uncertainty for parents of ill infants.* Unpublished doctoral dissertation, University of Alabama, Birmingham.

Evans, R. L., Matlock, A., Bishop, D. S., Stranahan, E., & Pederson, C. (1988). Family intervention after stroke: Does counseling or education help? *Stroke, 19,* 1243-1249.

Ezell, M. P., Paolucci, B., & Bubolz, M. J. (1984). Developing family properties. *Home Economics Research Journal, 12*(4), 563-574.

Failla, S., & Jones, L. (1991). Families of children with developmental disabilities: An examination of family hardiness. *Research in Nursing and Health, 14,* 41-50.

Family Nursing Unit. (1988). *Fundamentals of family systems nursing, family systems interventions.* Calgary, Alberta, Canada: University of Calgary Communications Media.

Faux, S. A. (1984). Sibling and maternal perceptions of having a child with a craniofacial or cardiac anomaly in the family. (Doctoral dissertation, University of Illinois, Chicago). *Dissertation Abstracts International, 46,* 1115B-1116B.

Faux, S., Walsh, M., & Deatrick, J. (1988). Intensive interviewing with children and adolescents. *Western Journal of Nursing Research, 10,* 180-194.

Faux, S. A. (1991). Sibling relationships in families of congenitally impaired children. *Journal of Pediatric Nursing, 6,* 175-184.

Fawcett, J. (1975). The family as a living open system: An emerging conceptual framework for nursing. *International Nursing Review, 22,* 113-116.

Fawcett, J. (1978). The relationship between theory and research: A double helix. *Advances in Nursing Science, 1*(1), 49-62.

Fawcett, J. (1984a). *Analysis and evaluation of conceptual models of nursing.* Philadelphia: F. A. Davis.

Fawcett, J. (1984b). The metaparadigm of nursing: Present status and future refinements. *Image, 16,* 84-87.

Fawcett, J. (1989). *Analysis and evaluation of conceptual models of nursing* (2nd ed.). Philadelphia: F. A. Davis.

Fawcett, J., & Whall, A. (1990). Family theory development in nursing: State of the art and science. In J. Bell, W. Watson, & L. Wright (Eds.), *The cutting edge of family nursing* (pp. 17-23). Calgary, Alberta, Canada: Family Nursing Unit Publications.

Feetham, S. (1984). Family research: Issues and directions for nursing. In H. Werley & J. J. Fitzpatrick (Eds.), *Annual review of nursing research* (Vol. 2, pp. 3-25). New York: Springer.

Feetham, S. L. (1986). Hospitals and home care: Inseparable in the '80s. *Pediatric Nursing, 12*(5), 383-386.

Feetham, S. (1990). Conceptual and methodological issues in research of families. In J. Bell, W. Watson, & L. Wright (Eds.), *The cutting edge of family nursing* (pp. 35-49). Calgary, Alberta, Canada: Family Nursing Unit Publications.

Feetham, S. (1991). Conceptual and methodological issues in research of families. In A. Whall & J. Fawcett (Eds.), *Family theory development in nursing: State of the science and art* (pp. 55-68). Philadelphia: F. A. Davis.

Feetham, S. L. (in press). *Family outcomes: Conceptual and methodological issues.* In P. Mortiz (Ed.) *Proceedings of Patient Outcomes Research: Examining the effectiveness of nursing practice.* Bethesda, MD: National Center for Nursing Research, National Institutes of Health.

Feetham, S. L., & Humenick, S. S. (1982). Feetham Family Functioning Survey. In S. S. Humenick (Ed.), *Analysis of current assessment strategies in the health care of young children and childbearing families* (pp. 259-268). New York: Appleton-Century-Crofts.

Ferketich, S., & Verran, J. (1986). Exploratory data analysis introduction. *Western Journal of Nursing Research, 8*(4), 464-467.

Ferraro, A. R., & Longo, D. C. (1985). Nursing care of the family with a chronically ill, hospitalized child: An alternative approach. *Image, XVII,* 77-81.

Fife, B. L. (1985). A model for predicting the adaptation of families to medical crisis: An analysis of role integration. *Image, XVII,* 108-112.

Fife, B. L., Huhman, M., & Keck, J. (1986). Development of a clinical assessment scale: Evaluation of the psychosocial impact of childhood illness on the family. *Issues in Comprehensive Pediatric Nursing, 9,* 11-31.

Figley, C., & McCubbin, H. (1983). *Stress and the family.* New York: Brunner/Mazel.

Filsinger, E. E. (1990). Empirical typology, cluster analysis, and family-level measurement. In T. W. Draper & A. C. Marcos (Eds.), *Family variables conceptualization, measurement, and use* (pp. 90-104). Newbury Park, CA: Sage.

First, R. J., Toomey, B. G., & Rife, J. C. (1990). *Preliminary findings on rural homelessness in Ohio.* Columbus: Ohio State University.

Fisher, L., Terry, H. E., & Ranson, D. C. (1990). Advancing a family perspective in health research: Models and methods. *Family Process, 29,* 177-189.

Fitzpatrick, J. J. (Ed.). *Annual Review of Nursing Research* (Vol. 2, pp. 3-25). New York: Springer.

Flaskerud, J. H. (1989). *AIDS/HIV infection: A reference guide for nursing professionals.* Philadelphia: W. B. Saunders.

Flint, M., & Walsh, M. (1988). Visiting policies in pediatrics: Parents' perceptions and preferences. *Journal of Pediatric Nursing, 3,* 237-245.

Frankenburg, W. F., Dick, N. P., & Carland, J. (1975). Development of preschool-aged children of different social and ethnic groups: Implications for developmental screening. *Journal of Pediatrics, 87,* 125-132.

Freeman, H. E., Blendon, R. J., Aiken, L. H., Sudman, S., Mullinix, C. F., & Corey, C. R. (1990). Americans report their access to health care. In P. R. Lee & C. L. Estes (Eds.), *The nation's health* (pp. 309-319). Boston: Jones & Bartlett.

Frey, M. A. (1989). Social support and health: A theoretical formulation derived from King's conceptual framework. *Nursing Science Quarterly, 2,* 138-148.

Frey, M. A., & Denyes, M. J. (1989). Health and illness self-care in adolescents with IDDM: A test of Orem's theory. *Advances in Nursing Science, 12*(1), 67-75.

Frey, M. A., & Fox, M. A. (1990). Assessing and teaching self-care to youths with diabetes mellitus. *Pediatric Nursing, 16,* 597-599.

Friedemann, M. L. (1989). The concept of family nursing. *Journal of Advanced Nursing, 14,* 211-216.

Friedman, E. (1991). The uninsured: From dilemma to crisis. *Journal of the American Medical Association, 265*(19), 2491-2495.

Friedman, M. (1986). *Family nursing: Theory and assessment* (2nd ed.). New York: Appleton-Century-Crofts.

Friedman, M. (1990). Transcultural family nursing. In J. M. Bell, W. L. Watson, & L. M. Wright (Eds.), *The cutting edge of family nursing* (pp. 51-66). Calgary, Alberta, Canada: Family Nursing Unit Publications.

Froman, R. D., & Owen, S. V. (1989). Infant care self-efficacy. *Scholarly Inquiry for Nursing Practice: An International Journal, 3*(3), 199-210.

Frost, H. (1939). *Nursing in sickness and health.* New York: Macmillan.

Furstenberg, F. F., Jr. (1991). As the pendulum swings: Teenage childbearing and social concern. *Family Relations, 40,* 127-138.

Furstenberg, F. F., Jr. (1992). Teenage childbearing and cultural rationality: A thesis in search of evidence. *Family Relations, 41,* 239-243.

Gadow, S. (1980). Existential advocacy: Philosophical foundations of nursing. In S. Spicker & S. Gadow (Eds.), *Nursing: Images and ideals* (pp. 00-00). New York: Springer.

Gagliardi, B. A. (1989). *Three families' experience of living with a child diagnosed with Duchenne muscular dystrophy.* Unpublished doctoral dissertation, New York University, New York.

Gallo, A. M. (1990). Family management style in juvenile diabetes: A case illustration. *Journal of Pediatric Nursing, 5,* 23-32.

Gallo, A. M., Breitmayer, B. J., Knafl, K. A., & Zoeller, L. H. (1991). Stigma in childhood chronic illness: A well sibling perspective. *Pediatric Nursing, 17*(1), 21-25.

Ganong, L. (1987). Integrative reviews of nursing research. *Research in Nursing and Health, 10,* 1-11.

Geary, M. (1979). Supporting family coping. *Supervisor Nurse, 10,* 52-59.

Gelles, R. J. (1974). *The violent home: A study of physical aggression between husbands and wives.* Beverly Hills, CA: Sage.

Gelles, R. J. (1978). Methods for studying sensitive family topics. *American Journal of Orthopsychiatry, 48*(3), 408-424.

Gelles, R. J. (1987). *The violent home* (rev. ed.). Newbury Park, CA: Sage.

Gerber, J., Wolff, J., Klores, W., & Brown, G. (1989). *Lifetrends: The future of baby boomers and other aging Americans.* New York: Macmillan.

Geronimus, A. T. (1991). Teenage childbearing and social and reproductive disadvantages: The evolution of complex questions and the demise of simple answers. *Family Relations, 40,* 463-471.

Gerominus, A. T. (1992). Teenage childbearing and social disadvantage: Unprotected discourse. *Family Relations, 41,* 244-248.

Gewirtzman, R., & Fodor, I. (1987). The homeless child at school: From welfare hotel to classroom. *Child Welfare, 66,* 237-245.

Giger, J. N., & Davidhizar, R. E. (Eds.). (1991). *Transcultural nursing.* St. Louis: C. V. Mosby.

Gill, K. M. (1987). Parent participation with a family health focus: Nurses' attitudes. *Pediatric Nursing, 13,* 94-99.

Gilliss, C. (1983). The family as a unit of analysis: Strategies for the nurse researcher. *Advances in Nursing Science, 5*(3), 50-59.

Gilliss, C. (1989a). Family research in nursing. In C. L. Gilliss, B. L. Highley, B. M. Roberts, & I. M. Martinson (Eds.), *Toward a science of family nursing* (pp. 37-63). Menlo Park, CA: Addison-Wesley.

Gilliss, C. (1989b). What is family nursing? In C. L. Gilliss, B. L. Highley, B. M. Roberts, & I. M. Martinson (Eds.), *Toward a science of family nursing* (pp. 64-73). Menlo Park, CA: Addison-Wesley.

Gilliss, C. (1989c). Why family health care? In C. L. Gilliss, B. L. Highley, B. M. Roberts, & I. M. Martinson (Eds.), *Toward a science of family nursing* (pp. 3-8). Menlo Park, CA: Addison-Wesley.

Gilliss, C. (1990). Foreword. In J. M. Bell, W. L. Watson, & L. M. Wright (Eds.), *The cutting edge of family nursing* (pp. iii-v). Calgary, Alberta, Canada: Family Nursing Unit Publications.

Gilliss, C. (1991). Family nursing research, theory, and practice. *Image, 23*(1), 19-22.

Gilliss, C., Campbell, T., & Patterson, J. (1989, November). *Family health as viewed by three disciplines: Agenda for the 1990s.* Paper presented at the National Conference of Family Relations, New Orleans, LA.

Gilliss, C., & Davis, L. (1991). *Family nursing interventions: An integrative review and meta-analysis.* Paper presented at the International Nursing Research Conference, American Nurses Association Council of Nurse Researchers, Los Angeles.

Gilliss, C., & Davis, L. L. (1992). Family nursing research: Precepts from paragons and peccadilloes. *Journal of Advanced Nursing, 17,* 28-33.

Gilliss, C., Highley, B. L., Roberts, B. M., & Martinson, I. M. (Eds.). (1989). *Toward a science of family nursing.* Menlo Park, CA: Addison-Wesley.

Gilliss, C., Neuhaus, J., & Hauck, W. (1990). Improving family functioning after cardiac surgery: A randomized trial. *Heart and Lung, 19,* 648-654.

Gillon, J. E. (1972). Family stresses when a child has congenital heart disease. *Maternal-Child Nursing Journal, 1,* 265-272.

Glaser, B., & Strauss, A. (1967). *The discovery of grounded theory: Strategies for qualitative research.* Chicago: Aldine.

Glenn, M. W. (1987). *Mental retardation: A parental perspective.* Unpublished doctoral dissertation, University of Illinois, Chicago.

Goodrich, T. J. , Rampage, C., Ellman, B., & Halstead, K. (1988). *Feminist family therapy: A casebook.* New York: Norton.

Gordon, D. R. (1984). Research application: Identifying the use and misuse of formal models in nursing practice. In P. Benner (Ed.), *From novice to expert: Excellence and power in clinical nursing practice* (pp. 225-243). Menlo Park, CA: Addison-Wesley.

Gordon, M. (1988-1989). *The manual of nursing diagnosis.* St. Louis: C. V. Mosby.

Gortner, S. R. (1983, September). *Knowledge for a practice discipline: Philosophy and pragmatics.* Unpublished keynote address for the Annual Meeting of the American Academy of Nursing, Minneapolis.

Gortner, S. R., Gilliss, C. L., Shinn, J. A., Sparacino, P. A., Rankin, S., Leavitt, M., Price, M., & Hudes, M. (1988). Improving recovery following cardiac surgery: A randomized clinical trial. *Journal of Advanced Nursing, 13,* 649-661.

Gortner, S. R., & Schultz, P. R. (1988). Approaches to nursing science methods. *Image, 20,* 22-24.

Goss, S. (1990). *Relationships between parental health-promoting behaviors, family time and routines, family sociodemographic factors, and school-aged children's health self-concept.* Unpublished master's thesis. University of Wisconsin, School of Nursing, Madison.

Gottlieb, L., & Rowat, K. (1987). The McGill model of nursing: A practice-derived model. *Advances in Nursing Science, 9*(4), 51-61.

Govoni, L. A. (1988, December). Psychosocial issues of AIDS in the nursing care of homosexual men and their significant others. *Nursing Clinics of North America, 23*(4), 749-765.

Gray, E., & Cosgrove, J. (1985). Ethnocentric perception of childrearing practices in protective services. *Child Abuse and Neglect, 9,* 389-396.

Gruetzner, H. (1988). *Alzheimer's: A caregiver's guide and sourcebook.* New York: John Wiley.

Gudermuth, S. (1975). Mothers' reports of early experiences of infants with congenital heart disease. *Maternal-Child Nursing Journal, 4,* 155-164.

Haas, S. (1986). *A survey of staff nurse perceptions of proposed outcomes of clinical ladder performance appraisal systems.* Unpublished doctoral dissertation, University of Illinois, Chicago.

Hagestad, G. O. (1981). Problems and promises in the social pychology of intergenerational relations. In R. W. Fogel, E. Hatfield, S. B. Kiesler, et al. (Eds.), *Aging: Stability and change in the family* (pp. 11-46). New York: Academic Press.

Ham, L. M., & Chamings, P. A. (1983). Family nursing: Historical perspectives. In I. W. Clements & F. B. Roberts (Eds.), *Family health: A theoretical approach to nursing care* (pp. 33-43). New York: John Wiley.

Hanson, S., & Bozett, F. (1987). *Family nursing curriculum survey.* Unpublished manuscript, Oregon Health Sciences University, Portland.

Haque, R. (1989). A family's experience with AIDS. In J. H. Flaskerud (Ed.), *AIDS/HIV infection: A reference guide for nursing professionals* (pp. 230-240). Philadelphia: W. B. Saunders.

Harding, S. (1987a). Conclusion: Epistemological questions. In S. Harding (Ed.), *Feminism and methodology: Social science issues* (pp. 181-190). Bloomington: Indiana University Press.

Harding, S. (1987b). Introduction: Is there a feminist method? In S. Harding (Ed.), *Feminism and methodology: Social science issues* (pp. 1-14). Bloomington: Indiana University Press.

Harper, S., & Lund, D. A. (1990). Wives, husbands, and daughters caring for institutionalized and noninstitutionalized dementia patients: Toward a model of caregiver burden. *International Journal on Aging and Human Development, 30*(4), 241-262.

Harter, S. (1985). *Manual for the self-perception profile for children.* Denver, CO: University of Denver.

Hartman, A. (1978). Diagrammatic assessment of the family. *Social Casework, 59*(8), 465-476.

Hartman, A. (1979). *Finding families: An ecological approach to family assessment in adoption.* Beverly Hills, CA: Sage.

Hartwig, F., & Dearing, B. (1979). *Exploratory data analysis.* Beverly Hills, CA: Sage.

Harwood, A. (Ed.). (1981). *Ethnicity and medical care.* Cambridge, MA: Harvard University Press.

Hayes, V. E., & Knox, J. E. (1984). The experience of stress in parents of children hospitalized with long-term disabilities. *Journal of Advanced Nursing, 9,* 333-341.

Hazelrigg, M. D., Cooper, H. M., & Borduin, C. M. (1987). Evaluating the effectiveness of family therapies: An integrative review and analysis. *Psychology Bulletin, 101*(3), 428-442.

Hazlett, D. E. (1989). A study of pediatric home ventilator management: Medical, psychosocial, and financial aspects. *Journal of Pediatric Nursing, 4,* 284-294.

Heatherington, L., Friedlander, M. L., & Johnson, W. F. (1989). Informed consent in family therapy research: Ethical dilemmas and practical problems. *Journal of Family Psychology, 2*(3), 373-385.

Hedges, L., & Olkin, I. (1985). *Statistical methods for meta-analysis.* New York: Academic Press.

Hedrick, G. (1979). Mothering conjoined twins. *Maternal-Child Nursing Journal, 8,* 125-133.

Henderson, G., & Primeaux, M. (1981). *Transcultural health care.* Reading, MA: Addison-Wesley.

Herberg, P. (1989). Theoretical foundations of transcultural nursing. In J. S. Boyle & M. M. Andrews (Eds.), *Transcultural concepts in nursing care* (pp. 3-92). Glenview, IL: Scott, Foresman.

Hill, R. (1949). *Families under stress.* New York: Harper & Row.

Hill, R. (1958). Generic features of families under stress. *Social Casework, 39,* 139-150.

Hinds, C. (1985). The needs of families who care for patients with cancer at home: Are we meeting them? *Journal of Advanced Nursing, 10*(6), 575-581.

Hirschfeld, M. J. (1991, May). *Health for all in the year 2000: The role of family nursing.* Paper presented at the Second International Family Nursing Conference, Portland, OR.

Hoaglin, D. C., Mosteller, F., & Tukey, J. W. (1983). *Understanding robust and exploratory data analysis.* New York: John Wiley.

Hodges, L. C., & Parker, J. (1987). Concerns of parents with diabetic children. *Pediatric Nursing, 13,* 22-24, 68.

Hoerlin, B. Y. (1989). *Connecting: Challenges in Health and Human Services in the Philadelphia region.* Philadelphia: Pew Charitable Trusts.

Holaday, B. (1987). Patterns of interaction between mothers and their chronically ill infants. *Maternal-Child Nursing Journal, 16,* 29-46.

Hopkins, L. J. (1973). A basis for nursing care of the terminally ill child and his family. *Maternal-Child Nursing Journal, 2,* 93-100.

Hopper, K., & Hamberg, J. (1984). *The making of America's homeless: From skid row to new poor: 1945-1984.* New York: Grune & Stratton.

Horowitz, A. (1985) Family caregiving to the frail elderly. *Annual Review of Gerontology and Geriatrics, 5,* 194-246.

Hu, D. J., Covell, R. M., Morgan, J., & Arcia, J. (1989). Health care needs for children of the recently homeless. *Journal of Community Health, 14,* 1-8.

Hughes, L. (1951). *The panther and the lady.* New York: Knopf.

Hymovich, D. P. (1981). Assessing the impact of chronic childhood illness on the family and parent coping. *Image, 13*(3), 71-74.

Hymovich, D. P. (1984). Development of a chronicity impact and coping impact instrument: Parent questionnaire (CICI: PQ). *Nursing Research, 33,* 218-222.

Iles, P. (1979). Children with cancer: Siblings' perceptions during the illness experience. *Cancer Nursing, 2,* 371-377.

Institute of Medicine. (1988). *Homeless, health, and human needs.* Washington, DC: National Academy Press.

Irvine, S. H., & Carroll, W. K. (1980). Testing and assessment across cultures: Issues in methodology and theory. In H. C. Triandis & J. W. Berry (Eds.), *Handbook of cross-cultural psychology* (Vol. 2, pp. 181-244). Boston: Allyn & Bacon.

Jacobsen, B., & Meininger, J. (1985). The design and methods of published nursing research: 1956-83, *Nursing Research, 34,* 306-312.

Jacobsen, B., Tulman, L., & Lowrey, B. (1991). Three sides of the same coin: The analysis of paired data from dyads. *Nursing Research, 40*(6), 359-363.

Jaggar, A. M., & Rothenberg, P. S. (1984). *Feminist frameworks: Alternative theoretical accounts of the relations between women and men* (2nd ed.). New York: McGraw-Hill.

Jay, S. S. (1975). The impact of a boy's head injury on his parents. *Maternal-Child Nursing Journal, 4,* 49-56.

Johnson, B. H. (1990). The changing role of families in health care. *Children's Health Care, 19,* 234-241.

Johnson, B. S. (1988). Parenting children with disabilities. Unpublished doctoral dissertation, Texas Woman's University, Denton.

Johnson, D. E. (1974). Development of theory: A requisite for nursing as a primary health profession. *Nursing Research, 23,* 372-377.

Johnson, J. V., & Hall, E. M. (1988). Job strain, work place social support, and cardiovascular disease: A cross-sectional study of a random sample of the Swedish working population. *American Journal of Public Health, 78*(10), 1336-1342.

Jones, D. A., & Vetter, N. J. (1984). A survey of those who care for the elderly at home: Their problems and their needs. *Social Science and Medicine, 19*(5), 511-514.

Jones, E. F., Forrest, J. D., Goldman, N., Henshaw, S. K., Lincoln, R., Rosoff, J. I., Westoff, C. F., & Wulf, D. (1985). Teenage pregnancy in developed countries: Determinants and policy implications. *Family Planning Perspectives, 17,* 53-63.

Kane, C. F. (1988). Family social support: Toward a conceptual model. *Advances in Nursing Science, 10*(2), 19-25.

Kelly, R. F., & Ramsey, S. H. (1991) Poverty, children, and public policy. *Journal of Family Issues, 12,* 388-403.

Kikuchi, J. F. (1980). Assimilative and accommodative responses of mothers to their newborn infants with congenital defects. *Maternal-Child Nursing Journal, 9*(3),141-221.

King, I. (1981). *A theory for nursing: Systems, concepts, process.* New York: John Wiley.

Kitson, G. C., Sussman, M. B., Williams, G. K., Zeehandelaar, R. B., Shickmanter, B. K., & Steinberger, J. L. (1982). Sampling issues in family research. *Journal of Marriage and the Family, 44,* 965-981.

Klein, D. (1981, October). *The problem of multiple perceptions in family research.* Paper presented at the National Council of Family Relations, Milwaukee, WI.

Kleinman, A. (1980). *Patients and healers in the context of culture.* Berkeley: University of California Press.

Kluckhohn, F. R. (1976). Dominant and variant value orientations. In P. Brink (Ed.), *Transcultural nursing* (pp. 63-81). Englewood Cliffs, NJ: Prentice-Hall.

Knafl, K. A. (1982). Parents' views of the response of siblings in a pediatric hospitalization. *Research in Nursing and Health, 5,* 13-20.

Knafl, K. A. (1985). How families manage a pediatric hospitalization. *Western Journal of Nursing Research, 7,* 151-176.

Knafl, K., Breitmayer, B., Gallo, A., & Zoeller, L. (1987). *How families define and manage a child's chronic illness.* Funded by the National Center for Nursing Research, Public Health Service (Grant #NR01594).

Knafl, K., Breitmeyer, B., Gallo, A., & Zoeller, L. (1990, April). *How parents manage a child's chronic illness: The work of creating a normal family life.* Paper presented at the meeting of the Midwest Nursing Research Society, Indianapolis, IN.

Knafl, K. A., Cavallari, K. A., & Dixon, D. M. (1988). *Pediatric hospitalization: Family and nurse perspectives.* Glenview, IL: Scott, Foresman.

Knafl, K. A., & Deatrick, J. (1986). How families manage chronic conditions: An analysis of the concept of normalization. *Research in Nursing and Health, 9,* 215-222.

Knafl, K. A., & Deatrick, J. A. (1990). Family management style: Concept analysis and development. *Journal of Pediatric Nursing, 5*(1), 4-14.

Knafl, K. A., Deatrick, J. A., & Kodadek, S. (1982). How parents manage jobs and a child's hospitalization. *MCN: American Journal of Maternal/Child Nursing, 7,* 125-127.

Knafl, K. A., & Dixon, D. M. (1983). The role of siblings during pediatric hospitalization. *Issues in Comprehensive Pediatric Nursing, 6*(1), 13-22.

Knafl, K. A., & Dixon, D. M. (1984). The participation of fathers in their children's hospitalization. *Issues in Comprehensive Pediatric Nursing, 7,* 269-281.

Knafl, K. A., & Howard, M. J. (1984). Interpreting and reporting qualitative research. *Research in Nursing and Health, 7,* 17-24.

Knox, J. E., & Hayes, V. E. (1983). Hospitalization of a chronically ill child: A stressful time for parents. *Issues in Comprehensive Pediatric Nursing, 6,* 217-226.

Kobasa, S. (1979). Stressful life events, personality, and health: An inquiry into hardiness. *Journal of Personality and Social Psychology, 37,* 1-11.

Kobasa, S. C. O., Maddi, S. R., Puccetti, M. C., & Zola, M. A. (1985). Effectiveness of hardiness, exercise, and social support as resources against illness. *Journal of Psychometric Research, 29*(5), 525-533.

Kodadek, S. M. (1985). *Family management for home care for the handicapped child.* Unpublished doctoral dissertation, University of Illinois, Chicago.

Kodadek, S., & Haylor, M. (1990). Using interpretive methods to understand family caregiving when a child is blind. *Journal of Pediatric Nursing, 5,* 42-49.

Korbin, J. (1977). Anthropological contributions to the study of child abuse. *Child Abuse and Neglect, 1*(1), 7-24.

Kotlowitz, A. (1991). *There are no children here.* New York: Doubleday.

Kovacs, M. (1985). Children's Depression Inventory. *Psychopharmacology Bulletin, 21,* 995-999.

Kozol, J. (1988). *Rachel and her children: Homeless families in America.* New York: Crown.

Kravitz, M., & Frey, M. A. (1989). Allen nursing model. In J. J. Fitzpatrick & A. L. Whall (Eds.), *Conceptual models of nursing: Analysis and application* (pp. 313-329). Norwalk, CT: Appleton & Lange.

Kroeber, T. (1964). *Ishi, last of his tribe.* New York: Bantam.

Krulik, T. (1980). Successful "normalizing" tactics of parents of chronically ill children. *Journal of Advanced Nursing, 5,* 573-578.

Kuhn, T. S. (1970). *The structure of scientific revolutions.* Chicago: University of Chicago Press.

Kviz, F. J. (1977). Toward a standard definition of response rate. *Public Opinion Quarterly, 41,* 265-267.

Ladner, J. (1971). *Tomorrow's tomorrow.* New York: Doubleday.

Lambert, C. E., Jr., & Lambert, V. A. (1987). Hardiness: Its development and relevance to nursing. *Image: Journal of Nursing Scholarship, 19*(2), 92-95.

Lapp, C. A., Diemert, C. A., & Enestvedt, R. (1990). Family-based practice: Discussion of a tool merging assessment with intervention. *Family and Community Health, 12*(4), 21-28.

LaRossa, R. L., Bennett, L. A., & Gelles, R. J. (1981). Ethical dilemmas in qualitative family research. *Journal of Marriage and the Family, 43,* 303-313.

Larson, A., & Olson, D. (1990). Capturing the complexity of family systems: Integrating family theory, family scores, and family analysis. In T. W. Draper & A. C. Marcos (Eds.), *Family variables: Conceptualization, measurement, and use* (pp. 19-47). Newbury Park, CA: Sage.

Lash, M. E. (1991). Community health nursing in a minority setting. In B. W. Spratley (Ed.), *Readings in community health nursing* (pp. 512-520). Philadelphia: J. B. Lippincott.

Lavee, Y., McCubbin, H., & Patterson, J. (1985). Double ABCX model of stress and adaptation: An empirical test by analysis of structural equations with latent variables. *Journal of Marriage and the Family, 47,* 811-825.

Lawton, M. P., Kleban, M. H., Moss, M., Rovine, M., & Glieksman, A. (1989). Measuring caregiving appraisal. *Journal of Gerontology, 44*(3), 61-71.

Lazarsfeld, P., & Menzel, H. (1969). On the relation between individual and collective properties. In A. Etzioni (Ed.), *Sociological reader on complex organizations* (2nd ed., pp. 499-516). New York: Holt, Rinehart & Winston.

Leahey, M., & Wright, L. M. (1987a). *Families and life-threatening illness.* Springhouse, PA: Springhouse.

Leahey, M., & Wright, L. M. (1987b). *Families and psychosocial problems.* Springhouse, PA: Springhouse.

Lederman, R. P., Weingarten, C. T., & Lederman, E. (1981). Postpartum Self-Evaluation Questionnaire: Measures of maternal adaptation. *Birth Defects: Original Article Series, 17*(6), 201-231.

Lee, H. J. (1983). Analysis of a concept: Hardiness. *Oncology Nursing Forum, 10*(4), 32-35.

Leet, H. E., & Dunst, C. J. (1988). Family Resource Scale. In C. J. Dunst, C. M. Trivette, & A. G. Deal (Eds.), *Enabling and empowering families: Principle and guidelines for practice* (p. 141). Cambridge, MA: Brookline.

Leininger, M. (1978). Becoming aware of types of health practitioners and cultural imposition. In M. Leininger (Ed.), *Transcultural nursing* (pp. 139-154). New York: John Wiley.

Leininger, M. M. (1988). Leininger's theory of nursing: Cultural care diversity and universality. *Nursing Science Quarterly, 1*(4), 152-160.

Leonard, V. W. (1989). A Heideggerian phenomenologic perspective on the concept of the person. *Advances in Nursing Science, 11*(4), 40-55.

Lewandowski, L. A. (1980). Stresses and coping styles of parents of children undergoing open heart surgery. *Critical Care Quarterly, 3,* 75-84.

Lewis, F. (1985). The impact of cancer on the family: A critical analysis of the research literature. *Patient Education and Counseling, 8,* 269-289.

Lewis, O. (1966, October). The culture of poverty. *Scientific American 215*(4), 19-25.

Leyn, R. M. (1972). A mother's reactions to her son's fatal illness. *Maternal-Child Nursing Journal, 1,* 231-241.

Leyn, R. M. (1976). Terminally ill children and their families: A study of the variety of responses to fatal illness. *Maternal-Child Nursing Journal, 5,* 179-188.

Liddle, H. A., Breunlin, D. C., & Schwartz, R. C. (1988). Family therapy training and supervision: An introduction. In H. A. Liddle, D. C. Breunlin, & R. C. Schwartz (Eds.), *Handbook of family therapy training and supervision* (pp. 3-9). New York: Guilford.

Liddle, H. A., & Saba, G. (1985). The isomorphic nature of training and therapy: Epistemologic foundation for a structural-strategic training paradigm. In J. Schwartzman (Ed.), *Families and other systems* (pp. 27-47). New York: Guilford.

Light, R., & Pillemer, D. (1984). *Summing up: The science of reviewing research.* Cambridge, MA: Harvard University Press.

Lincoln, Y. S., & Guba, E. G. (1985). *Naturalistic inquiry.* Beverly Hills, CA: Sage.

Lindsey, A. M. (1989). Health care for the homeless. *Nursing Outlook, 32,* 78-81.

Lipman, T., & Deatrick, J. (in progress). *Enhancing specialist preparation for the next century.*

Lipman-Blumen, J. (1984). *Gender roles and power.* Englewood Cliffs, NJ: Prentice-Hall.

Long, K. A., & Weinert, C. (1989). Rural nursing: Developing the theory base. *Scholarly Inquiry for Nursing Practice, 3,* 113-127.

Lonner, W. J., & Berry, J. W. (Eds.). (1986). *Field methods in cross-cultural research.* Beverly Hills, CA: Sage.

Louis, M., & Kertvelyessy, A. (1989). The Neuman model in nursing research. In B. Neuman (Ed.), *The Neuman systems model* (pp. 99-103). Norwalk, CT: Appleton & Lange.

Loveland-Cherry, C. J., Youngblut, J. M., & Leidy, N. W. K. (1989). A psychometric analysis of the Family Environment Scale. *Nursing Research, 38,* 262-266.

Luepnitz, D. A. (1988). *The family interpreted: Feminist theory in clinical practice.* New York: Basic Books.

Lundberg, G. D. (1991). National health care reform: An aura of inevitability is upon us. *Journal of the American Medical Association, 265*(19), 2566-2567.

MacIntyre, A. (1984). *After virtue: A study in moral theory* (2nd ed.). Notre Dame, IN: University of Notre Dame Press.

MacPhee, D. (1984). The pediatrician as a source of information about child development. *Journal of Pediatric Psychology, 9*(1), 87-100.

Maheady, D. C. (1986). Cultural assessment of children. *Maternal-Child Nursing Journal, 11,* 128.

Mair, M. (1988). Psychology as storytelling. *International Journal of Personal Construct Psychology, 1,* 125-138.

Maj, M. (1991). Psychological problems of families and health care workers who deal with people infected with human immunodeficiency virus 1. *Acta-Psychiatr-Scand, 83*(3), 161-168.

Malach, R. S., & Segal, N. (1990). Perspectives on health care delivery systems for American Indian families. *Children's Health Care, 19,* 219-228.

Mardiros, M. (1982). Mothers of disabled children: A study of parental stress. *Nursing Papers, 14*(3), 47-56.

Mardiros, M. Z. (1987). *Understanding parents of children with disabilities: Developing a meaning-centered approach.* Unpublished doctoral dissertation, University of Texas, Austin.

Martin, M. E., & Henry, M. (1991). Cultural relativity and poverty. In B. W. Spratley (Ed.), *Readings in community health nursing* (pp. 521-531). Philadelphia: J. B. Lippincott.

Martinson, I. (1976). *Home care for the dying child: Professional and family perspectives.* New York: Appleton-Century-Crofts.

Martinson, I. M., Gillis, C., Colaizzo, D. C., Freeman, M., & Bossert, E. (1990). Impact of childhood cancer on healthy school-age siblings. *Cancer Nursing, 13,* 183-190.

Maturana, H. (1978). Biology of language: The epistemology of reality. In G. Miller & E. Lenneberg (Eds.), *Psychology and biology of language and thought: Essays in honor of Eric Lenneberg* (pp. 27-63). New York: Academic Press.

Maturana, H. (1983). What is it to see? *Archives of Biological Medicine, 16,* 255-269.

Maturana, H. (1985). Comment by Humberto R. Maturana: The mind is not in the head. *Journal of Social and Biological Structure, 8,* 308-311.

Maturana, H. [Speaker]. (1987). *The sin of certainty* [Videotape]. Calgary, Alberta, Canada: University of Calgary.

Maturana, H. (1988). Reality: The search for objectivity or the quest for a compelling argument. *Irish Journal of Psychology, 9*(1), 25-83.

Maturana, H. R., Lettvin, J. Y., McCulloch, W. S., & Pitts, W. H. (1960). Anatomy and physiology of vision in the frog (*Rana pipiens*). *Journal of General Physiology, 43*(6), 129-175.

Maturana, H. R., Uribe, G., & Frenk, S. (1968). A biological theory of relativistic color coding in the primate retina. *Archivos de Biolgia y Medicin Experimentales,* (Suppl. 1), 1-30.

Maturana, H., & Varela, F. (1987). *The tree of knowledge: The biological roots of human understanding.* Boston: New Science Library.

May, W. (1983). *The physician's covenant.* Philadelphia: Westminster.

McArt, E. W., & McDougal, L. W. (1985). Secondary data analysis: A new approach to nursing research. *Image: Journal of Nursing Scholarship, XVII*(2), 54-57.

McCausland, M. P., & Burgess, A. W. (1989). The home visit for data collection. *Applied Nursing Research, 2*(1), 54-55.

McCubbin, H., & Figley, C. R. (Eds.). (1983). *Stress and the family. Volume I: Coping with normative transitions.* New York: Brunner/Mazel.

McCubbin, H., & McCubbin, M. A. (1988). Typologies of resilient families: Emerging roles of social class and ethnicity. *Family Relations, 37*(3), 247-254.

McCubbin, H., McCubbin, M., Patterson, J., Cauble, A., Wilson, L., & Warwick, W. (1983). CHIP-Coping Health Inventory for parents in the care of the chronically ill child. *Journal of Marriage and the Family, 45,* 359-370.

McCubbin, H., McCubbin, M., & Thompson, A. (1991). FTRI: Family Time and Routines Index. In H. McCubbin & A. Thompson (Eds.), *Family assessment inventories for research and practice* (pp. 137-146). Madison: University of Wisconsin.

McCubbin, H., McCubbin, M., & Thompson, A. (in press). Resiliency in families: The role of family schema and appraisal in family adaptation to crises. In T. Brubaker (Ed.), *Family relationships: Current and future directions.* Newbury Park, CA: Sage.

McCubbin, H., Needle, R., & Wilson, M. (1985). Adolescent health risk behaviors: Family stress and adolescent coping as critical factors. *Family Relations, 34,* 51-62.

McCubbin, H., Nevin, R., Cauble, A., Larsen, A., Comeau, J., & Patterson, J. (1982). Family coping with chronic illness: The case of cerebral palsy. In H. McCubbin, A. Cauble, & J. Patterson (Eds.), *Family stress, coping, and social support* (pp. 169-188). Springfield, IL: Charles C. Thomas.

McCubbin, H. I., Olson, D. H., & Larsen, A. S. (1987). F-COPES, Family Crises Oriented Personal Evaluation Scales. In H. I. McCubbin & A. I. Thompson (Eds.), *Family assessment inventories for research and practice* (pp. 195-207). Madison: University of Wisconsin.

McCubbin, H., & Patterson, J. (1983). The family stress process: The Double ABCX model of adjustment and adaptation. In M. Sussman, H. McCubbin, & J. Patterson (Eds.), *Social stress and the family: Advances and developments in family stress theory and research* (pp. 7-37). New York: Haworth.

McCubbin, H., Patterson, J., & Cauble, E. (1981). *Systematic assessment of family stress, resources, and coping: Tools for research, education, and clinical interventions.* Minneapolis: University of Minnesota.

McCubbin, H., & Thompson, A. (1987). *Family assessment inventories.* Madison: University of Wisconsin.

McCubbin, H., & Thompson, A. (1989). *Balancing work and family life on Wall Street: Stockbrokers and families coping with economic instability.* Minneapolis: Burgess.

McCubbin, H., & Thompson, A. (1991). Family typologies and family assessment. In H. McCubbin & A. Thompson (Eds.), *Family assessment inventories for research and practice* (pp. 35-49). Madison: University of Wisconsin.

McCubbin, H., Thompson, A., Pirner, P., & McCubbin, M. (1988). *Family types and strengths: A life cycle and ecological perspective.* Minneapolis: Burgess.

McCubbin, M. (1988). Family stress, resources, and family types: Chronic illness in children. *Family Relations, 37,* 203-210.

McCubbin, M. (1989a). *Family hardiness and mastery of complex home care regimens.* Paper presented at the National Conference on Family Nursing, Portland, OR.

McCubbin, M. (1989b). Family stress and family strengths: A comparison of single- and two-parent families with handicapped children. *Research in Nursing and Health, 12,* 101-110.

McCubbin, M. (1990). *Children's chronic illness: Parent and family adaptation* (5 R29-NRO2563-02). Bethesda, MD: National Institutes of Health, National Center for Nursing Research.

McCubbin, M. (1991). CHIP-Coping Health Inventory for parents. In H. McCubbin & A. Thompson (Eds.), *Family assessment inventories for research and practice* (pp. 181-199). Madison: University of Wisconsin.

McCubbin, M. (1987). Coping Health Inventory for parents. In H. I. McCubbin & A. I. Thompson (Eds.), *Family assessment inventories for research and practice* (pp. 175-192). Madison: University of Wisconsin.

McCubbin, M., & Huang, S. (1989). Family strengths in the care of handicapped children: Targets for intervention. *Family Relations, 38,* 436-443.

McCubbin, M., & McCubbin, H. (1989). Theoretical orientations to family stress and coping. In C. Figley (Ed.), *Treating stress in families* (pp. 3-43). New York: Brunner/Mazel.

McCubbin, M., & McCubbin, H. (1991). Family stress theory and assessment: The resiliency model of family stress, adjustment, and adaptation. In H. McCubbin & A. Thompson (Eds.), *Family assessment inventories for research and practice* (pp. 3-32). Madison: University of Wisconsin.

McCubbin, M., & McCubbin, H. (in press). Family coping with health crisis: The Resiliency Model of Family Stress, Adjustment, and Adaptation. In C. Danielson, B. Hamel-Bissell, & P. Winstead-Fry (Eds.), *Families, health, and illness.* St. Louis: C. V. Mosby.

McCubbin, M., McCubbin, H., & Thompson, A. (1988). *Family Problem Solving Communication Index.* Madison: University of Wisconsin.

McCubbin, M., McCubbin, H., & Thompson, A. (1991). FHI: Family Hardiness Index. In H. McCubbin & A. Thompson (Eds.), *Family assessment inventories for research and practice* (pp. 127-133). Madison: University of Wisconsin.

McDaniel, S. H., Campbell, T. L., & Seaburn, D. B. (1990). *Family oriented primary care.* New York: Springer-Verlag.

McKeever, P. T. (1981). Fathering the chronically ill child. *American Journal of Maternal/Child Nursing, 6*(2), 124-128.

Medicus. (1980). *An evaluation of the levels of practice system.* Chicago: Rush-Presbyterian-St. Luke's Medical Center.

Meier, P. P. (1978). A crisis group for parents of high-risk infants. *Maternal-Child Nursing Journal, 7,* 21-30.

Meisenhelder, J. B., & LaCharite, C. (1989, Spring). Fear of contagion: The public response to AIDS. *Journal of Nursing Scholarship, 21*(1), 7-9.

Meister, S. (1984). Family well-being. In J. Campbell & J. Humphreys (Eds.), *Nursing care of victims of family violence* (pp. 53-73), Reston, VA: Reston.

Meister, S. B. (1989a). Family health policy: A perspective on its development and trends for the future. In L. G. Krentz (Ed.), *National conference on family nursing: Proceedings* (pp. 65-76). Portland: Oregon Health Sciences University, Department of Family Nursing.

Meister, S. B. (1989b). Health care financing, policy, and family nursing practice: New opportunities. In C. L. Gilliss, B. L. Highley, B. M. Roberts, & I. M. Martinson (Eds.), *Toward a science of family nursing* (pp. 146-155). Menlo Park, CA: Addison-Wesley.

Meleis, A. I. (1987). International nursing research. In J. J. Fitzpatrick & R. L. Taunton (Eds.), *Annual review of nursing research* (pp. 205-227). New York: Springer.

Mendez, C. L., Coddou, F., & Maturana, H. (1988). The bringing forth of pathology. *Irish Journal of Psychology, 9*(1), 144-172.

Menke, E. M. (1987). The impact of a child's chronic illness on school-aged siblings. *Children's Health Care, 15,* 132-140.

Mercer, R. T. (1974). Mothers' responses to their infants with defects. *Nursing Research, 23,* 133-137.

Mercer, R. T. (1989). Theoretical perspectives on the family. In C. L. Gilliss, B. L. Highley, B. M. Roberts, & I. M. Martinson (Eds.), *Toward a science of family nursing* (pp. 9-36). Menlo Park, CA: Addison-Wesley.

Mercer, R. T., & Ferketich, S. L. (1990). Predictors of family functioning eight months following birth. *Nursing Research, 39,* 76-82.

Mercer, R. T., Ferketich, S. L., DeJoseph, J., May, K. A., & Sollid, D. (1988). Effect of stress on family functioning during pregnancy. *Nursing Research, 37*(5), 268-275.

Mercer, R. T., May, K. A., Ferketich, S., & DeJoseph, J. (1986). Theoretical models for studying the effect of antepartum stress on the family. *Nursing Research, 35,* 339-346.

Merves, E. S. (1986). *Conversations with homeless women: A sociological examination.* Unpublished doctoral dissertation, Ohio State University, Columbus.

Miles, M., & Huberman, A. M. (1984). *Qualitative data analysis: A sourcebook of new methods.* Beverly Hills, CA: Sage.

Miller, B., & Montgomery, A. (1990). Family caregivers and limitations in social activities. *Research on Aging, 12*(1), 72-93.

Miller, H. G., Turner, C., & Moses, L. E. (1990). *AIDS: The second decade.* Washington, DC: National Academy Press.

Miller, S. R., & Winstead-Fry, P. (1982). *Family systems theory in nursing practice.* Reston, VA: Reston.

Millett, K. (1970). *Sexual politics.* New York: Ballantine.

Minuchin, S. (1974). *Families and family therapy.* Cambridge, MA: Harvard University Press.

Minuchin, S., & Fishman, H. C. (1981). *Family therapy techniques.* Cambridge, MA: Harvard University Press.

Mishel, M. H., & Murdaugh, C. L. (1987). Family adjustment to heart transplantation: Redesigning the dream. *Nursing Research, 36,* 332-338.

Mitchell, E. S. (1986). Multiple triangulation: A methodology for nursing science. *Advances in Nursing Science, 8,* 18-26.

Moffatt, B. C. (1986). *When someone you love has AIDS.* New York: NAL Penguin.

Mohatt, G., McDiarmid, G. W., & Montoya, V. (1988). Societies, families, and change: The Alaskan example. In S. M. Manson & N. G. Dinges (Eds.), *Behavioral health issues among American Indians and Alaska Natives: Explorations on the frontiers of the biobehavioral sciences* (Vol. 1, pp. 325-365). Monograph 1. Denver, CO: National Center for American Indian and Alaska Native Mental Health Research.

Monette, P. (1988). *Borrowed time.* New York: Avon.

Moody, L. E., Wilson, M. E., Smyth, K., Schwartz, R., Tittle, M., & Van Cott, M. L. (1988). Analysis of a decade of nursing research: 1977-1986. *Nursing Research, 37,* 374-379.

Moos, R. H., & Moos, B. S. (1986). *Family Environment Scale manual.* Palo Alto, CA: Consulting Psychologists.

Moriarty, H. J. (1990). Key issues in the family research process: Strategies for nurse researchers. *Advances in Nursing Science, 12*(3), 1-14.

Moriarty, H. J. (1991). The relationship of family cohesion, family adaptability, and time postdeath to parental bereavement reactions after the death of a child. *Dissertation Abstracts International, 51,* 3315b-3316b. (University Microfilms No. 902662)

Moritz, D. J., Kasl, S. V., & Berkman L. F. (1989). The health impact of living with a cognitively impaired elderly spouse: Depressive symptoms and social functioning. *Journal of Gerontology, 44*(1), S17-27.

Moses, E. B. (1990). Profile of contemporary nursing population. In National League for Nursing (Ed.), *Perspectives in nursing, 1989-1991* (pp. 33-44). New York: National League for Nursing.

Moynihan, D. P. (1986). *Family and nation.* Orlando, FL: Harcourt Brace Jovanovich.

Munet-Vilaro, F., & Egan, M. (1990). Reliability issues of the Family Environment Scale for cross-cultural research. *Nursing Research, 39,* 244-247.

Munhall, P. L., & Oiler, C. J. (1986). Philosophical foundations of qualitative research. In P. L. Munhall & C. J. Oiler (Eds.), *Nursing research: A qualitative perspective* (pp. 47-63). New York: Appleton-Century-Crofts.

Murphy, K. L. (1989). *Threatened perinatal loss: Defining and managing strategies used by parents of critically ill infants.* Unpublished doctoral dissertation, University of Illinois, Chicago.

Murphy, K. M. (1990). Interactional styles of parents following the birth of a high-risk infant. *Journal of Pediatric Nursing, 5,* 33-41.

Murphy, S. (1986). Family study and nursing research. *Image, 18,* 170-174.

Musick, J. S. (1987). Adolescents as mothers: The being and the doing. *Zero to Three, 8*(2), 7-8, 23-28.

Natapoff, J. N., & Essoka, G. C. (1990). Homeless families. In J. N. Natapoff & R. Wieczoreck (Eds.), *Maternal-child health policy: A nursing perspective* (pp. 203-220). New York: Springer.

National Center for Family-Centered Care. (1990). *Physician education forum report.* Bethesda, MD: Association for the Care of Children's Health.

Nelson, E. C., & Simmons, J. J. (1983). Health promotion—The second public health revolution: Promise or threat. *Family and Community Health, 5*(2), 1-15.

Nightingale, F. (1979). *Cassandra.* New York: Feminist Press. (Original work written in 1852.)

Noelker, L. S., & Poulshock, S. W. (1982). *The effects on families of caring for impaired elderly in residence.* Final report submitted to the Administration on Aging, Margaret Blenker Research Center for Family Studies, Benjamin Rose Institute, Cleveland, OH.

Norbeck, J. S. (1984). Norbeck Social Support Questionnaire. In K. E. Barnard, P. A. Brandt, B. S. Raff, & P. Carroll (Eds.), *Social support and families of vulnerable infants* (pp. 45-57). New York: March of Dimes Birth Defects Foundation.

Nowak, K. M. (1986). Type A, hardiness, and psychological distress. *Journal of Behavioral Medicine, 9,* 537-548.

Nygarrd, H. A. (1988). Strain on caregivers of demented elderly people living at home. *Scandinavian Journal of Primary Health Care, 6,* 33-37.

Oberst, M., Hughes, S., Chang, A., & McCubbin, M. (1991). Self-care burden, stress appraisal, and mood among persons receiving radiotherapy. *Cancer Nursing, 14,* 71-78.

Oberst, M., & Scott, D. (1988). Postdischarge distress in surgically treated cancer patients and spouses. *Research in Nursing and Health, 11,* 223-233.

O'Brien, E. L. (1987). Living with chronically ill siblings: A developmental study. (Doctoral dissertation, Catholic University of America, Washington, DC). *Dissertation Abstracts International, 47,* 5075B.

Ogilvie, L. (1990). Hospitalization of children for surgery: The parents' view. *Children's Health Care, 19,* 49-56.

Olson, D. (1989). Circumplex model of family systems VIII: Family assessment and intervention. In D. Olson, C. Russell, & D. Sprenkle (Eds.), *Circumplex model: Systemic assessment and treatment of families* (pp. 7-49). New York: Haworth.

Olson, D. H., & Hanson, M. K. (1990). *2001: Preparing families for the future.* Minneapolis: National Council on Family Relations.

Olson, D., & Killorin, E. (1984). *Clinical rating scale for circumplex model.* St. Paul: University of Minnesota, Family Social Science.

Olson, D., McCubbin, H., Barnes, H., Larson, A., Muxen, M., & Wilson, M. (1983). *Families: What makes them work.* Beverly Hill, CA: Sage.

Olson, D. H., Portner, J., & Lavee, Y. (1985). *FACES III.* St. Paul: University of Minnesota, Family Social Science.

Olson, D. H., et al. (1989). *Families: What makes them work.* Newbury Park, CA: Sage.

Orem, D. H. (1985). *Nursing concepts of practice* (3rd ed.). New York: McGraw-Hill.

Orque, M. S., Bloch, B., & Monrroy, L. S. A. (1983). *Ethnic nursing care: A multicultural approach.* St. Louis: C. V. Mosby.

Orr, R., Cameron, S., & Day, D. (1991). Coping with stress in families with children with developmental disabilities: An evaluation of the Double ABCX model using path analysis. *American Journal of Mental Retardation, 95,* 444-450.

Ortner, S. B. (1974). Is female to male as nature is to culture? In M. Z. Rosaldo & L. Lamphere (Eds.), *Women, culture, and society* (pp. 67-87). Stanford, CA: Stanford University Press.

Packer, M. J. (1985). Hermeneutic inquiry in the study of human conduct. *American Psychologist, 40,* 1081-1093.

Palazzoli, M. S., Boscolo, L., Cecchin, G., & Prata, G. (1980). Hypothesizing-circularity-neutrality. Three guidelines for the conductor of the session. *Family Process, 19,* 3-12.

Parkerson, G. R., Michener, J. L., Wu, L. R., Finch, J. M., Broadhead, W. W., Muhlbaier, L. J., Magruder-Habib, K., Lelms, M. J., Kertesz, J. W., Clapp-Channing, N., & Jokerst, E. (1989). The effect of a telephone family assessment intervention on the functional health of patients with elevated family stress. *Medical Care, 27,* 680-693.

Passo, S. (1978). Parents' perceptions, attitudes, and needs regarding sex education for the child with myelomeningocele. *Research in Nursing and Health, 1,* 53-90.

Patterson, G. R. (1988). Family process: Loops, levels, and linkages. In N. Bolger, A. Caspi, G. Downey, & M. Moorehouse (Eds.), *Persons in context* (pp. 114-151). Cambridge, UK: Cambridge University Press.

Patterson, J. M. (1990). Family and health research in the 1980s: A family scientist's perspective. *Family Systems Medicine, 8,* 421-434.

Patterson, J., & McCubbin, H. (1983). The impact of family life events on the health of the chronically ill child. *Family Relations, 32,* 255-264.

Pearlin, L. I., Semple, S., & Turner, H. (1988). Stress of AIDS caregiving: A preliminary overview of the issues. *Death Studies, 12,* 501-517.

Pender, N. J. (1987). *Health promotion in nursing practice* (2nd ed.). Norwalk, CT: Appleton & Lange.

Perkins, M. T. (1988). *Caregiving identity emergence in the parents of hospitalized disabled children.* Unpublished doctoral dissertation, University of California, San Francisco.

Peszencker, B. (1984). The poor: A population at risk. *Public Health Nursing, 1,* 237-249.

Pinch, W. J., & Spielman, M. L. (1989). Parental voices in the sea of neonatal ethical dilemmas. *Issues in Comprehensive Pediatric Nursing, 12,* 423-435.

Pinch, W. J., & Spielman, M. L. (1990). The parents' perspective: Ethical decision making in neonatal intensive care. *Journal of Advanced Nursing, 15,* 712-719.

Pinyerd, B. J. (1983). Siblings of children with myelomeningocele: Examining their perceptions. *Maternal-Child Nursing Journal, 12,* 61-70.

Pirrotta, S., & Cecchin, G. (1988). The Milan training program. In H. A. Liddle, D. C. Breunlin, & R. C. Schwartz (Eds.), *Handbook of family therapy training and supervision* (pp. 38-61). New York: Guilford.

Pittman, D. C. (1989). Nursing case management: Holistic care for the deinstitutionalized chronically mentally ill. *Journal of Psychosocial Nursing, 27,* 23-27.

Piven, F. F., & Cloward, R. A. (1971). *Regulating the poor: The functions of public welfare.* New York: Vintage.

Pollock, S. E. (1989). The hardiness characteristic: A motivation factor in adaptation. *Advances in Nursing Science, 11*(2), 53-62.

Pollock, S. E., Christian, B. J., & Sands, D. (1990). Responses to chronic illness: Analysis of psychological and physiological adaptation. *Nursing Research, 39*(5), 300-304.

Poortinga, Y. H. (1975). Some implications of three different approaches to intercultural comparison. In J. W. Berry & W. J. Lonner (Eds.), *Applied cross-cultural psychology* (pp. 327-332). Amsterdam: Swetsand Zeitlinger B.V.

Porter, A. (1987). *A clinical ladder system in nursing: A program evaluation.* Unpublished doctoral dissertation, Northwestern University, Evanston, IL.

Poster, M. (1978). *Critical theory of the family.* New York: Seabury.

Poulshock, J. W., & Deimling, G. T. (1984). Families caring for elders in residence: Issues in the measurement of burden. *Journal of Gerontology, 39*(2), 230-239.

Powell-Cope, G., & Brown, M. A. (1992). Going public as an AIDS family caregiver. *Social Science and Medicine, 34*(5), 571-580.

Pratt, J. W., & Zeckhauser, R. J. (1985). Principals and agents: An overview. In J. W. Pratt & R. J. Zeckhauser (Eds.), *Principals and agents: The structure of business* (pp. 1-35). Boston: Harvard Business School Press.

Pridham, K., Martin, R., Sondel, S., & Fluczek, A. (1989). Parental issues in feeding young children with bronchopulmonary dysplasia. *Journal of Pediatric Nursing, 4,* 177-185.

Prins, M. M. (1989). The effect of family visits on intercranial pressure. *Western Journal of Nursing Research, 11,* 281-297.

PROJECT SERVE. (1985). *New directions: Serving children with special health care needs in Massachusetts.* Boston: Massachusetts Health Research Institute.

Pruchno, R. A., & Resch, N. L. (1989). Aberrant behaviors and Alzheimer's disease: Mental health effects on spouse caregivers. *Journal of Gerontology, 44*(5), S177-182.

Puskar, K. R. (1989). Families on the move: Promoting health through family relocation adaptation. *Family and Community Health, 11*(4), 52-62.

Quint, J. C. (1967). The case for theories generated from empirical data. *Nursing Research, 16*(2), 109-114.

Rabinow, P., & Sullivan, W. M. (1987). The interpretive turn: A second look. In P. Rabinow & W. M. Sullivan (Eds.), *Interpretive social science: A second look* (pp. 1-30). Berkeley: University of California Press.

Rabins, P. V., Fitting, M. D., Eastham, J., & Fetting, J. (1990). The emotional impact of caring for the chronically ill. *Psychosomatics, 31*(3), 331-336.

Rafferty, M. (1989). Standing up for America's homeless. *American Journal of Nursing, 89,* 1614-1617.

Ransom, D. C. (1988). Family therapists teaching in family practice settings: Issues and experiences. In H. A. Liddle, D. C. Breunlin, & R. C. Schwartz (Eds.), *Handbook of family therapy training and supervision* (pp. 290-302). New York: Guilford.

Ransom, D., Fisher, L., Phillips, S., Kokes, R., & Weiss, R. (1990). The logic of measurement in family research. In T. W. Draper & A. C. Marcos (Eds.), *Family variables: Conceptualization, measurement, and use* (pp. 48-63). Newbury Park, CA: Sage.

Rapping, E. (1990). The future of motherhood: Some unfashionably visionary thoughts. In K. V. Hansen & I. J. Philipson (Eds.), *Women, class, and the feminist imagination: A socialist-feminist reader* (pp. 537-548). Philadelphia: Temple University Press.

Rawlins, P. S., Rawlins, T. D., & Horner, M. (1990). Development of the Family Needs Assessment Tool. *Western Journal of Nursing Research, 12,* 201-214.

Reed, S. B. (1990). Potential for alteration in family process: When a family has a child with cystic fibrosis. *Issues in Comprehensive Pediatric Nursing, 13,* 15-23.

Region X Nursing Network. (1990). *Prenatal and child health nursing standards.* Unpublished manuscript available from Kathryn Barnard, R.N., Ph.D., Associate Dean and Professor, School of Nursing, University of Washington, Seattle, WA 98195.

Reidy, M., & Thibaudeau, M. F. (1984). Evaluation of family functioning: Development and validation of a scale which measures family competence in matters of health. *Nursing Papers, 16*(3), 42-56.

Reiss, D. (1981). *The family's construction of reality.* Cambridge, MA: Harvard University Press.

Reiss, D., Gonzalez, S., & Kramer, N. (1986). Family process, chronic illness, and death: On the weakness of strong bonds. *Archives of General Psychiatry, 43,* 795-804.

Richmond, J. B., & Kotelchuck, M. L. (1983). Political influences: Rethinking national health policy. In C. H. McGuire, R. P. Foley, A. Gorr, R. W. Richards, & Associates (Eds.), *Handbook on health professions education* (pp. 386-404). San Francisco: Jossey-Bass.

Riehl, J. P., & Roy, S. C. (1980). *Conceptual models for nursing practice.* New York: Appleton-Century-Crofts.

Rix, S. E. (1990). *The American woman 1990-1991: A status report.* (Report by the Women's Research and Education Institute). New York: Norton.

Roberts, C., & Feetham, S. L. (1982). Assessing family functioning across three areas of relationships. *Nursing Research, 31*(4), 231-235.

Robinson, C. A. (1984). When hospitalization becomes an "everyday thing." *Issues in Comprehensive Pediatric Nursing, 7,* 363-370.

Robinson, C. A. (1985). Parents of hospitalized chronically ill children: Competency in question. *Nursing Papers, 17*(2), 59-68.

Robinson, C. A. (1987). Roadblocks to family-centered care when a chronically ill child is hospitalized. *Maternal-Child Nursing Journal, 16,* 181-194.

Robinson, C. A., & Thorne, S. E. (1984). Strengthening family "interference." *Journal of Advanced Nursing, 9,* 597-602.

Rodick, J., Henggeler, S., & Hanson, C. (1986). An evaluation of Family Adaptability and Cohesion Evaluation Scales (FACES) and the Circumplex Model. *Journal of Abnormal Child Psychology, 14,* 77-87.

Rolland, J. (1987). Family systems and chronic illness: A topological model. *Journal of Psychotherapy and the Family, 3*(3), 143-168.

Rolland, J. (1988). Family systems and chronic illness: A typological model. In F. Walsh & C. Anderson (Eds.), *Chronic disorders and the family* (pp. 143-168). New York: Haworth.

Roman, L. A. (1988). Creating mothering for preterm infants: A grounded theory of veteran parent support initiated in a neonatal intensive care setting. Unpublished doctoral dissertation, Michigan State University, East Lansing.

Roper, R. H., & Boyer, R. (1987). Perceived health status among the new urban homeless. *Social Science Medicine, 34,* 669-678.

Rose, L. E. (1985). Responses of families to the treatment setting. *Nursing Papers, 17*(2), 72-84.

Rose, M. H., & Thomas, R. B. (Eds.). (1987). *Children with chronic conditions: Nursing in a family and community context.* New York: Grune & Stratton.

Rosenman, M., & Stein, M. (1990). Homeless children: A new vulnerability. *Child and Youth Services, 14,* 89-109.

Ross, B., & Cobb, K. L. (1988). *Family nursing: A nursing process approach.* Redwood City, CA: Addison-Wesley Nursing.

Ross, C. E. (1991). Marriage and the sense of control. *Journal of Marriage and the Family, 53,* 831-838.

Rossi, P. (1989). *Without shelter.* New York: Priority.

Roth, D., Bean, J., Lust, N., & Saveanu, T. (1985). *Homelessness in Ohio: A study of people in need.* Columbus: Ohio Department of Mental Health.

Rushton, C. H. (1990a). Family-centered care in the critical care setting: Myth or reality? *Children's Health Care, 19,* 68-78.

Rushton, C. H. (1990b). Strategies for family-centered care in the critical care setting. *Pediatric Nursing, 16,* 195-199.

Ryan, W. (1971/1976). *Blaming the victim.* New York: Vintage.

Salmon, M. E. (1989). Public health nursing: The neglected specialty. *Nursing Outlook, 37*(5), 26-29.

Sandelowski, M. (1986). The problem of rigor in qualitative research. *Advances in Nursing Science, 8*(3), 27-37.

Sandven, K., & Resnick, M. D. (1990). Informal adoption among black adolescent mothers. *American Journal of Orthopsychiatry, 60,* 210-224.

Scharer, K., & Dixon, D. (1989). Managing chronic illness: Parents with a ventilator-dependent child. *Journal of Pediatric Nursing, 4,* 236-247.

Schilling, R., Schinke, S., & Kirkham, M. (1985). Coping with a handicapped child: Differences between mothers and fathers. *Social Science and Medicine, 21,* 857-863.

Schorr, L. B., & Schorr, D. (1988). *Within our reach: Breaking the cycle of disadvantage.* New York: Doubleday.

Schultz, P. R. (1987). When the client is more than one: Extending the foundational concept of "person." *Advances in Nursing Science, 10*(1), 71-86.

Schumm, W. R. (1982). Integrating theory, measurement, and data analysis in family studies survey research. *Journal of Marriage and the Family, 44,* 983-998.

Schumm, W. R., Barnes, H. L., Bollman, S. R., Jurich, A. P., & Milliken, G. A. (1985). Approaches to the statistical analysis of family data. *Home Economics Research Journal, 14*(1), 112-122.

Seidel, J. (1988). *Ethnograph Version 3.0* [computer program]. Littleton, CO: Qualis Research Associates.

Shadish, W. R., & Sweeney, R. B. (1991). Mediators and moderators in meta-analysis: There's a reason we don't let Dodo birds tell us which psychotherapies should have prizes. *Journal of Consulting and Clinical Psychology, 59*(6), 883-893.

Shelton, T. L., Jeppson, E. S., & Johnson, B. H. (1987). *Family-centered care for children with special health needs.* Washington, DC: Association for the Care of Children's Health.

Shilts, R. (1987). *And the band played on: Politics, people, and the AIDS epidemic.* New York: St. Martin's.

Sidel, R. (1986). *Women and children last: The plight of poor women in affluent America.* New York: Penguin.

Silva, M. C. (1977). Philosophy, science, and theory: Interrelationship and implications for nursing research. *Image, 9,* 59-63.

Silva, M. C. (1986). Research testing nursing theory: State of the art. *Advances in Nursing Science, 9*(1), 1-11.

Silva, M. C. (1990). Ethics decision framework. In M. C. Silva (Ed.), *Ethical decision making in nursing administration* (pp. 109-126). Norwalk, CT: Appleton & Lange.

Simon, R. (1985). A frog's eye view of the world. *Family Therapy Networker, 9*(3), 32, 34-35.

Smilkstein, G. (1978). The family APGAR: A proposal for a family function test and its use by physicians. *Journal of Family Practice, 6,* 1231-1239.

Smith, A. B. (1989). *Development of a behavioral observation instrument to identify orientation of the nurse toward parents of hospitalized children.* Unpublished doctoral dissertation, Texas Woman's University, Denton.

Smith, M. C., & Stullenbarger, E. (1989). Meta-analysis: An overview. *Nursing Science Quarterly, 2*(3), 114-115.

Smith, M. L., & Glass, G. V. (1977). Meta-analysis of psychotherapy outcome studies. *American Psychologist, 32*(9), 752-760.

Sommers, T., & Shields, L. (1987). *Women take care: The consequences of caregiving in today's society.* Gainesville, FL: Triad.

Special Populations Task Force of the President's Commission on Mental Health. (1978). *Task panel reports submitted to the President's Commission on Mental Health: Vol. 3.* Washington, DC: Government Printing Office.

Spector, R. E. (1985). *Cultural diversity in health and illness* (2nd ed.). New York: Appleton-Century-Crofts.

Speer, J. J., & Sachs, B. (1985). Selecting the appropriate family assessment tool. *Pediatric Nursing, 11,* 349-355.

Spencer, M. B. (1990). Development of minority children: An introduction. *Child Development, 61*(2), 267-269.

Sprott, J. (1990, October). *One person's "spoiling" is another's "freedom to become": Interpreting Alaska Native parenting.* Paper presented at the 16th Annual Transcultural Nursing Society Conference, Seattle, WA.

Sprott, J. (in press). *Alaska native parents in Anchorage: Perspectives on parenting.* Lanham, MD: University Press of America.

Stacey, J. (1986). Are feminists afraid to leave home? The challenge of conservative pro-family feminism. In J. Mitchell & A. Oakley (Eds.), *What is feminism?* (pp. 208-237). New York: Pantheon.

Stack, C. G. (1974). *All our kin: Strategies for survival in a black community.* New York: Harper & Row.

Stanitis, M. A., & Ryan, J. (1982). Noncompliance: An unacceptable diagnosis? *American Journal of Nursing, 6,* 941-942.

Stark, M. (1979). Introduction. In F. Nightingale, *Cassandra* (pp. 1-23). New York: Feminist Press.

Stein, R., & Jessop, D. J. (1982). A noncategorical approach to chronic childhood illness. *Public Health Reports, 97*(4), 354-362.

Stein, R., & Jessop, D. (1984). Does pediatric home care make a difference for children with chronic illness? Findings from the pediatric ambulatory care treatment study. *Pediatrics, 73*(6), 845-853.

Stengel, J. C., Echeveste, D. W., & Schmidt, G. C. (1985). Problems identified by registered nurse students in families with apnea-monitored infants. *Family and Community Health, 8*(3), 52-61.

Stephens, M. A. P., & Kenney, J. M. (1989). Caregiving stress instruments: Assessment of content and measurement quality. *Gerontology Review, 2*(1), 40-54.

Stetz, K., Lewis, F., & Primomo, J. (1986). Family coping strategies and chronic illness in the mother. *Family Relations, 35,* 515-522.

Stetz, K. M. (1987) Caregiving demands during advanced cancer: The spouse's needs. *Cancer Nursing, 10*(5), 260-268.

Stetz, K. M. (1989). The relationship among background characteristics, purpose in life, and caregiving demands on perceived health of spouse caregivers. *Scholarly Inquiry for Nursing Practice, 3*(2), 133-153.

Stevens, M. S. (1990). A comparison of mothers' and fathers' perceptions of caring for an infant requiring home cardio-respiratory monitoring. *Issues in Comprehensive Pediatric Nursing, 13,* 81-95.

Straus, M. A. (1964). Measuring families. In H. T. Christensen (Ed.), *Handbook of marriage and the family* (pp. 335-400). Skokie, IL: Rand McNally.

Straus, M. A., & Gelles, R. J. (1990). How violent are American families? Estimates from the National Family Violence Re-survey and other studies. In M. A. Straus & R. J. Gelles (Eds.), *Physical violence in American families* (pp. 95-112). New Brunswick, NJ: Transactions.

Strauss, A. L. (1987). *Qualitative analysis for social scientists.* Cambridge, UK: Cambridge University Press.

Strauss, S. S., & Munton, M. (1985). Common concerns of parents with disabled children. *Pediatric Nursing, 11,* 371-375.

Strong, B., & DeVault, C. (1989). *The marriage and family experience* (4th ed.). New York: West.

Stuifbergen, A. K. (1987). The impact of chronic illness on families. *Families and Community Health, 9*(4), 43-51.

Stuifbergen, A. K. (1990). Patterns of functioning in families with a chronically ill parent: An exploratory study. *Research in Nursing and Health, 13,* 35-44.

Stull, M., & Deatrick, J. (1986). Measuring parental participation: Part I. *Issues in Comprehensive Pediatric Nursing, 9,* 157-165.

Stullenbarger, B., Norris, J., Edgil, A. E., & Prosser, M. J. (1987). Family adaptation to cystic fibrosis. *Pediatric Nursing, 13,* 29-31.

Sturner, R. A., Green, J. A., & Funk, S. G. (1985). Preschool Denver Developmental Screening Test as a predictor of later school problems. *Journal of Pediatrics, 87,* 125-132.

Sudman, S., & Bradburn, N. M. (1974). *Response effects in surveys: A review and synthesis.* Chicago: Aldine.

Sue, S., & Zane, N. (1987). The role of culture and cultural techniques in psychotherapy. *American Psychologist, 42*(1), 37-45.

Sweeney, L. B. (1988). Impact on families caring for an infant with apnea. *Issues in Comprehensive Pediatric Nursing, 11,* 1-15.

Swoiskin-Schwartz, S., Deatrick, J. A., & Hanson, D. (1989). Parents' views about having a child after a SIDS death. *Journal of Pediatric Nursing, 3,* 24-28.

Szasz, T. S. (1973). *The second sin.* New York: Anchor.

Taylor, C. (1989). *Sources of the self: The making of the modern identity.* Cambridge, MA: Harvard University Press.

Taylor, S. C. (1980). The effect of chronic childhood illnesses upon well sibling. *Maternal-Child Nursing Journal, 9,* 109-116.

Thomas, R. B. (1986). *Ventilator dependency consequences for child and family.* Unpublished doctoral dissertation, University of Washington, Seattle.

Thomas, R. B. (1987). Methodological issues and problems in family health care research. *Journal of Marriage and the Family, 49,* 65-70.

Thomas, R. B. (1990). A foundation for clinical family assessment. *Children's Health Care, 19,* 224-250.

Thomas, R. B., & Barnard, K. E. (1986). Understanding families: A look at measures and methodologies. *Zero to Three, 6*(5), 11-14.

Thomas, R. B., Barnard, K. E., & Sumner, G. A. (1989). *Tools for family-centered care.* Paper presented at the National Center for Clinical Infants Program Sixth Biennial National Training Institute, Washington, DC.

Thompson, L. (1987, November). *Objectivity and subjectivity in feminist and family science.* Paper presented at the Pre-Conference Workshop on Theory Construction and Research Methodology, National Council on Family Relations, Atlanta, GA.

Thompson, R. H. (1985). *Psychosocial research on pediatric hospitalization and health care.* Springfield, IL: Charles C. Thomas.

Thorne, B. (1982). Feminist rethinking of the family: An overview. In B. Thorne with M. Yalom (Eds.), *Rethinking the family: Some feminist questions* (pp. 1-24). New York: Longman.

Thorne, S. E., & Robinson, C. A. (1988). Health care relationships: The chronic illness perspective. *Research in Nursing and Health, 11,* 293-300.

Thorne, S. E., & Robinson, C. A. (1989). Guarded alliance: Health care relationships in chronic illness. *Image, 21*(3), 153-157.

Tibler, K. (1987). Intervening with families of young adults with AIDS. In M. Leahey & L. M. Wright (Eds.), *Families and life-threatening illness* (pp. 255-270). Springhouse, PA: Springhouse.

Tomm, K. (1984a). One perspective on the Milan systemic approach: Part 1. Overview of development, theory, and practice. *Journal of Marital and Family Therapy, 10,* 113-125.

Tomm, K. (1984b). One perspective on the Milan systemic approach: Part 2. Description of session format, interviewing style, and interventions. *Journal of Marital and Family Therapy, 10,* 253-271.

Tomm, K. (1987a). Interventive interviewing: Part 1. Strategizing as a fourth guideline for the therapist. *Family Process, 26,* 3-13.

Tomm, K. (1987b). Interventive interviewing: Part 2. Reflexive questioning as a means to enable self-healing. *Family Process, 26*, 167-183.

Tomm, K. (1988). Interventive interviewing: Part 3. Intending to ask lineal, circular, strategic questions and reflexive questions? *Family Process, 27*, 1-15.

Tripp-Reimer, T., Brink, P., & Saunders, J. M. (1984). Cultural assessment: Content and process. *Nursing Outlook, 32,*(2), 78-82.

Tripp-Reimer, T., & Fox, S. S. (1990). Beyond the concept of culture. In J. McCloskey & H. Grace (Eds.), *Current issues in nursing* (pp. 542-546). St. Louis: C. V. Mosby.

Tukey, J. W. (1977). *Exploratory data analysis.* Menlo Park, CA: Addison-Wesley.

Uphold, C. R., & Harper, D. C. (1986). Methodological issues in intergenerational family nursing research. *Advances in Nursing Science, 8*(3), 38-49.

Uphold, C. R., & Strickland, O. L. (1989). Issues related to the unit of analysis in family nursing research. *Western Journal of Nursing Research, 11*(4), 405-417.

U.S. Congress, Office of Technological Assessment. (1990). *Health care in rural America* (OTA-H-434). Washington, DC: Government Printing Office.

U.S. Department of Health and Human Services: Public Health Services. (1990). *Healthy People 2000* (pp. 29-39). DHHS pub. # (PHS) 91-50212. Government Printing Offfice.

Valentine, C. A. (1968). *Culture and poverty.* Chicago: University of Chicago Press.

Veatch, R. (1981). *A theory of medical ethics.* New York: Basic Books.

Ventura, J. (1986). Parent coping: A replication. *Nursing Research, 35,* 77-80.

Verran, J. A., & Ferketich, S. (1987). Exploratory data analysis—Examining single distributions. *Western Journal of Nursing Research, 9*(1), 142-149.

Videka-Sherman, L. (1982). Coping with the death of a child: A study over time. *American Journal of Orthopsychiatry, 52*(4), 688-698.

Wagner, J., & Menke, E. M. (1988). *Homeless women and their families.* Columbus: Ohio State University.

Wagner, J., & Menke, E. M. (1991). Stressors and coping behaviors of homeless, poor, and low-income mothers. *Journal of Community Health Nursing, 8,* 75-84.

Walker, C. L. (1986). *Coping in siblings of childhood cancer patients.* Unpublished doctoral dissertation, University of Utah, Salt Lake City.

Walker, C. L. (1988). Stress and coping in siblings of childhood cancer patients. *Nursing Research, 37,* 208-212.

Walker, S. N., Sechrist, K. R., & Pender, N. J. (1987). The health promoting lifestyle profile: Development and psychometric characteristics. *Nursing Research, 36*(2), 76-81.

Walters, L. H., Pittman, J. F., & Norrell, J. E. (1984). Development of a quantitative measure of a family from self-reports of family members. *Journal of Family Issues, 5*(4), 497-514.

Watson, A. (1972). A study of family attitudes to children with diabetes. *Community Health, 128,* 122-125.

Weibe, D. J., & McCallum, D. M. (1986). Health practices and hardiness as mediators in the stress-illness relationship. *Health Psychology, 5,* 425-438.

Weichler, N. K. (1990). Information needs of mothers of children who have had liver transplants. *Journal of Pediatric Nursing, 5,* 88-96.

Weinstein, M. C., & Fineberg, H. V. (1980). *Clinical decision analysis.* Philadelphia: W. B. Saunders.

Whall, A. (1980). Congruence of existing theories of family functioning and nursing theories. *Advances in Nursing Science, 3,* 59-67.

Whall, A. (1982). Family systems theory: Relationship to nursing conceptual models. In J. J. Fitzpatrick, A. L. Whall, R. L. Johnson, & J. A. Floyd (Eds.), *Nursing models and their psychiatric mental health applications* (pp. 69-94). Bowie, MD: Brady.

Whall, A. (1984). *The relationship of theory to family research.* Paper presented at the First Wingspread Conference: Advancing Family Research in Nursing, Racine, WI.

Whall, A. L. (1986). The family as the unit of care in nursing: A historical review. *Public Health Nursing, 3,* 240-249.

Whall, A. L., & Fawcett, J. (1991a). An anthology of nursing perspectives on the family: Introduction. In A. L. Whall & J. Fawcett (Eds.), *Family theory development in nursing: State of the science and art* (pp. 87-90). Philadelphia: F. A. Davis.

Whall, A. L., & Fawcett, J. (1991b). The family as a focal phenomenon in nursing. In A. L. Whall & J. Fawcett (Eds.), *Family theory development in nursing: State of the science and art* (pp. 7-29). Philadelphia: F. A. Davis.

Whall, A. L., & Fawcett, J. (1991c). *Family theory development in nursing: State of the science and art.* Philadelphia: F. A. Davis.

Whall, A., & Loveland-Cherry, C. (in press). Family unit research in nursing. *Annual Review of Nursing Research.* New York: Springer.

White, L. K., & Brinkerhoff, D. B. (1977). Measurement problems in family research: A critical note on units of analysis. *International Journal of Sociology of the Family, 7,* 171-179.

Williams, C. A. (1990). Biopsychosocial elements of empathy: A multidimensional model. *Issues in Mental Health Nursing, 11*(2), 155-173.

Wills, J. M. (1983). Concerns and needs of mothers providing home care for children with tracheostomies. *Maternal-Child Nursing Journal, 12,* 89-108.

Wilson, H. S. (1989). Family caregiving for a relative with Alzheimer's dementia: Coping with negative choices. *Nursing Research, 38,* 94-98.

Wilson, W. J. (1991). Public policy research and "The truly disadvantaged." In C. Jenks & P. E. Peterson (Eds.), *The urban underclass* (pp. 460-481). Washington, DC: Brookings Institution.

Wolcott, D. L., Fawzy, F. I., Landsverk, J., et al. (1986). AIDS patients' needs of psychosocial services and their use of community service organizations. *Journal of Psychosocial Oncology, 4*(1), 135-146.

Wolf, F. (1986). *Meta-analysis: Quantitative methods for research synthesis.* Newbury Park, CA: Sage.

Woodham-Smith, C. (1951). *Florence Nightingale.* New York: Avon.

Woods, J. H., & Browning, M. (1990, October). *A dialogue between colleagues: Cross-cultural communication of caregivers.* Unpublished paper presented at the University of Michigan National Conference on Partnerships, Ann Arbor.

Woods, N. F. (1988). Women's health. In J. Fitzpatrick, R. Taunton, & J. Benoliel (Eds.), *Annual review of nursing research* (Vol. 6, pp. 209-236). New York: Springer.

Woods, N. F., Yates, B. C., & Primomo, J. (1989). Supporting families during chronic illness. *Image, 21,* 46-50.

Wright, J. D. (1987). The National Health Care for the Homeless Program. In R. Bingham, R. E. Green, & S. B. White (Eds.), *The homeless in contemporary society* (pp. 150-170). Newbury Park, CA: Sage.

Wright, J. D. (1989). *Address unknown: The homeless in America.* New York: Aldine de Gruyter.

Wright, J. D., & Weber, E. (1987). *Homelessness and health.* New York: McGraw-Hill.

Wright, L. M., & Bell, J. (1989). A survey of family nursing education in Canadian universities. *Canadian Journal of Nursing Research, 21*(3), 59-74.

Wright, L. M., & Leahey, M. (1984). *Nurses and families: A guide to family assessment and intervention.* Philadelphia: F. A. Davis.

Wright, L. M., & Leahey, M. (1987). *Families and chronic illness.* Springhouse, PA: Springhouse.

Wright, L. M., & Leahey, M. (1988). Nursing and family therapy training. In H. A. Liddle, D. C. Breunlin, & R. C. Schwartz (Eds.), *Handbook of family therapy training and supervision* (pp. 278-289). New York: Guilford.

Wright, L. M., & Leahey, M. (1990). Trends in nursing of families. In J. Bell, W. Watson, & L. Wright (Eds.), *The cutting edge of family nursing* (pp. 5-16). Calgary, Alberta, Canada: University of Calgary.

Wright, L. M., & Nagy, J. C. (in press). Death: The most troublesome family secret of all. In E. I. Black (Ed.), *Secrets in families and family therapy.* New York: Norton.

Wright, L. M., & Simpson, P. (1991). A systemic belief approach to epileptic seizures: A case of being spellbound. *Contemporary Family Therapy: An International Journal, 13*(2), 165-181.

Wright, L. M., & Watson, W. L. (1988). Systemic family therapy and family development. In C. J. Falicov (Ed.), *Family transitions: Continuity and change over the life cycle* (pp. 407-430). New York: Guilford.

Wright, L. M., Watson, W. L., & Bell, J. M. (1990). The family nursing unit: A unique integration of research, education, and clinical practice. In J. M. Bell, W. L. Watson, & L. M. Wright (Eds.), *The cutting edge of family nursing* (pp. 95-112). Calgary, Alberta, Canada: Family Nursing Unit Publications.

Wuest, J., & Stern, P. N. (1990a). Childhood otitis media: The family's endless quest for relief. *Issues in Comprehensive Pediatric Nursing, 13*, 25-39.

Wuest, J., & Stern, P. N. (1990b). The impact of fluctuating relationships with the Canadian health care system on family management of otitis media with effusion. *Journal of Advanced Nursing, 15*, 556-563.

Wuest, J., & Stern, P. N. (1991). Empowerment in primary health care: The challenge for nurses. *Qualitative Health Research, 1*, 80-99.

Yaffe, M. J. (1988, February 1). Implications of caring for an aging parent. *CMAJ, 138*, 231-235.

Youssef, F. A. (1987). Discharge planning for psychiatric patients: The effect of a family-patient teaching programme. *Journal of Advanced Nursing, 12*, 611-616.

Zeckhauser, R. J. (1986). The middle responsibilities of public and private America. In W. Knowlton & R. J. Zeckhauser (Eds.), *American society: Public and private responsibilities* (pp. 45-78). Cambridge, MA: Harvard University Press.

About the Contributors

Lioness Ayres, MS, RN, is a PhD candidate at the University of Illinois, Chicago. She is completing her dissertation, a grounded theory study of family caregiving, and is especially interested in the use of computers in qualitative research.

Kathryn E. Barnard, PhD, RN, PAAN, is the Associate Dean for Academic Affairs and a Professor in the School of Nursing, University of Washington, Seattle. Her interests have centered on the ecology of the developing child; this naturally involves the family. She currently is investigating the issue of maternal depression and how to modify the impact on parenting and on the child's behavior and development.

Sharon Jackson Barton, MS, RN, is a PhD candidate at Loyola University of Chicago and a Clinical Nurse Manager at Children's Memorial Hospital in Chicago.

Janice M. Bell, PhD, RN, is Research Coordinator, Family Nursing Unit, and Associate Professor, Faculty of Nursing, University of Calgary. Her research and clinical interests include families with cancer, effectiveness of family systems nursing interventions, and the teaching and learning of family systems nursing skills. She is the senior editor of *The Cutting Edge of Family Nursing,* a book of selected papers from the First International Family Nursing Conference.

Bonnie J. Breitmayer, PhD, RN, is an Associate Professor in the Department of Psychiatric Nursing at the University of Illinois, Chicago. Her research interest focuses on processes that ameliorate or exacerbate developmental problems of children at risk.

Marie Annette Brown, PhD, RN, is an Associate Professor in the Department of Community Health Care Systems and Coordinator of the Primary Health Care Programs in the School of Nursing at the University of Washington, Seattle. She currently facilitates a support group for families and significant others of people with AIDS. She also serves on the Board of Directors for Shanti, an organization that provides emotional support for persons and families affected by AIDS.

Marta A. Browning, MSN, RN, is an Assistant Professor in the Department of Nursing, College of Allied Health Profession, Temple University, Philadelphia. Her professional experience has centered around developing and providing care to underserved clients. She has worked in health departments both as staff nurse and as supervisor and has served as Director of Professional Services for the Visiting Nurse Association of San Diego. Her research and publications focus on special clinical needs of underserved population groups, which include older adults, pregnant inner-city teens, and the poor.

Mary Burman, PhD, RN, is Assistant Professor, University of Wyoming, School of Nursing, College of Health Services, Laramie. She was a doctoral candidate and Research Assistant with Dr. Carol Loveland-Cherry at the School of Nursing, University of Michigan, when the work reported in this volume was done.

Mary M. Cardwell, MS, RN, is a doctoral student and Research Assistant at Wayne State University, College of Nursing, Detroit. Her areas of interest include feminism, families, mental illness, the abuse of women, and theory development in nursing.

Ruth Carroll, PhD, RN, is an Assistant Professor in Mental Health Nursing at Villanova University, Villanova, Pennsylvania. Her program of research is directed to bereavement in families.

Catherine A. Chesla, DNSc, RN, is an Assistant Professor in the Department of Family Health Care Nursing at the University of California, San Francisco, where she teaches family theory and family intervention to graduate family nurse practitioner students. She has been instrumental in starting a Family Nursing Clinic in which families experiencing new or changed health conditions are seen for brief family counseling. Her research focuses on how families in the community cope with and care for a chronically ill member.

Margaret Cotroneo, PhD, RN, CS, is an Associate Professor and Program Director, Psychiatric-Mental Health Nursing Program, School of Nursing, University of Pennsylvania, Philadelphia. She holds secondary appointments in the Department of Psychiatry, School of Medicine, University of Pennsylvania, and in the Department of Mental Health Sciences, Hahnemann University. She is a family therapist in private practice. Her research interests include studies of family processes in child custody disputes and intrafamilial abuse, and the study and application of relational ethics.

Linda L. Davis, PhD, ANP, RN, is a Professor and Research Consultant for the Center for Nursing Research at the University of Alabama School of Nursing, Birmingham. She has taught nursing theory, research, and clinical issues for undergraduate and graduate nursing students. She is an adult nurse practitioner, and her personal research program focuses on individual and family members with acute illness.

Janet A. Deatrick, PhD, RN, FAAN, received her PhD in Nursing from the University of Illinois, Chicago. She is currently Associate Professor and Program Director, Nursing of Children Division, University of Pennsylvania School of Nursing, Philadelphia. Her current research focuses on the day-to-day work involved in the care of children with chronic conditions and the contribution of qualitative research to an understanding of those phenomena.

Jeri W. Dunkin, PhD, RN, is Director, Rural Health Nursing Specialty, College of Nursing, University of North Dakota, Grand Forks.

Barbara A. Durand, EdD, RNC, FAAN, is a Professor and Chairperson, Department of Maternal-Child Nursing, Rush-Presbyterian-St. Luke's Medical Center and Rush University in Chicago. During her professional career, she has played a significant role nationally in advocating for and promoting the nurse practitioner movement and advanced nursing practice. Her 18 years (1970-1988) with the Pediatric Nurse Practitioner Program at the University of California, San Francisco, included serving as Director from 1976-1988. She is co-author of *Handbook of Pediatric Primary Care,* an American Journal of Nursing (AJN) Book of the Year award winner. She is the only nurse elected to office in the Ambulatory Pediatric Association. She is a member of the Executive Committee of the Council on Maternal-Child Nursing of the American Nurses Association.

Sandra A. Faux, PhD, RN, is Associate Professor, University of Western Ontario in London, Ontario, Canada. Her research expertise is in qualitative methods, specifically grounded theory. Her program of research focuses on how families of chronically ill children define and manage the illness experience, particularly the siblings of the affected child. She currently is funded to evaluate the effectiveness of community nurse specialists in managing the health of developmentally disabled adults in the community.

Suzanne L. Feetham, PhD, RN, FAAN, is Chief, Office of Planning Analysis and Evaluation, National Center for Nursing Research, National Institutes of Health, and Professor, Associated Faculty, School of Nursing, University of Pennsylvania, Philadelphia. Her program of research focuses on the families of children with health problems. She also has directed her research to examining measurement issues in research of families.

Maureen A. Frey, PhD, RN, is an Assistant Professor in Parent-Child Nursing, School of Nursing, University of Michigan, Ann Arbor. Her research interests are in the areas of family and child health, illness care and management, and social support in children with chronic conditions. Of particular interest is testing nursing conceptual frameworks and theories, including King's framework, Orem's self-care theory, family stress theory, and Pender's health promotion model.

Judy Friedrichs, MS, RN, is Assistant Unit Leader, Special Care Nursery, Rush-Presbyterian-St. Luke's Medical Center, Chicago. She has been a neonatal intensive care unit nurse for 14 years, during which time she started the Parent-to-Parent Program in 1979 for families experiencing the crisis of a critically ill infant. She has coordinated the Bereavement Support Program at Rush-Presbyterian-St. Luke's Medical Center since its inception 11 years ago, following 160 families a year. She is also a certified bereavement counselor and death educator.

Agatha M. Gallo, PhD, RN, is an Associate Professor in the Department of Maternal Child Nursing at the University of Illinois, Chicago. Her recent research has focused on how families define and manage a child's chronic illness and on sibling response to chronic illness.

Catherine L. Gilliss, DNSc, RN C, FAAN, is Associate Professor and Director of the Primary Health Care Nurse Practitioner Core Curriculum in the School of Nursing, University of California, San Francisco. She also serves as Director of the Family Nursing Service in the Department of Family Health Care Nursing, a unit developed to promote the education of nurses in the care of families experiencing a disruption in health. Her long-standing interest in families and health is perhaps best known through her award-winning, co-edited text, *Toward a Science of Family Nursing* (Gilliss, Highley, Roberts, & Martinson, 1989).

Kim Guyer, MSN, RN, is a nurse clinician for Paidos Healthcare, Inc., in Paoli, Pennsylvania. She is also a Clinical Instructor, Nursing of Children Division, at the University of Pennsylvania School of Nursing in Philadelphia.

Sheila A. Haas, PhD, RN, is an Associate Professor at Loyola University in the Marcella Niehoff School of Nursing in Chicago.

Virginia E. Hayes, PhD, RN, is an Assistant Professor in the School of Nursing at the University of British Columbia, Vancouver. Her recent clinical, educational, and research work has focused on chronically ill children and families.

Laura Hayman, PhD, RN, FAAN, is Associate Professor and Chair, Nursing of Children Division, University of Pennsylvania School of Nursing in Philadelphia. Her program of research incorporates a longitudinal twin-family design and focuses on the determinants of risk for cardiovascular disease during the developmental transition from childhood to adolescence.

Colleen Holzwarth, PNP, RN, is a Nurse Practitioner at Merit Care Midwest Clinic, Jamestown, North Dakota, and a graduate student in the College of Nursing, University of North Dakota, Grand Forks.

304 NURSING OF FAMILIES

Mary Horan, PhD, RN, is Professor and Director, Kirkhof School of Nursing, Grand Valley State University, Allendale, Michigan. She and Dr. Loveland-Cherry were co-investigators of the research of families of preterm infants from which data in this volume were taken.

Kathleen A. Knafl, PhD, is a Professor in the Department of Psychiatric Nursing and Associate Dean for Research in the College of Nursing, University of Illinois, Chicago. Her research interests focus on family response to illness and disability. She is principal investigator on a study entitled "How Families Define and Manage a Child's Chronic Illness."

Maribelle B. Leavitt, DNSc, RN, is on the clinical faculty of the Department of Family Health Care Nursing at the University of California, San Francisco, where she teaches in the Family Nurse Practitioner Masters Degree Program. She is also a Faculty Clinician for the Family Nursing Service, which specializes in helping families manage effectively new or long-standing illness in the family. Previously she was a member of the Faculty of Nursing at the University of San Francisco and maintained a private practice of individual and family therapy until she began doctoral studies at the University of California, San Francisco. She is the author of *Families at Risk* (1982) and numerous articles in the field of family health care.

Anne Marie C. Levac, MN, RN, is a Family Nursing Specialist at Alberta Children's Hospital, Calgary, Alberta, Canada. She is interested in clinical practice with children and their families experiencing psychosocial problems from an interactional perspective.

Carol J. Loveland-Cherry, PhD, RN, is an Associate Professor and Specialty Head, Community Health Nursing, University of Michigan, Ann Arbor. She and Dr. Mary Horan were co-principal investigators for the larger study from which data in this volume were taken.

Marilyn A. McCubbin, PhD, RN, is an Associate Professor and Co-Program Director of the Master's Option in Community Health Nursing at the School of Nursing, University of Wisconsin, Madison. She is currently the principal investigator for "Children's Chronic Illness: Parent and Family Adaptation," a 5-year longitudinal study.

Susan B. Meister, PhD, RN, FAAN, is a member of the Working Group on Early Life and Adolescent Health Policy, Division of Health Policy Research and Education, Harvard University, Cambridge, Massachusetts. She is also a Trustee of the Foundation for Seacoast Health in New Hampshire. As the Director of Health Services Research at Children's Hospital in San Diego, she was the first Director of the consortium, six-hospital (California Association of Children's Hospitals) project in quantifying nursing resource consumption in children's hospitals. She was the principal investigator of a San Diego/Chicago project—Children's Hospitals REACH Out. She serves on technical advisory panels for the Health Care Financing Administration, including the Quality of Medicaid Study. Her research focuses on health policies for children, with particular emphasis on health care financing.

Edna M. Menke, PhD, RN, is an Associate Professor and Associate Dean at the College of Nursing, The Ohio State University, Columbus. She has been involved actively in family research for the past 15 years. She has conducted research regarding siblings of chronically ill children and transitions in parenthood. For the past 5 years, her research has focused on home- less families.

Carol Murphy Moore, MSN, RN, received her MSN from the University of Pennsylvania in Nursing of Children. She previously was employed as a staff nurse at the Children's Hospital of Philadelphia and is currently Instructor of Nursing in Pediatrics at Bloomsburg University in Bloomsburg, Pennsylvania.

Helene J. Moriarty, PhD, RN, CS, is an Assistant Professor in the College of Nursing, Villanova University, Villanova, Pennsylvania. She also is a Clinical Nurse Specialist at the Pennsylvania Sudden Infant Death Syndrome Center. She is certified by the American Nurses Association as a Clinical Nurse Specialist in Adult Psychiatric and Mental Health Nursing. She is engaged in research with families experiencing severe stressors, specifically death of a child, intrafamilal abuse, and child custody disputes.

Mary Perkins, DNSc, RN, is currently the Director of Nursing Education, Staff Development and Training, Children's National Medical Center, Washington, DC. Her research focuses on the caregiving behaviors of parents of chronically ill children and the development of education models to enable parent caregiving in health care settings.

Kathy Rigney, MSN, RN, is currently an Advanced Clinical Educator in Nursing Education, Staff Development, and Training, Children's National

Medical Center, Washington, DC. She also coordinates the development of patient and family education materials at Children's National Medical Center.

Willard Rodgers, PhD, is a Research Scientist in the Survey Research Center, Institute for Social Research, University of Michigan, Ann Arbor. He was the statistician with co-principal investigators Carol Loveland-Cherry and Mary Horan for the project on families with preterm infants, described in this volume.

Teresa A. Savage, MS, RN, is Practitioner and Teacher, Maternal-Child Nursing, College of Nursing, Rush University, and Rush-Presbyterian-St. Luke's Medical Center, Chicago. She has extensive clinical experience with critically ill and chronically ill children. Much of her professional career has been focused on ethical issues and the nurse's role. Her research interests are nursing attitudes and beliefs toward the Do Not Resuscitate order, the nurse's perspective on withholding food and fluid, and on comfort measures for the dying patients. She is pursuing her PhD in nursing with an emphasis on ethics and ethical decision making.

Jeanne F. Slack, DNSc, RN, is the Associate Chairperson in the Department of Maternal-Child Nursing and Assistant Professor at Rush University and Rush-Presbyterian-St. Luke's Medical Center, Chicago. She has more than 15 years of experience in pediatric nursing in a variety of positions, including staff nurse, supervisor, critical care, and clinical nurse specialist. She has published on organizational systems and pediatric pain management issues and is co-investigator on a study of nursing interventions for pain management in cancer patients.

Lee SmithBattle, DNSC, RN, recently completed her disseratation at the School of Nursing at the University of California, San Francisco. Her research investigates teenage mothering as shaped and organized by family practices from a phenomenological perspective. She is currently employed part-time as a high-risk infant nurse at Golden Gate Regional Center in San Francisco in a home visiting program that provides nursing services to children from birth to 3 years of age and their families.

Arlene M. Sperhac, PhD, RN, is Director of the Department of Nursing Education and Research at Children's Memorial Hospital in Chicago. She has co-edited the award-winning text, *Nursing Care of Children and Families* (Mott, James, & Sperhac, 1990).

Julie E. Sprott, PhD, RN, CPNP, has taught 4 years as an Assistant Professor at the School of Nursing, University of Alaska, Anchorage, and most recently worked as a Nursing Consultant and Pediatric Nurse Practitioner with Public Health Nursing, Maniilaq Association, the Health Corporation for the Inupiat Eskimo of Northwest Alaska.

Terry Stratton, MA, is Research Analyst at the University of North Dakota Center for Rural Health, Grand Forks.

Georgina A. Sumner, MSN, RN, is Director of the N.C.A.S.T. Program, School of Nursing, University of Washington, Seattle. She continues to be vitally interested in the dissemination of research to nurses to enrich and in some cases change their practice. She has fostered communication about family assessment through the *NCAST National News.*

Robin B. Thomas, PhD, RN, is in private practice as an individual, couple, and family therapist in Seattle. She continues to study clinical family assessment and is interested in investigating the relationship between family of origin and individual self-concept and functioning.

Janet D. Wagner, PhD, RN, is an Assistant Professor at the College of Nursing, The Ohio State University, Columbus. She helped establish a homeless families foundation in Columbus and is a board member of two community organizations that work with the homeless. She has undertaken several research studies regarding homeless families.

Ann L. Whall, PhD, RN, FAAN, has master's preparation in both public health nursing, and psychiatric mental health nursing. She has continued to practice throughout her academic career and currently is certified as a psychiatric mental health nurse specialist in Michigan. She conducts group and individual therapy with elders and their families. Three of her five published textbooks deal with family theory research and practice, as do many of her published articles.

Jean H. Woods, PhD, RNCS, is an Associate Professor and Chairperson of the Department of Nursing in the College of Allied Health Professions at Temple University, Philadelphia. She is certified by the ANA as a Clinical Specialist in Child and Adolescent Psychiatric Mental Health Nursing. She is currently in private practice as a family therapist and counselor. Her research interests are in the areas of child abuse issues affecting child development; developmental issues affecting children over time who have been exposed to substances in utero; and as an educator, meeting the teaching and learning needs of culturally diverse students.

Lorraine M. Wright, PhD, RN, is Director of the Family Nursing Unit and Professor in the Faculty of Nursing at the University of Calgary, Calgary, Alberta, Canada. Her current clinical research interests include family belief systems and families experiencing difficulties with physical/emotional health problems.

JoAnne Youngblut, PhD, RN, is Assistant Professor, Frances Payne Bolton School of Nursing, Case Western Reserve University, Cleveland. She was a doctoral candidate and Research Assistant at the School of Nursing, University of Michigan, Ann Arbor, when work for this volume was done.

Linda H. Zoeller, MPH, RNC, is an Assistant Professor in the Department of Public Health Nursing at the University of Illinois, Chicago. She is a doctoral candidate in the School of Public Health at the University of Illinois, Chicago. Her research interests focus on the interface between the family and the health care system and nursing's role in meeting family health care needs.